Management of Patients at High Risk for Breast Cancer

Management of Patients at High Risk for Breast Cancer

Edited by

Victor G. Vogel, MD
Director, Comprehensive Breast Program
Professor of Medicine and Epidemiology
Magee-Women's Hospital
University of Pittsburgh School of Medicine
Pittsburgh, Pennsylvania

Blackwell
Science

Editorial Offices:
Commerce Place, 350 Main Street, Malden, Massachusetts 02148, USA
Osney Mead, Oxford OX2 0EL, England
25 John Street, London WC1N 2BL, England
23 Ainslie Place, Edinburgh EH3 6AJ, Scotland
54 University Street, Carlton, Victoria 3053, Australia

Other Editorial Offices:
Blackwell Wissenschafts-Verlag GmbH, Kurfürstendamm 57, 10707 Berlin, Germany
Blackwell Science KK, MG Kodenmacho Building, 7-10 Kodenmacho Nihombashi, Chuo-ku, Tokyo 104, Japan

Distributors:

USA

    Blackwell Science, Inc.
    Commerce Place
    350 Main Street
    Malden, Massachusetts 02148
    (Telephone orders: 800-215-1000 or 781-388-8250; fax orders: 781-388-8270)

Canada

    Login Brothers Book Company
    324 Saulteaux Crescent
    Winnipeg, Manitoba, R3J 3T2
    (Telephone orders: 204-837-2987)

Australia

    Blackwell Science Pty, Ltd.
    54 University Street
    Carlton, Victoria 3053
    (Telephone orders: 03-9347-0300; fax orders: 03-9349-3016)

Outside North America and Australia

    Blackwell Science, Ltd.
    c/o Marston Book Services, Ltd.
    P.O. Box 269
    Abingdon
    Oxon OX14 4YN
    England
    (Telephone orders: 44-01235-465500; fax orders: 44-01235-465555)

Acquisitions: Chris Davis
Development: Julia Casson
Production: Louis C. Bruno, Jr.
Manufacturing: Lisa Flanagan
Director of Marketing: Lisa Larsen
Marketing Manager: Anne Stone
Interior design by Lou C. Bruno, Jr.
Cover design by Linda Dana Willis
Typeset by Laser Words
Printed and bound by Sheridan Books

Printed in the United States of America
00 01 02 03 5 4 3 2 1

Library of Congress Cataloging-in-Publication Data

Management of patients at high risk for breast cancer / edited by Victor G. Vogel.
   p. ; cm.
   ISBN 0-632-04323-7
   1. Breast — Cancer — Risk factors. 2. Health risk assessment. 3.
Breast — Cancer — Prevention. 4. Breast — Cancer — Chemoprevention. I. Vogel, Victor G.
   [DNLM: 1. Breast Neoplasms. 2. Risk Factors. WP 870 M266 2001]
   RC280.B8 M335 2001
   616.99′449 — dc21

                                   00-030391

For Naoma and Matilda and Margaret:
That their deaths were not in vain

Contents

Preface

He is the better physician that keeps diseases off us than he that cures them being on us. Prevention is so much better than healing because it saves the labor of being sick.

Thomas Adams
17th-century British physician

The twentieth century saw remarkable advances both in the treatment of breast cancer and in our understanding of the etiology of the disease. As we stand on the threshold of a new century, we are the privileged heirs of the knowledge that was painstakingly gained by those who have gone before us. Advances in epidemiology, molecular biology, genetics, pharmacology, and diagnostic imaging have all produced the tools we need to manage breast cancer risk.

Breast cancer risk management is a composite task that is similar to many other clinical risk-reduction skills such as cholesterol lowering, hypertension management, osteoporosis prevention, and cervical or colorectal cancer screening. Breast cancer risk management is supported by specific information and skills that define it as a unique clinical discipline. This book was designed to provide clinicians with information that creates the foundation for clinical breast cancer risk management. We review behavioral and epidemiologic risk factors that have been shown conclusively and repeatedly to be associated with increased risk of breast cancer. We identify the qualitative and quantitative methods that are available to assess risk accurately and to communicate risk clearly. We highlight the significant advances that have been made in genetic counseling and molecular testing for the disorders and syndromes that increase risk of breast cancer. We review the diagnostic imaging strategies that are currently available for women who are at increased risk, particularly those younger women for whom no specific imaging guidelines exist. We devote considerable attention to chemoprevention strategies that

are now available, as well as exploring the option of prophylactic surgery.

Throughout our discussions, the focus is on the development of those critical skills and orientation that enable physicians who are unfamiliar with risk assessment and prevention to add these important clinical skills to their diagnostic and management capabilities. We believe that a great number of competent clinicians are simply not familiar with the techniques described within this book and that they have little experience in evaluating and managing the risk of breast cancer in a systematic way. Recognizing both the novelty of the information and the potential uncertainties of the likely readers, we have made a concerted effort to avoid technical jargon or hypothetical and theoretical discussions. The goal of this book is to educate clinicians in the foundations of risk management for the reduction of breast cancer risk and to provide them with specific tools that can be incorporated into their daily clinical practices as they regularly attend to the health-care needs of adult women. We believe that patients will demand the clinical services that we describe in this book and that clinicians will need to be familiar with the principles and practices described by the experts who have contributed to this work.

Epidemiology is the basic science that underlies all of clinical cancer prevention. Dr. Kuller reviews factors known to be associated with increased risk of breast cancer, and he lays the foundation for many chapters that follow. Thorough knowledge of the diverse genetic syndromes that are now known to increase the risk of breast cancer is essential to adequate risk management. Dr. Rubinstein reviews these syndromes in considerable detail and discusses the challenges and limitations of current genetic testing technology. She also describes the components of competent genetic counseling in this context. Dr. Narod reviews the clinical characteristics of genetically determined breast cancer so that clinicians might be vigilant in the identification of women who have the characteristics of genetically based syndromes.

The validation of the quantitative risk assessment model developed by Dr. Mitchell Gail and his colleagues and the availability of the model both in print and on the Internet have made it imperative that physicians be familiar with the use and limitations of the model. Several other models also have been developed recently and facilitate risk evaluation in myriad clinical circumstances. Available models allow more accurate evaluation of the impact of family history on the risk of developing breast cancer, permit estimation of the likelihood that a woman is a carrier of a specific genetic mutation, and aid in estimation of the likelihood of developing breast cancer within a number of possible genetic scenarios. The chapter by Ms. O'Neill carefully instructs the reader who is unfamiliar with these models in their intricate details and use.

Because several of the genetic syndromes that increase the risk of breast cancer also increase the risk of ovarian cancer, Drs. Shaw, Deavers, and Mills provide information about the characteristics of genetically determined ovarian cancer that will assist clinicians in identifying women who are at increased risk for both breast and ovarian cancer. To provide further assistance, Drs. Sit and Edwards review the information that is available on genetic screening for ovarian cancer risk.

Evaluation of risk is of limited practical benefit if no plan for risk management is provided. The second half of the book is devoted to strategies that have been shown to be effective in the management of breast cancer risk. Dr. Harris begins with a thorough review of available breast cancer imaging techniques. Recognizing that imaging often leads to the need for breast biopsy, Drs. Sumkin and Harris review in detail the techniques of minimally invasive breast biopsy that lessen substantially the

physical and emotional burden on the patient and facilitate accurate diagnosis of both benign and malignant conditions. Drs. Sumkin and Hardesty review emerging technologies for breast screening and diagnosis (including magnetic resonance imaging techniques) and show how these new approaches may be useful in the management of women who are at increased risk.

Many clinical environments are currently not configured to provide either accurate and efficient cancer risk assessment or to offer management prescriptions. Dr. Hughes and colleagues outline a successful strategy that has been used both in their institution and in many others to create and structure an effective risk assessment clinic.

Complete management of breast cancer risk includes quantitative risk assessment, genetic counseling and testing, discussions of the possible need for prophylactic mastectomy, offering chemopreventive interventions where appropriate, and managing the psychological burden of knowing that one is at increased risk. Drs. Shestak, Medalie, and Williams review the indications for prophylactic mastectomy as well as the accepted surgical techniques for performing the procedure. They also review the indications for and the limitations of the procedure, and they define how it is part of a comprehensive set of management options for women at increased risk.

The dramatic findings from the Breast Cancer Prevention Trial led to the approval of tamoxifen by the Food and Drug Administration for breast cancer risk reduction. Tamoxifen and raloxifene, a second generation selective estrogen receptor modulator, are currently being studied in a clinical trial to identify the relative merits of each agent. In my chapter, I review in considerable detail the basic science data and the findings from clinical trials that have made breast cancer chemoprevention a clinical reality. I also review the design and objectives for the Study of Tamoxifen and Raloxifene (STAR) trial, and I identify women who are ideal candidates for whom to consider breast cancer risk reduction using chemoprevention.

Identifying women who are at increased risk for breast cancer carries with it a psychological burden for these women. Labeling women as being at increased risk carries with it the obligation that clinicians support the patient at risk by providing both reassurance and credible management options to deal with a patient's heightened awareness of her risk. Drs. Posluszny and Baum offer useful guidelines and directives for dealing with this psychological burden. In addition to this burden of increased risk, unique legal and ethical issues surround the management of these women. Drs. Parker, Meisel, and Hogan concisely and expertly review these challenging questions. Their consideration of the issues will offer reassurance to patients and their clinicians who are understandably concerned about the legal and ethical consequences of being identified as members of a high-risk group.

Of equal importance are the concerns of hospital and clinic administrators as well as public policy planners who may question whether risk-assessment and risk-reduction strategies are cost effective. Dr. Hughes and April Levine demonstrate that risk assessment clinics and the provision of breast cancer risk-management services within typical clinical environments is, indeed, cost effective.

Finally, Drs. Dietz, Love, and Newcomb review strategies that can result in reduction of breast cancer risk within entire populations. These considerations offer additional opportunities for public health-care planners, health-plan administrators, and politicians who may be interested in developing risk-reduction programs within large populations at risk.

Taken together, the expert contributors have defined the new clinical subspecialty of breast cancer risk management. Readers of this book will acquire the skills they need to offer competent risk assessment and management to all the patients in their clinical practices who are concerned about their risk of developing breast cancer and who seek effective strategies to reduce and manage their risk.

Victor G. Vogel

Contributors

Andrew Baum, PhD
Professor, Departments of Psychology and
  Psychiatry
University of Pittsburgh School of Medicine;
Director, Behavioral Medicine Clinical Service
University of Pittsburgh Cancer Institute
Pittsburgh, Pennsylvania

Michael T. Deavers, MD
Assistant Professor of Pathology
University of Texas Medical School at
  Houston;
Staff Pathologist, Department of Pathology
M.D. Anderson Cancer Center
Houston, Texas

Robert P. Edwards, MD
Assistant Professor, Department of Obstetrics,
  Gynecology, and Reproductive Services
University of Pittsburgh School of Medicine;
Director, Division of Gynecologic Oncology
Magee-Womens Hospital
Pittsburgh, Pennsylvania

Lara A. Hardesty, MD
Assistant Professor, Department of Radiology
University of Pittsburgh School of Medicine;
Staff Radiologist, Department of Radiology
Magee-Womens Hospital
Pittsburgh, Pennsylvania

Kathleen M. Harris, MD, FACR
Associate Professor, Department of Radiology
University of Pittsburgh School of Medicine;
Staff Radiologist, Breast Imaging Division
Magee-Womens Hospital
Pittsburgh, Pennsylvania

Melissa J. Hogan, JD
Bass, Berry & Sims
Nashville, Tennessee

Kevin S. Hughes, MD
Assistant Clinical Professor, Department of
  Surgery
Tufts Medical School
Boston, Massachusetts;
Director, The Breast Center
Lahey Clinic
Burlington, Massachusetts

Lewis H. Kuller, MD, DrPH
Professor and Chair
Department of Epidemiology
University of Pittsburgh Graduate School of
  Public Health
Pittsburgh, Pennsylvania

April Levine, BS
Director, Quality and Performance
  Improvement
Quality Resource Department
Lahey Clinic
Burlington, Massachusetts

Richard R. Love, MD
Professor of Medicine and Family Medicine
University of Wisconsin Medical School
Madison, Wisconsin

Michele R. Lucas, LICSW
Social Worker
Lahey Clinic
Peabody, Massachusetts

Daniel A. Medalie, MD
Assistant Professor of Plastic Surgery
University of Kentucky College of Medicine
Lexington, Kentucky

Alan Meisel, JD
Dickie, McCanney and Chilcote Professor of
   Bioethics,
   and Professor of Law and Psychiatry
Center for Bioethics and Health Law
University of Pittsburgh
Pittsburgh, Pennsylvania

Gordon B. Mills, MD, PhD
Professor, Division of Medicine
University of Texas Medical School at
   Houston;
Chairman, Department of Molecular
   Oncology
M.D. Anderson Cancer Center
Houston, Texas

Steven A. Narod, MD
Associate Professor, Department of Public
   Health Sciences
University of Toronto Faculty of Medicine;
Chair of Breast Cancer Research
The Centre for Research in Women's Health
Sunnybrook & Women's College Health
   Science Centre
Toronto, Ontario, Canada

Polly A. Newcomb, PhD, MPH
Senior Scientist
University of Wisconsin Medical School
Madison, Wisconsin;
Member
Fred Hutchinson Cancer Research Center
Seattle, Washington

Suzanne O'Neill, MA, MS, CGC
Doctoral Candidate, Department of Human
   Genetics
University of Pittsburgh Graduate School of
   Public Health;
Certified Genetic Counselor, Comprehensive
   Breast Program
University of Pittsburgh Cancer
   Institute/Magee-Womens Hospital
Pittsburgh, Pennsylvania

Lisa S. Parker, PhD
Associate Professor of Human Genetics,
   and Director of Graduate Education
Center for Bioethics and Health Law
University of Pittsburgh
Pittsburgh, Pennsylvania

Donna M. Posluszny, MS
Faculty Member, Department of Psychology
   and Behavioral Medicine Clinical Service
University of Pittsburgh Cancer Institute
Pittsburgh, Pennsylvania

Constance A. Roche, MSN, RNCS
Coordinator, Risk Assessment Clinic
Lahey Clinic
Peabody, Massachusetts

Wendy S. Rubinstein, MD, PhD
Assistant Professor, Department of Medicine
   and Human Genetics,
   and Department of Obstetrics, Gynecology,
   and Reproductive Sciences
University of Pittsburgh School of Medicine;
Director, Cancer Genetics Program,
and Medical Geneticist, Comprehensive
   Breast Program
Magee-Womens Hospital
Pittsburgh, Pennsylvania

Patricia A. Shaw, MD, FRCPC
Assistant Professor, Department of
   Laboratory Medicine and Pathobiology
University of Toronto Faculty of Medicine;
Gynecologic Pathologist, Department of
   Pathology
Sunnybrook & Women's College Health
   Science Centre
Toronto, Ontario, Canada

Kenneth C. Shestak, MD
Associate Professor, Department of Plastic
   Surgery
University of Pittsburgh School of Medicine;
Chief of Plastic Surgery
Magee-Womens Hospital
Pittsburgh, Pennsylvania

Anita S. Y. Sit, MD
Instructor, Department of Obstetrics,
   Gynecology, and Reproductive Services
University of Pittsburgh School of Medicine;
Staff Member, Division of Gynecologic
   Oncology
Magee-Women's Hospital
Pittsburgh, Pennsylvania

Jules Sumkin, DO
Associate Professor of Radiology and Interim
  Chairman,
Department of Radiology
University of Pittsburgh School of Medicine;
Chief of Radiology
Magee-Womens Hospital
Pittsburgh, Pennsylvania

Amy Trentham-Dietz, PhD
Assistant Scientist
University of Wisconsin Comprehensive
  Cancer Center
Madison, Wisconsin

Scott L. Williams, MD
Professor of Surgery
University of Pittsburgh School of Medicine
Pittsburgh, Pennsylvania

Victor G. Vogel, MD, MHS
Professor of Medicine and Epidemiology
University of Pittsburgh School of Medicine;
Director, Comprehensive Breast Program
University of Pittsburgh Cancer
  Institute/Magee-Womens Hospital
Pittsburgh, Pennsylvania

1

Epidemiology of Breast Cancer

Lewis H. Kuller

Epidemiology is the study of the determinants and distribution of disease in populations. These determinants may be the direct cause of a specific disease such as breast cancer, a marker in the causal pathway of a disease, or unrelated to the cause of disease (i.e., an association). It is likely that there are many associations that are not causal to the risk of breast cancer sharing only a common distribution in the environment with the risk of breast cancer. For example, upper-social-class women have a higher risk of postmenopausal breast cancer. Any variable whose distribution is greater in upper-social-class or in better-educated women probably will be associated with a risk of breast cancer (1).

The most important approach to determining a causal association of a variable and disease is through *human experimentation*, either natural experiments or clinical trials. An example of a natural experiment is the well-known substantial variation in breast cancer incidence and mortality among countries (2) and the increase in breast cancer when women migrate from countries with low to higher breast cancer rates (3). The increase in death and incidence rates of disease among migrants is overwhelming evidence that the large geographic differences in breast cancer incidence and mortality are not primarily due to genetic factors; that is, the gene pool could not possibly change within one generation (3). Major lifestyle or environmental causes of breast cancer probably account for much of the geographic variations in breast cancer among countries. The fundamental question in epidemiology, therefore, is to clearly identify these determinants of disease.

A second natural experiment is the effects of changing lifestyles on incidence or mortality of disease over time (i.e., temporal trends) (4–7). A change in mortality rates can be due to better treatment or to change in the incidence of disease. An increase or decrease in incidence of disease can be due to improved detection methods or changes in environmental risk factors of disease. For example, breast cancer incidence rates have increased dramatically among postmenopausal women. This increase is probably due to better detection and the higher percentage of women having mammography (8). The mortality rates have begun to decline, primarily among premenopausal but also among younger (i.e., under 60 years old) postmenopausal women (4–5). This is probably due to a combination of early detection, mammography, and better treatment of breast cancer. It is difficult to judge the effects of various therapies because the mortality from breast cancer often occurs many years after the incident diagnosis, and thus deaths from breast cancer at the current time may be related to incident cases and treatment 5, 8, or 10 years in the past. The 5-year survival percentage has improved dramatically for breast cancer over time (6).

The improved treatments of breast cancer may not have any major affect on breast cancer mortality rates for perhaps the next 5 or even 10 years. Thus it is not useful to compare current mortality rates or even recent trends with current therapies.

The increased incidence in older age groups and declining case-fatality rate have resulted in a very substantial increase in the number of women currently living with breast cancer or prevalence

of breast cancer. The age-standardized prevalence of breast cancer has increased 32% between
1982 and 1994 (9). There is a growing population
of women at high risk of second primary breast
cancer.

Natural History of Breast Cancer and Recent Secular Trends

The development of clinical breast cancer from
initial neoplastic changes to clinical diagnosis,
either by mammography or clinical examination,
requires numerous divisions of the cells (i.e.,
doubling times), perhaps up to 8 years among
postmenopausal women. A recent introduction,
for example, of an environmental carcinogen or
protective dietary factor or a new diagnostic
procedure may not have an impact on breast
cancer incidence rates for years, unless the effect
is to modify the time to detection of breast cancer
(but not the initial neoplastic changes). Such an
introduction also could be related to an apparent
rapid change in breast cancer rates because it
modifies the ability for early detection of breast
cancer (i.e., detection bias) or the frequency
in which diagnostic tests are performed (i.e.,
monitoring) (10–12).

Examination of normal breast tissue at
autopsy has shown that up to 20% of women
may have undetected ductal carcinoma in situ
(DCIS) at the time of their death (13). We do

not know how many of these cancers would
have been diagnosed clinically if the woman had
survived longer, had been exposed to better techniques for early diagnosis of breast cancer, or
perhaps had been exposed to an environmental
agent that increased the doubling time of the
neoplastic cells to clinical diagnosis. The women
would have had diagnosed breast cancer prior to
death from another cause.

If we assume that 20% of postmenopausal
women (i.e., 20 million) had subclinical breast
cancer (i.e., 4 million), and if we further hypoth-
esize that these 4 million women could be identified at equal frequencies per year between the
ages of 55 and 75 years, then each year there could
be another 200,000 new cases of breast cancer
among these 20 million women, or about 1% per
year. The average annual incidence of breast cancer is only about half (4–5/1000 per year) among
postmenopausal women. Therefore, any variable
that either increases or decreases the likelihood
of detection will have a major effect on breast
cancer incidence rates (14–15).

The trends in premenopausal breast cancer
also have very important implications. There has
been a decline in both the incidence and the
mortality of breast cancer among premenopausal
women (4). The decline in incidence has been
noted for at least 5 years and has been relatively consistent within each 5-year age group
of premenopausal women. The decrease in

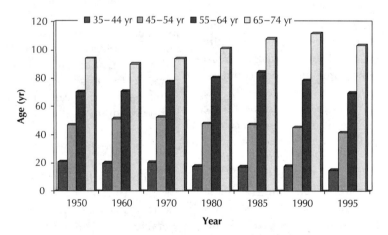

Figure 1-1. Death rates for malignant neoplasm of the breast for women by age — United States, selected
years 1950–1995. (Reproduced from National Center for Health Statistics. Health, United States, 1996–97
and injury chartbook. DHHS publication no. PHS97-1232. Hyattsville, MD: U.S. Department of Health and
Human Services, 1997.)

mortality is likely due to better treatment (i.e., improved survivorship), but the decrease in incidence is almost certainly related to changes in lifestyle, since it is unlikely that early detection and screening could result in a decrease in incidence (4) (Figs. 1-1 and 1-2).

Two hypotheses have been proposed to explain the decline:

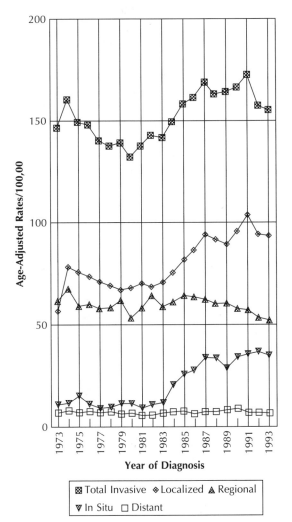

Figure 1-2. Age-adjusted breast cancer incidence rates by extent of disease at diagnosis for white women, standardized to the 1970 U.S. population 40 to 49 years of age. (Reproduced with permission from Chu KC, Tarone RE, Kessler LG, et al. Recent trends in U.S. breast cancer incidence, survival, and mortality rates. J Natl Cancer Inst 1996;88:1571–1579.)

1. A cohort effect (i.e., older age at first pregnancy) of cohorts from the low-birth-rate years around the great depression. Women born in the 1930s have now become postmenopausal, and women born in the 1940s and 1950s who have had higher birth rates and earlier age at first pregnancy are now moving through the premenopausal period of their lives (6). Since these women had an earlier age at first pregnancy, they are therefore at lower risk of breast cancer than women born in the 1930s. This is a very intriguing and important observation. Important behavioral changes can have a major effect on potential population levels of disease (i.e., breast cancer incidence) (16).

The reason why age at first pregnancy is associated with a lower risk of breast cancer is not certain. The effect is limited to women with full-term pregnancies and not to those with spontaneous or induced abortions, in whom there may be a slight increase. The most plausible hypothesis is that pregnancy is associated with a greater differentiation of breast glandular tissue and that development of this glandular tissue reduces the susceptibility to carcinogens that are related to breast cancer (17).

2. The alternative hypotheses is that there has been an increase in the prevalence of obesity in recent years among premenopausal women. There is a direct association between the frequency of anovulatory cycling (i.e., menstrual irregularities) and obesity among premenopausal women. Furthermore, there is some evidence that obesity is associated with a reduced risk of premenopausal breast cancer. There is some evidence that irregular or longer menstrual cycling also may be associated with lower risk of breast cancer. Two hypotheses (i.e., earlier age at first pregnancy and obesity) also may be linked to greater weight gain after pregnancy (18–20).

Colon cancer, interestingly enough, also has been decreasing in the United States and other countries. The decrease has been greater in women than in men and does not appear to be related to use of hormone replacement therapy (21). The decline in both breast (premenopausal) and colon cancer also may suggest some common environmental change. Dietary variables such as the amount of dietary fat, fiber, calcium, etc. may be important. There has been a modest decrease in the percentage of fat calories in the diet but an actual increase in the number of fat grams. There has been a substantial decrease in egg consumption and a modest decrease in the consumption of meat and high-fat dairy products. These foods are the primary source of arachidonic acid in the diet. An increase in arachidonic acid in the diet has been associated with increasing fatty acid ester arachidonic acid levels as well as with higher levels of arachidonic acid in platelet membranes.

Arachidonic acid is the major precursor of eicosanoids, and higher levels of several of the eicosanoids have been related to increased risk of both breast and colon cancer. It is possible that the substantial declines in coronary heart disease and colon cancer as well as in premenopausal breast cancer incidence are related to changes in the amount of arachidonic acid in the diet.

The use of non-steroidal anti-inflammatory agents also has increased in recent years. There is fairly strong evidence that anti-inflammatory agents are associated with lower risks of colon cancer. Their association with breast cancer is less impressive. The decline in incidence of breast cancer in premenopausal women, if it continues, provides an excellent natural experiment to determine changes in risk factors for premenopausal breast cancer (22). Women who migrate from countries with a low risk of breast cancer to countries with a higher risk of breast cancer have a significant change in their rates of breast cancer within the first generation. The Japanese migrant population has been studied most extensively (3). The rates of breast cancer increase in the first generation of migration to the United States. The increase is greater for subsequent generations born in the United States. The rates do not approach those of white women in the United States, but they are substantially higher than those for Japanese women in Japan.

The increase in rates within the first generation obviously cannot be due to genetic factors. The most likely hypotheses relate the changes in diet and weight gain and in reproductive history, menstrual cycling, etc. Both pre- and postmenopausal breast cancer rates are increasing in Japan, as well as in many other countries that originally had relatively low breast cancer

incidence and mortality rates (18). This, again, reflects the importance of recent environmental changes on the risk of breast cancer.

Models for the Etiology of Breast Cancer

The geographic and temporal trends should provide important clues to the etiology of breast cancer. The next step in epidemiologic studies is to develop a testable model of the etiology of breast cancer. The model should be based on the previously described ecological (i.e., natural) experiments, descriptive epidemiology, animal experimental studies, and pathophysiology.

The most plausible and parsimonious model for the etiology of breast cancer presumes four or five key factors: 1) that there is an initial exposure to a carcinogen that modifies the DNA of breast epithelial cells, 2) that the initial response to the carcinogen is related to age at exposure, host susceptibility (i.e., genetic factors), and metabolism of the carcinogen, 3) that the likelihood of growth of a neoplasm to clinical disease is a function of hormone levels, estrogens, and possibly androgens and their interaction with the intracellular nuclear receptors and post-transcription of various growth factors, 4) that the risk of clinical disease is further importantly determined by genetic host susceptibility factors, and 5) that the probability of metastatic disease may be related to mutation of a clone of cells during increased mitotic activity secondary to the initial neoplastic changes or exposure to other carcinogens later in the development of the disease. The model presumes that the effect of estrogen is to enhance cell division (i.e., it is a mitogen). There is also some evidence that metabolites of estrogen may act as mutagens (18).

This model is compatible with both clinical and epidemiologic data. First, women at very low risk of breast cancer can be identified (1,16,18,23). These include women with early age at first pregnancy, such as before age 20. Second, premenopausal hormone levels are kept very low, that is, oophorectomy at an early age, late age of menarche, or irregular or long menstrual cycles (24). Third, there is no family history of breast cancer. And finally, postmenopausal or late premenopausal hormone levels are very low.

Unfortunately, it is not feasible to use many of these approaches in the prevention of breast cancer for most women. Therefore, we have to develop approaches that mimic some of these preventive approaches but also would be acceptable within the context of good health in our society.

Factors that Increase the Risk of Breast Cancer

The only specific breast carcinogen that has been clearly identified to increase breast cancer is radiation to breast tissue (25–26). The risk is directly related to the age at exposure to radiation, especially if exposure occurred prior to menarche and first pregnancy. Later-age exposure to similar doses of radiation have a much smaller impact on the incidence of disease. There is clearly an increased risk of breast cancer among children treated with thoracic radiation for childhood malignancy (26). It is clear that radiation exposure to breast tissue should be avoided, if at all possible, early in life. Whether there is any increased risk of breast cancer associated with mammography in premenopausal women has been a hotly debated subject.

Xenoestrogens are chemicals that may bind the estrogen receptor and can be mitogens (i.e., cause cell division) and mutagens (i.e., cause DNA changes) (27–31). Polychlorinated biphenyls (such as DDT) are considered to be xenoestrogens. There has been a great deal of interest in whether these compounds, especially pesticides in the general environment or occupational exposures, can be associated with an increased risk of breast cancer.

These chemicals are stored in fat tissue for long periods of time, and metabolism of these chemicals by type 1 and type 2 metabolic enzymes may play an important role in any potential risk of breast cancer. Initial studies had shown a relationship between either blood levels or levels in fat and risk of breast cancer. These observations have not been substantiated by later studies (30). The apparent geographic variations in breast cancer in the United States are most closely linked to socioeconomic factors than to exposure to pesticides. The risk of breast cancer among women with very high occupational exposures to pesticides has not been tested in any great detail. There is still some potential that, at high levels, some of these chemicals may be important breast carcinogens.

The real absence of any major geographic variations in breast cancer in the United States, except related to socioeconomic factors, plus the higher rates in upper-social-class women (especially postmenopausal women), would seem to be fairly strong evidence against a major single environmental carcinogen, unless the carcinogen is in the food chain and is widely distributed in the United States. Breast glandular tissue may concentrate and secrete many carcinogens that can be identified in breast secretions. It is possible, therefore, that many carcinogens "cause breast cancer but with low relative and attributable risk" (31).

The modifiable risk associated with any single carcinogen may be small (i.e., relative risk) either because of low carcinogenicity of the agent (i.e., mutagen), variations in the metabolism of the agent, or differences in host susceptibility. It also is possible that the primary mutagens are metabolites of estrogens. The levels of the "mutagenic" estrogen metabolites could be related to activation of both type 1 and type 2 metabolizing enzymes or genetic variations of the enzymes (32–33). Recent reports have suggested, for example, that null genotypes of glutathione-*S*-transferase (a type 2 metabolizing enzyme) may be associated with an increased risk of breast cancer (34). Variations in P450 type 1 metabolizing enzymes also have been related to an increased risk of breast cancer (35).

Lupus erythematosus is an inflammatory tissue disease that is seen much more frequently in women than in men and has been linked to possible aberrant estrogen metabolism. Women with lupus have increased symptomology associated with estrogen exposure and pregnancy. They have higher rates of premature premenopausal cardiovascular disease (42). There is preliminary evidence that they have an increased risk of breast cancer. If the specific abnormality of estrogen metabolism can be identified, and if there is a true increased risk of breast cancer, then the disease would be a model of an estrogen metabolite as a mutagen.

Cigarette smoking is an example of a powerful environmental carcinogen. Chemicals associated with cigarette smoke such as cotinine can be identified easily in breast secretions. There is, however, a very weak association between cigarette smoking and the risk of breast cancer. Variations in the genetic polymorphisms of these type 1 and type 2 enzymes could, in part, determine the association between exposure to environmental carcinogen and the risk of breast cancer (36).

Hormonal factors clearly play a crucial role in the etiology of breast cancer (18,37–38). Menopause (oophorectomy) at an early age results in a very substantial reduction in both pre- and postmenopausal breast cancer (18). Oophorectomy reduces the levels of both estrogens and androgens. Early age at menarche is a risk factor for breast cancer by increasing the length of exposure to sex steroid hormones from the pre- to the postmenopausal years. The age at menarche deceased in the United States over time, probably due to the increase in body size. Later age at menarche is characteristic of populations with low rates of breast cancer. The age at menarche decreases with greater body size due to increased protein and probably fat in the diet. Big, taller girls and an early age at menarche are probably important determinants of the risk of breast cancer.

Factors that May Decrease the Risk of Breast Cancer

Breast feeding, probably by increasing the length of time of anovulation following pregnancy (i.e., postpartum), is associated with a small reduction in the risk of breast cancer, primarily premenopausal breast cancer (39).

Increasing physical activity may modify menstrual cycling, increasing the length of the cycles and possibly decreasing peak estrogen levels secondary to the hypothalamic-pituitary-ovarian axis. Increased physical activity also may be associated with a later age at menarche. Observational studies have reported that increased physical activity is more frequent in control individuals than in premenopausal breast cancer patients. It is unclear what amount of physical activity is required to modify the risk of breast cancer. The effects of physical activity, for example, also may be modified (in part) by changes in body weight with high levels of physical activity, associated with substantial reductions or very low body weight, and result in hypothalamic-pituitary-ovarian failure and amenorrhea (40–41).

Unfortunately, if substantial physical activity with decreases in body weight and lengthening of menstrual cycling or amenorrhea reduced the risk of breast cancer, it probably also would increase the number of women with low bone mineral density and osteoporosis and possibly also increase the risk of cardiovascular disease. There are no clinical trials at present that document that exercise results in a reduction in breast cancer in either pre- or postmenopausal women.

Lower-intensity activities that are acceptable to much of the population could be an approach to the prevention of breast cancer without adverse effects on osteoporosis or cardiovascular disease.

Several diseases may be associated with changes in menstrual cycling or premenopausal hormone levels and reduced risk of breast cancer (24,42). The most common disease associated with abnormal menstrual cycling is polycystic ovary disease. Women with this condition frequently have anovulatory menstrual cycling and elevated insulin, testosterone, and estrone levels but low peak estradiol and progesterone levels. Such women also have increased intra-abdominal fat. Whether they have an increased or decreased risk of breast cancer is controversial (18).

Turner syndrome affects 50 in 100,000 women and is due to absence, total or partial, of one X chromosome and absence of female sex hormones (43). Reduced bone mineral density and short stature are common in this syndrome. Sex hormone replacement therapy is a major component of therapy. A study from the Danish Cytogenic Central Registry (N = 594) reported that the risks of both heart disease and bone fracture were increased, but there was no difference between observed and expected risk of breast cancer. The number of patients, however, was very similar (43).

Gene-Environment Interactions

The genetics of breast cancer are discussed in detail in Chapter 2. It is very important to separate major gene effects with very high relative risk (i.e., *BRCA1* or *BRCA2*) from genetic polymorphisms that are more frequent but have lower relative risks. A better understanding of how abnormalities of *BRCA1* and *BRCA2* increase the risk of breast cancer could have important implications for understanding the etiology of breast cancer. Both *BRCA1* and *BRCA2* are apparently tumor-suppressor genes. Whether a function of the "normal" *BRCA* genes is to moderate increased mitotic activity secondary to sex steroid hormone exposure at the breast or moderate mutagenic DNA changes is not certain. If *BRCA1* or *BRCA2* functions to suppress mitogenic stimulation, then oophorectomy, by substantially lowering endogenous estrogen levels, may reduce the risk of breast cancer. The Breast Cancer Prevention Trial recently has reported about a 40% to 50% decrease in the risk of breast cancer among high-risk women using the drug tamoxifen (14). A percentage of the women were at risk because of strong family history of breast cancer (i.e., *BRCA1, BRCA2*). It will be very important to determine whether selective estrogen receptor modulators (SERMs), such as tamoxifen, can reduce the risk of breast cancer among women who are carriers of *BRCA1* or *BRCA2* abnormalities and are at high risk of breast cancer (44–45).

The genetic polymorphisms are much more frequent than major gene effects and are associated with lower relative risks. These polymorphisms are of very great importance in epidemiologic studies because they possibly play a major role in determining host susceptibility to environmental agents and lifestyles. There are likely to be many genetic polymorphisms of estrogen production, receptors, protein synthesis (especially growth factors), estrogen metabolism, other hormone and growth factors, inflammation and immune response, and metabolism of carcinogens (46–48).

The identification of the interaction between genetic polymorphisms and environmental host, lifestyle exposures, and risk of breast cancer is a very important approach for identifying high-risk women candidates for chemopreventive therapies.

Postmenopausal breast cancer occurs among women in an environment of much lower endogenous estrogen production than premenopausal breast cancer (18). The major source of postmenopausal estrogens is from adrenal androgens and aromatization of androstenedione to estrone, primarily in adipose tissue. Of the 43,644 breast cancer deaths in the United States in 1994, 32,750 (75%) occurred among postmenopausal women aged 55+ and about one-third among women over the age of 75. Approximately 1 (0.44%) in 27 women will develop incident breast cancer from birth to age 40, whereas 1 (about 4%) in 25 women develop breast cancer between the ages of 40 and 59 and 1 (6.9%) in 15 between the ages of 60 and 79. The incidence of breast cancer is about 40 per 100,000 among women aged 30 to 39 years, 150 per 100,000 among women aged 40 to 49, and 500 per 100,000 among women aged 65+, a 10-fold greater risk than among those aged 30 to 39. By definition, therefore, older postmenopausal women are a high-risk group for breast cancer (21).

Postmenopausal breast cancer patients probably should be further divided into two subgroups: those with early postmenopausal breast cancer (i.e., probably prior to age 55 or 60) and those with later-age postmenopausal breast cancer (i.e., over age 60). The time from early neoplastic changes to clinical breast cancer detection, even by mammography, may be as long as 10 years, especially among postmenopausal women. The breast cancers in the early postmenopausal period may have already begun to develop during the pre- to peri- to postmenopausal period. The risk factors related to high estrogens or estrogen/progestins during the late peri- and early postmenopausal period when there is still residual ovarian function may play an important role in the development of early postmenopausal breast cancer. Women who develop incident breast cancer early after menopause may be at risk because of late age at menopause or continued high estrogen production by the ovaries during or just after menopause. The majority of breast cancers that develop after age 60+ are probably determined, to a considerable degree, by the postmenopausal hormone environment.

Measurable Determinants of Breast Cancer Risk

There is overwhelming evidence now that postmenopausal breast cancer is determined primarily by sex steroid hormone levels and metabolism. There is solid evidence from longitudinal epidemiologic studies that higher blood levels of sex steroid hormones, including androstenedione, estrone, estradiol, and testosterone, are associated with a substantial increased risk of breast cancer. The risks are in the neighborhood of three- to fourfold or even greater in many of the more recent large studies and are of the same magnitude as is the relationship of many of the cardiovascular risk factors and coronary heart disease (49–53) (Fig. 1-3).

Bone mineral density, a probable marker of higher estrogen levels, also has been associated with a substantial increased risk of breast cancer, at least within the first 3 to 4 years after the bone mineral density measurements (54–55). Greater

breast density, which also is apparently related to higher estrogen levels, is also a marker for increased risk of breast cancer, even among postmenopausal women (Fig. 1-4).

Postmenopausal obesity is associated with higher levels of estrone and estradiol, lower sex hormone–binding globulin, and a greater risk of breast cancer (18,56–57). Weight gain just before and just after menopause is also a significant independent risk factor for breast cancer, even after adjustment for current body mass index (20).

The important recent results of trials of selective estrogen receptor modulators such as tamoxifen (14) and raloxifene (58) documented that these drugs substantially reduce the incidence of both pre- and postmenopausal breast cancer and do so within a relatively short period of time. This is certainly very strong evidence for an important role of estrogen and estrogen metabolism in the etiology of clinical breast cancer.

Long-term postmenopausal exogenous estrogen or estrogen/progesterone therapy has been associated with at least a 50% increase in the risk of breast cancer. It has not been determined, however, whether the combination of estrogen and progesterone as compared with estrogen alone or the specific type of estrogen is related to the increased risk of breast cancer (59).

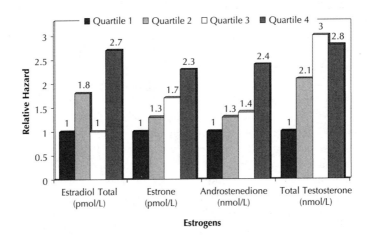

Figure 1-3. Relative hazard of breast cancer by level of sex steroid hormone. (Reproduced with permission from Cauley JA, Lucas FL, Kuller LH, et al. for the Study of Osteoporotic Fractures Research Group. Elevated serum estradiol and testosterone concentrations are associated with a high risk of breast cancer. Arch Intern Med 1999 (in press).)

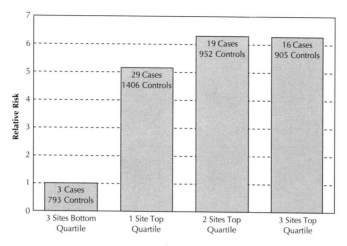

Figure 1-4. Relative risk of breast cancer by bone mineral density. Women with top quartile BMD at one, two, or three sites compared with women with lowest BMD at three sites. (Reproduced with permission from Kuller LH, Cauley JA, Lucas L, et al. Sex steroid hormones, bone mineral density, and risk of breast cancer. Environ Health Perspect 1997;105(suppl 3):593–599.)

The primary source of postmenopausal estrone and testosterone, as noted earlier, is the adrenal androgens (57,60). Increased levels of androstenedione have been associated with a greater risk of breast cancer in longitudinal studies (51–52). The primary determinants of the production and levels of androstenedione are not known (61–62). There is little evidence, for example, that adrenocorticotropic hormone (ACTH) stimulation raises androstenedione production by the adrenal gland. Levels of androstenedione decline with age in both men and women (62). It is very possible that women may be at higher risk of breast cancer if the levels of androstenedione do not decline substantially with increasing age. There is very little longitudinal data on changes in androstenedione levels over time in relationship to risk of breast cancer. There also may be an inverse relationship between the production of stress-related glucocorticoids and androstenedione production in the adrenal gland (61).

Genetic polymorphisms of enzyme metabolism as well as the effects of environmental factors or drugs on the activity of these enzymes may be important in the production of androstenedione in the adrenal gland (63).

The conversion of androstenedione to estrone, that is, aromatization, occurs primarily in fat cells (63). The aromatase activity increases with age in women (60). There is also an increase in body fat and a decrease in both bone and muscle mass in women. The aromatase activity in women increases with advancing age, independent of increases in body fat.

There is also an increase in visceral or abdominal fat in women as they age as compared with lower body or thigh fat, the usual site of fat storage in women (64–65). This increase in visceral fat is related to higher levels of insulin (insulin resistance), higher free fatty acid flux, especially to the liver, and an increase in tumor necrosis factor (TNFα) and interleukin 6 (IL6). Some studies have suggested that increased waist circumference, a measure of visceral fat, is also an independent risk factor for breast cancer (66). Weight gain just before to just after menopause is probably associated with an increase in visceral fat. There is no consistent evidence that either diabetes or insulin level is a risk factor for breast cancer (67–69). Recent studies have suggsted that cytokines, particularly IL6 and TNFα, may play an important role in regulating estrogen synthesis in breast tissue. Both IL-6 and TNFα apparently stimulate aromatase and estradiol-17β-hydroxysteroid dehydrogenas type I) (E2DH) and estrone sulfatase (60). It is generally believed that local autocrine and paracrine effects in the breast account for increase in TNFα and IL-6 rather than peripheral production, that is, visceral fat. However, it is possible that elevated levels of these cytokines associated with increased visceral fat could contribute to the growth of breast cancer.

Another important factor related to increasing intra-abdominal fat is the decrease in the levels of sex hormone–binding globulin (SHBG). The lower levels of SHBG would result in an increase in circulating free and albumin-bound estradiol and testosterone levels. Testosterone is much more tightly bound to SHBG than is estradiol, and therefore, the increase in intra-abdominal fat and associated decrease in SHBG would likely shift the distribution toward higher free or albumin-bound testosterone levels as compared with free or albumin-bound estradiol levels (19).

A small amount of testosterone continues to be produced by the granulosa cells in the ovary. Epidemiologic studies have shown that blood levels of testosterone are associated with a greater risk of breast cancer, almost to the same extent as that for estradiol. Testosterone is metabolized to estradiol. A higher testosterone level therefore may contribute to higher estradiol levels. Whether the higher testosterone levels are related to increased production by the ovary or the adrenal and the decrease in SHBG is associated with increasing abdominal fat and greater free or albumin-bound testosterone are unknown.

The conversion of estrone to estradiol occurs in breast tissue by E2DH (60,70). This enzyme is found in breast tissue and in higher levels in breast tumor cells. As noted earlier, estrone sulfatase is also found in normal and malignant breast tissue and results in a conversion of estrone sulfate to estrone. A large percentage of estrone in breast tissue is from the effects of sulfatase on estrone sulfate. The level of estradiol in breast tissue is much higher than that in the serum. This has lead to a controversy about whether measurements of peripheral hormone levels such as estradiol or estrone truly reflect the activity within the breast and therefore can be used as a predictor of breast cancer. However, as noted earlier, recent large epidemiologic studies have shown a very strong association between peripheral blood estrogen levels and the subsequent risk of breast cancer. It is possible that these high levels of estradiol found in the

blood are a reflection of increasing production in breast tissue.

There is increasing evidence that cells of the immune system may play an important role as a source of stimulation of tumor estrogen synthesis in the breast. Inflammatory cells and cells of the immune system clearly infiltrate breast tumors. As noted earlier, it has been suggested that cytokines (both IL-6 and TNFα) may stimulate estrogen synthesis in breast tissue and probably other tissues as well. A major source of the IL-6 and TNFα may be the immune cells that infiltrate the breast tissue. Genetic polymorphisms, as well as systemic effects such as increased intra-abdominal fat or total fat, may contribute to high levels of cytokines and estradiol in the breast.

The ability to measure low levels of cytokines and various inflammatory markers in blood may provide another tool to identify women at high risk of breast cancer. Insulin-like growth factor I (IGF-I) also may stimulate estrogen synthesis in breast tissue. Recent studies have suggested that peripheral serum levels of IGF-I and insulin-like growth factor–binding protein III may be associated with an increased risk of prostate cancer (71). Similar data have not been published with regard to breast cancer. Again, it is difficult to determine whether the effects of these cytokines and growth factors, primarily autocrine and paracrine within the breast tissue, are secondary to the breast cancer or are a major factor potentiating the effects of estrogens on the development of breast cancer and whether peripheral endocrine rather than autocrine or paracrine effects are associated with increased estrogen synthesis and risk of at least the growth of breast cancer.

Role of Dietary Factors in the Etiology of Breast Cancer

There is little evidence to date that any dietary factors, except high fat intake and total calories, are an important risk factor for postmenopausal breast cancer (72). There is a high correlation with the amount of dietary fat in grams and total caloric intake (73). Animal experimental studies support an increased risk of breast cancer with both high dietary fat and total calories. It is extremely difficult to quantify total caloric intake using traditional nutrition survey methods (74). There is a very poor correlation between reported caloric intake and more objective measures of energy intake such as double-labeled water.

The estimated caloric intake is also biased. Obese individuals tend to grossly underestimate their caloric intake and especially fat consumption. Many epidemiologic studies have reported either an inverse or no relationship between measures of body weight, obesity, and caloric intake. This is not feasible, and such studies clearly have underestimated caloric intake as well as having substantial bias in their reporting of caloric intake. They are of little value.

Fat intake in a homogeneous population is also difficult to measure (72–74). Many studies in relatively homogeneous populations cannot measure fat consumption accurately. Thus the fact that some of these studies find no relationship between total fat, caloric intake, and risk of breast cancer is not unexpected given the relatively poor quality of the data (75–77). There are also questions about whether the specific type of fat may be related to the risk of breast cancer. Some investigators have suggested that polyunsaturated fat and linoleic acid are more important as risk factors than monounsaturated fat, and others have suggested that saturated fat also may be an important risk factor for breast cancer (78).

A high caloric intake — as well as a high fat intake and decreased energy expenditure — are important determinants of obesity and weight gain. Obesity and weight gain are clearly major risk factors for postmenopausal breast cancer. There is also a major genetic component related to obesity and distribution of body fat. This may contribute in part to the genetic risks of breast cancer. Current clinical trials such as the Women's Health Initiative (WHI) (72) and the Women's Intervention Nutrition Study (WINS) (79), a secondary prevention trial in women who already have breast cancer, will provide important information about the relationship between dietary fat and breast cancer.

There is little evidence at the present time of an association between any specific fat-soluble vitamins and the risk of breast cancer (80–81). However, the levels of the fat-soluble vitamins may not be the important variable, but rather whether substantial increases in fat-soluble vitamins, such as vitamin E, may be associated with a reduced risk of breast cancer. Recent studies have suggested that vitamin E supplementation in a clinical trial was associated with a decreased risk of prostate cancer (82). There are no completed vitamin E trials investigating reduction of the risk of breast cancer.

A high fiber intake may increase the excretion of estrogens in the feces and reduce blood estrogen levels. The effect, however, is relatively small (83). High intakes of fruits and vegetables have been suggested as a method of reducing overall risk of cancer. However, the effect seems to be stronger for epithelial cancers and especially for smoking-related cancers. Postmenopausal breast cancer has a direct relationship with socioeconomic status. There is a striking and direct relationship between the intake of fruits and vegetables and socioeconomic status. It is unlikely that major differences in the intake of fruits and vegetables are playing an important role in the etiology of postmenopausal breast cancer.

The intake of phytoestrogens, especially flavonoids from soy protein, has generated a great deal of interest with regard to the prevention of hormone-related cancers, including breast cancer (84–85). Higher intakes of soy proteins in such populations as the Japanese have been linked to their lower risks of breast cancer. High doses of phytoestrogens may compete for estrogen receptors with natural estrogens and, much like specialized estrogen receptor modulators (SERMs), reduce the risk of breast cancer. It is possible, although unproven, that high doses of phytoestrogens could be a nonpharmacologic approach to the prevention of breast cancer. Unfortunately, the amount of phytoestrogens that would be required from diet is substantial. If the phytoestrogens were to have any protective effect, they probably would have to be given in a concentrated pill form because of the high doses that are necessary. There are no clinical trials that document any benefit of the phytoestrogens in modifying the risk of breast cancer.

Leisure time physical activity among older women has been associated with a possible decrease in the risk of breast cancer (86).

Increased leisure time physical activity generally is associated with a decrease in the amount of intra-abdominal fat. Leisure time physical activity could reduce the risk of breast cancer by moderating the amount or activity of intra-abdominal fat. The ability to measure the amount of visceral fat by computed tomography (CT) or magnetic resonance imaging (MRI) may provide an important opportunity to understand the interrelationships between the amount of fat, location of fat, visceral fat, etc., hormones, growth factors, inflammatory markers, and breast cancer.

Alcohol consumption also has been related to an increased risk of both pre- and postmenopausal breast cancer (87). A recent meta-analysis of alcohol studies has suggested that an increase of one drink, approximately 10 gm of alcohol, per day is associated with a 9% increase in the risk of breast cancer. Adjustment for other risk factors for breast cancer did not eliminate the increased risk associated with alcohol intake. There is some evidence that women who consume alcohol have higher blood levels of estrone or estradiol both before and after menopause, as well as higher levels of estrone sulfate (18,88). Alcohol intake may be associated with elevation of liver enzymes and possibly increased production of estrone sulfate.

Other Etiologic Factors

Host susceptibility and genetic factors appear to play a less important role in the development of postmenopausal breast cancer as compared with early-age premenopausal breast cancer. About 8% to 10% of postmenopausal women with breast cancer probably have a first-degree family history of breast cancer. Concordance of breast cancer among older monozygotic twins is relatively low, and the risk associated with familial breast cancer from most of the recent studies is relatively modest, probably less than twofold for older postmenopausal women. Genetic polymorphisms of the metabolism of estrogens and of the effects of estrogen receptors could play a modest role in increasing host susceptibility to the development of breast cancer among postmenopausal women (89–90).

The recent discovery of two estrogen receptors, alpha and beta, that appear to have different distributions and functions in tissues has generated a great deal of interest in whether there is a potential interrelationship perhaps between environmental factors (i.e., xenoestrogens), natural estrogens, and the risk of breast cancer (91–93). The important role of these estrogen receptors, alpha and beta, in terms of the epidemiology of breast cancer is still not determined; however, future epidemiologic studies to identify high-risk women probably will have to evaluate both the alpha and beta estrogen receptors and specific polymorphisms of these receptors. To date, epidemiologic and genetic studies of the relationship between polymorphisms of estrogen receptors and the risk of breast cancer have been equivocal.

One of the most important new issues in identifying high-risk women for breast cancer is the evaluation of estrogen metabolic products and the risk of breast cancer. Cytochrome P450 enzymes that metabolize estrogens are found in breast and other tissues. They result in hydroxylated estrogens in the tissues that may be metabolically important in terms of the risk of breast cancer. These metabolic products may be determined, in part, by genetic variations in the P450 enzymes, as well as environmental factors including xenoestrogens (94).

Most interest in recent years has centered on the measurement of 2-, 4-, and 16-hydroxylated estrone in the urine (48,95,96). There is still controversy as to which metabolite is likely to be a potent mutagen or increase mitogenic activity. Some investigators have suggested that elevated 16-hydroxylation in the urine (as compared with 2-hydroxylation) is associated with an increased risk of breast cancer. Animal experimental studies would tend to support this hypothesis. Other investigators have suggested that 4-hydroxy estrone is a more potent carcinogen and that increased levels of 4-hydroxy estrone (but not 16-hydroxy estrone) are the primary risk factor for breast cancer (97).

A few epidemiologic studies have evaluated primarily the 2- to 16-hydroxy estrone ratio in the urines of both pre- and postmenopausal women, along with one case-control study (98) and one prospective study (99), and have shown that greater excretion of 16- as compared with 2-hydroxy estrone is associated with a greater risk of breast cancer. However, the sample sizes in these studies were small, and the results are not conclusive. There is no solid evidence that measurement of the urinary metabolites of estrogen will substantially enhance risk prediction. Further studies are indicated in this area.

O-Methylation of the 4-hydroxy catechol metabolite of estradiol also has been suggested as possibly contributing to the risk of breast cancer (100–101). The 4-hydroxy estradiol may be a direct mutagen, rather than just stimulating proliferation of breast neoplastic cells; that is, it may be a primary cause of the initial neoplastic transformation. *O*-Methylation of 4-hydroxy estradiol by the enzyme catechol-*o*-methyltransferase (COMT) inactivates the catechol estrogens. There are polymorphisms of this enzyme. Low levels of the enzyme therefore would result in higher levels of the 4-hydroxy estradiol and potentially a mutagenic effect. At least one study has suggested that among postmenopausal women with low production of the enzyme there is an increased risk of breast cancer (101). The increased risk was greater among more obese women. These studies are based on very small sample sizes but suggest the potential of identifying high-risk women especially in association with other risk factors such as obesity and high endogenous estrogen production.

An important issue is why the risk of breast cancer is not substantially higher among women on hormone replacement therapy, especially long-term users, given the much higher levels of estradiol among women on such therapy. We would expect a higher than a 1.5-fold increase in risk. The levels of estradiol among postmenopausal women on hormone replacement therapy are not nearly as high as levels before menopause, especially around the time of ovulation. There is also evidence that the greater percentage of the exogenous estrogens from hormone replacement therapy among postmenopausal women are metabolized by the 2- as opposed to the 16-hydroxy estrone pathway. The 2-hydroxy pathway may be less carcinogenic, accounting perhaps for the lower than expected increased risk of breast cancer in patients with hormone replacement therapy. It is also important to note that it is only recent cohorts of postmenopausal women (i.e., from the middle to 1980s) that have been on long-term estrogen replacement therapy other than for symptomology (i.e., low estrogen levels) or osteoporosis (102). It is possible that the risks of breast cancer among current long-term estrogen or estrogen/progesterone users may be substantially higher than reported from previous cohorts.

Summary

The incidence of premenopausal breast cancer is very low, that is, 1.5 cases per 1000 women per year. It is very unlikely that environmental or lifestyle factors will identify large numbers of high-risk premenopausal women. The focus for premenopausal women should be on identifying genetic determinants and interaction with lifestyle. Family history is the most important risk factor. It is possible that population changes in lifestyles will reduce the incidence of premenopausal breast cancer without identification of specific high-risk groups, that is, increased physical activity, decreased age at first pregnancy, increased prevalence of obesity, and anovulatory cycling.

For the majority of breast cancers occurring among postmenopausal women, the situation is very different. It is probable that the measurements of estrogen exposure, such as blood levels of sex steroid hormones, measurement of estrogen metabolites, bone mineral density, breast density, degree of obesity, body fatness, and distribution of body fat (i.e., visceral fat), will help to identify older women at very high risk of breast cancer who probably would be candidates for more aggressive pharmacologic therapy (i.e., with specialized receptor modifiers). There is less conclusive evidence that these measures will identify women who have more "malignant" breast cancer (i.e., likely to metastasize or cause serious morbidity and mortality).

The results of the Breast Cancer Prevention Trial of tamoxifen as compared with placebo demonstrated a substantial decrease in both node-negative and one- to three-node-positive breast cancer but no effect (11 versus 12) for women with four or more positive nodes nor for estrogen receptor–negative breast cancer. It is possible that such cancers are less associated with estrogen levels, estrogen receptors, or estrogen metabolites.

Long-term follow-up of the studies of estrogen receptor modifiers will be necessary to determine whether there is also a reduction in the morbidity and mortality associated with breast cancer.

It is extremely important to test whether these combined measures of identification of risk of postmenopausal breast cancer can identify high-risk women with both high relative and attributable risk (i.e., a high percentage of women who will develop breast cancer). The risk of breast cancer among postmenopausal women is 4 to 5 cases per 1000 women per year; a fivefold increased risk would increase the risk to 2% per year, a level at which pharmacologic therapies are recommended for prevention of disease, such as coronary heart disease.

Non-pharmacologic therapies, if proven in clinical trials to reduce the risk of breast cancer, may be the preferential therapy for average- or lower-risk postmenopausal women. The best candidates at present are a low-fat diet, increased physical activity, weight reduction and decreased intra-abdominal fat, decreased alcohol consumption, and increased consumption of phytoestrogens. It is very important to test these interventions with regard to breast cancer and other diseases. Lowering estrogen levels could prevent breast cancer at the expense of enhancing other diseases (e.g., osteoporosis, coronary heart disease, and dementia). On the other hand, SERMs may be the preferable approach to reducing breast cancer rather than attempting to lower endogenous estrogen levels with the accompanying increased risks of osteoporosis and coronary heart disease.

References

1. Krieger N. Social class and the black/white crossover in the age-specific incidence of breast cancer: a study linking census-derived data to population-based registry records. Am J Epidemiol 1990;131:804–814.
2. Hoel DG, Davis DL, Miller AB, et al. Trends in cancer mortality in 15 industrialized countries, 1969–1986. J Natl Cancer Inst 1992;84:313–320.
3. Ziegler RG, Hoover RN, Pike MC, et al. Migration patterns and breast cancer risk in Asian-American women. J Natl Cancer Inst 1993;85:1819–1827.
4. Chu KC, Tarone RE, Kessler LG, et al. Recent trends in the U.S. breast cancer incidence, survival, and mortality rates. J Natl Cancer Inst 1996;88:1571–1579.
5. Hankey BF. Breast. In: Miller BA, Ries LAG, Hankey BF, et al., eds. Cancer statistics review: 1973–1989 (NIH Publication No. 92-2789). Bethesda, MD: National Cancer Institute, 1992.
6. Feigelson HS, Henderson BE, Pike MC. Recent trends in U.S. breast cancer incidence, survival, and mortality rates. J Natl Cancer Inst 1997;89:1810.
7. Wingo PA, Ries LA, Rosenberg HM, Miller DS, Edwards BK. Cancer incidence and mortality, 1973–1995: a report card for the U.S. Cancer 1998;82:1197–1207.
8. U.S. Department of Health and Human Services. Use of mammography services by women aged equal to or greater than 65 years enrolled in Medicare — United States, 1991–1993. MMWR 1995;44:777–781.
9. Polednak AP. Estimating the prevalence of cancer in the United States. Cancer 1997;80:136–141.
10. Nandi S, Guzman RC, Yang J. Hormones and mammary carcinogenesis in mice, rats, and humans: a unifying hypothesis. Proc Natl Acad Sci USA 1995;92:3650–3657.
11. Peer PG, van Dijck JA, Hendriks JH, et al. Age-dependent growth rate of primary breast cancer. Cancer 1993;71:3547.
12. Harris JR, Hellman S. Natural history of breast cancer. In: Harris JR, Lippman ME, Morrow M, Hellman S, eds. Diseases of the breast, chap. 12. Philadelphia: Lippincott-Raven, 1996:375–391.
13. Welch HG, Black WC. Using autopsy series to estimate the disease "reservoir" for ductal carcinoma in situ of the breast: how much more breast cancer can we find? Ann Intern Med 1997;127:1023–1028.
14. Fisher B, Costantino JP, Wickerham DL, et al. Tamoxifen for prevention of breast cancer: report of the National Surgical Adjuvant Breast and Bowel Project P-1 study. J Natl Cancer Inst 1998;90:1371–1388.
15. Collaborative Group on Hormonal Factors in Breast Cancer. Breast cancer and hormone replacement therapy: collaborative reanalysis of data from 51 epidemiological studies of 52,705 women with breast cancer and 108,411 women without breast cancer. Lancet 1997;350:1047–1059.
16. Hunter DJ, Spiegelman D, Adami HO, et al. Non-dietary factors as risk factors for breast cancer, and as effect modifiers of the association

of fat intake and risk of breast cancer. Cancer Causes Control 1997;8:49–56.

17. Spicer DV, Pike MC. Sex steroids and breast cancer prevention. Monogr Natl Cancer Inst 1994;16:139–147.

18. Kuller LH. The etiology of breast cancer: from epidemiology to prevention. Public Health Rev 1995;23:157–213.

19. Azziz R. Reproductive endocrinologic alterations in female asymptomatic obesity. Fertil Steril 1989;52:703–725.

20. Huang Z, Hankinson SE, Colditz GA, et al. Dual effects of weight and weight gain on breast cancer risk. JAMA 1997;278:1407–1411.

21. Murphy GP, Holb AI, Garfinkel L, Cohen-Kligerman B, eds. Cancer Statistics 1998. Cancer J Clin 1998;48:3–63.

22. Ziegler J. Exposures and habits early in life may influence breast cancer risk. J Natl Cancer Inst 1998;90:187–188.

23. Gail MH, Brinton LA, Byar DP, et al. Projecting individualized probabilities of developing breast cancer for white females who are being examined annually. J Natl Cancer Inst 1989;81:1879–1886.

24. Garland M, Hunter DJ, Colditz GA, et al. Menstrual cycle characteristics and history of ovulatory infertility in relation to breast cancer risk in a large cohort of U.S. women. Am J Epidemiol 1998;147:636–643.

25. Land CE, Hayakawa N, Machado SG, et al. A case-control interview study of breast cancer among Japanese A-bomb survivors: II. Interactions with radiation dose. Cancer Causes Control 1994;5:167–176.

26. Kaste SC, Hudson MM, Jones DJ, et al. Breast masses in women treated for childhood cancer: incidence and screening guidelines. Cancer 1998;82:784–792.

27. Safe SH. Xenoestrogens and breast cancer. New Engl J Med 1997;337:1303–1304. Editorial.

28. Shekhar PVM, Werdell J, Basrur VS. Environmental estrogen stimulation of growth and estrogen receptor function in preneoplastic and cancerous human breast cell lines. J Natl Cancer Inst 1997;89:1774–1782.

29. Davidson NE, Yager JD. Pesticides and breast cancer: fact or fad? J Natl Cancer Inst 1997;89:1743–1744. Editorial.

30. Hunter DJ, Hankinson SE, Laden F, et al. Plasma organochlorine levels and the risk of breast cancer. New Engl J Med 1997;337:1253–1258.

31. Petrakis NL. Epidemiologic studies of mutagenicity of breast fluids: relevance to breast cancer risk. In: Pike MC, Sisiteri PK, Welsch CW, eds. Banbury report 8: Hormones and breast cancer. Cold Spring Harbor, NY: Cold Spring Harbor Laboratory 1981:243–255.

32. Talalay P. The role of enzyme induction in protection against carcinogenesis. In: Wattenberg LW, Lipkin M, Boone CW, Kelloff GJ, eds. Cancer chemoprevention. Boca Raton, FL: CRC Press, 1992:469–478.

33. Davis DL, Pongsiri MJ, Wolff M. Recent developments on the avoidable causes of breast cancer. In: Castagnetta L, Nenci I, Bradlow HL, eds. Basis for cancer management. New York: New York Academy of Science, 1996:513–523.

34. Helzlsouer KJ, Selmin O, Huang HY, et al. Association between glutathione S-transferase M1, P1, and T1 genetic polymorphisms and development of breast cancer. J Natl Cancer Inst 1998;90:512–518.

35. Kelsey KT, Wiencke JK. Growing pains for the environmental genetics of breast cancer: observations on a study of the glutathione S-transferases. J Natl Cancer Inst 1998;90:484–485. Editorial.

36. Ambrosone CB, Freudenheim JL, Graham S, et al. Cytochrome P4501A1 and glutathione S-transferase (M1) genetic polymorphisms and postmenopausal breast cancer risk. Cancer Res 1995;55:3483–3485.

37. Pike MC, Spicer DV, Dalmoush L, Press MF. Estrogens, progesterones, normal breast cell proliferation, and breast cancer risk. Epidemiol Rev 1993;15:17–35.

38. Pathak DR, Whittemore AS. Combined effects of body size, parity, and menstrual events on breast cancer incidence in seven countries. Am J Epidemiol 1992;135:153–168.

39. Newcomb PA, Storer BE, Longnecker MP, et al. Lactation and a reduced risk of premenopausal breast cancer. New Engl J Med 1994;330:81–87.

40. Bernstein L, Henderson BE, Hanisch R, et al. Physical exercise and reduced risk of breast cancer in young women. J Natl Cancer Inst 1994;86:1403–1408.

41. Frisch RE. Body fat, menarche, fitness and fertility. In: Frisch RE, ed. Adipose tissue and reproduction, vol. 14. Basel: Karger, 1990:1–26.

42. Baird DT. Amenorrhoea. Lancet 1997;350:275–279.

43. Gravholt CH, Juul S, Naeraa RW, Hansen J. Morbidity in Turner syndrome. Clin Epidemiol 1998;51:147–158.

44. Newman B, Mu H, Butler LM, et al. Frequency of breast cancer attributable to *BRCA1* in a population-based series of American women. JAMA 1998;279:915–921.

45. Malone KE, Daling JR, Thompson JD, et al. *BRCA1* mutations and breast cancer in the general population: analyses in women before age 35 years and in women before age 45 years with first-degree family history. JAMA 1998;279:922–929.

46. Southey MC, Batten LE, McCredie MRE, et al. Estrogen receptor polymorphism at codon 325 and risk of breast cancer in women before age forty. J Natl Cancer Inst 1998;90:532–536.

47. Layman LC, Lee EJ, Peak DB, et al. Delayed puberty and hypogonadism caused by mutations in the follicle-stimulating hormone b-subunit gene. New Engl J Med 1997;337:607–611.

48. Zhu BT, Conney AH. Functional role of estrogen metabolism in target cells: review and perspectives. Carcinogenesis 1998;19:1–27.

49. Toniolo PG, Levitz M, Zeleniuch-Jacquotte A, et al. A prospective study of endogenous estrogens and breast cancer in postmenopausal women. J Natl Cancer Inst 1995;87:190–197.

50. Dorgan JF, Longcope C, Stephenson HE Jr, et al. Relation of prediagnostic serum estrogen and androgen levels to breast cancer risk. Cancer Epidemiol Biomark Prev 1996;5:533–539.

51. Cauley JA, Lucas FL, Kuller LH, et al. Endogenous sex steroid hormone concentrations and bone mass predict breast cancer in older women. Presented at the Department of Defense Breast Cancer Research Program Meeting; "Era of Hope," October 31–November 4, 1997. In: Proceedings, vol. I. Washington: U.S. Government Printing Office, 1997:506–586.

52. Dorgan JF, Stanczyk FZ, Longcope C, et al. Relationship of serum dehydroepiandrosterone (DHEA), DHEA sulfate, and 5-androstene-317β-diol to risk of breast cancer in postmenopausal women. Cancer Epidemiol Biomar Prev 1997;6:177–182.

53. Zeleniuch-Jacquotte A, Bruning PF, Bonfrer JMG, et al. Relation of serum levels of testosterone and dehydroepiandrosterone sulfate to risk of breast cancer in postmenopausal women. Am J Epidemiol 1997;145:1030–1038.

54. Cauley JA, Lucas FL, Kuller LH, et al. Bone mineral density and risk of breast cancer in older women. JAMA 1996;276:1404–1408.

55. Zhang Y, Kiel DP, Kreger BE, et al. Bone mass and the risk of breast cancer among postmenopausal women. New Engl J Med 1997;336:611–617.

56. Cauley JA, Gutai JP, Kuller LH, et al. The epidemiology of serum sex hormones in postmenopausal women. Am J Epidemiol 1989;129:1120–1131.

57. Jaffe RB. The menopause and perimenopausal period. In: Yen SSC, Jaffe RB, eds. Reproductive endocrinology: Physiology, pathophysiology and clinical management. Philadelphia: WB Saunders, 1986.

58. Gustafsson JA. Raloxifene: Magic bullet for heart and bone? Nature Med 1998;4:152–153.

59. Beral V, Bull D, Doll R, et al. Breast cancer and hormone replacement therapy: collaborative reanalysis of data from 51 epidemiological studies of 52,705 women with breast cancer and 108,411 women without breast cancer. Lancet 1997;350:1047–1059.

60. Reed MJ, Purohit A. Breast cancer and the role of cytokines in regulating estrogen synthesis: an emerging hypothesis. Endocr Rev 1997;18:701–715.

61. Simpson ER, Waterman MR. Steroid hormone biosynthesis in the adrenal cortex and its regulation of adrenocorticotropin. In: DeGrott LJ, ed. Endocrinology. New York: Grune & Stratton, 1994:1630–1641.

62. Parker LN, ed. Adrenal androgens in clinical medicine. San Diego, Academic Press, 1989.

63. Kelloff GJ, Lubet RA, Lieberman R, et al. Aromatase inhibitors as potential cancer chemopreventives. Cancer Epidemiol Biomark Prev 1998;7:65–78.

64. Wing RR, Matthews KA, Kuller LH, et al. Waist to hip ratio in middle-aged women: associations with behavioral and psychosocial factors and with changes in cardiovascular risk factors. Arterioscler Thromb 1991;11:1250–1257.

65. Lapidus L, Bengtsson C, Larsson B, et al. Distribution of adipose tissue and risk of cardiovascular disease and death: a 12-year follow-up of participants in the population study of women in Gothenburg, Sweden. Br Med J 1984;289:1257–1261.

66. Schapira DV, Kumar NB, Lyman GH, et al. Upper-body fat distribution and endometrial cancer risk. JAMA 1991;266:1808–1811.

67. Sellers TA, Anderson KE, Olson JE, Folsom AR. Family histories of diabetes mellitus and breast cancer and incidence of postmenopausal breast cancer. Epidemiology 1998;9:102–105.

68. Bruning PF, Bonfrèr JMG, van Noord PA, et al. Insulin resistance and breast cancer risk. Int J Cancer 1992;52:511–516.

69. Sellers TA, Sprafka JM, Gapstur SM, et al. Does body fat distribution promote familial aggregation of adult onset diabetes mellitus and postmenopausal breast cancer? Epidemiology 1994;5:102–108.

70. Clarke R, Dickson RB, Lippman ME. Hormonal aspects of breast cancer: growth factors, drugs and stromal interactions. Crit Rev Oncol Hematol 1992;12:1–23.

71. Chan JM, Stampfer MJ, Giovannucci E, et al. Plasma insulin-like growth factor-I and prostate cancer risk: a prospective study. Science 1998;279:563–566.

72. Prentice RL, Kakar F, Hursting S, et al. Aspects of the rationale for the Women's Health Trial. J Natl Cancer Inst 1988;80:802–814.

73. Freedman LS, Clifford C, Messina M. Analysis of dietary fat, calories, body weight, and the development of mammary tumors in rats and mice: a review. Cancer Res 1990;50:5710–5719.

74. Kuller LH. Eating fat or being fat and risk of cardiovascular disease and cancer among women. Ann Epidemiol 1994;4:119–127.

75. Hunter DJ, Spiegelman D, Adami H-O, et al. Non-dietary factors as risk factors for breast cancer, and as effect modifiers of the association of fat intake and risk of breast cancer. Cancer Causes Control 1997;8:49–56.

76. Wynder EL, Cohen LA, Rose DP, Stellman SD. Dietary fat and breast cancer: where do we stand on the evidence? J Clin Epidemiol 1994;47:217–222.

77. Howe GR. High-fat diets and breast cancer risk: the epidemiologic evidence. JAMA 1992;268:2080–2081.

78. Ip C. Review of the effects of trans fatty acids, oleic acid, n-3 polyunsaturated fatty acids, and conjugated linoleic acid on mammary carcinogenesis in animals. Am J Clin Nutr 1997;66(suppl):1523S–1529S.

79. Ashley JM. Lipid biomarkers of adherence to low fat diets. In: Heber D, Kritchevsky D, eds. Dietary fats, lipids, hormones, and tumorigenesis: new horizons in basic research. New York: Plenum Press, 1996.

80. Longnecker MP, Newcomb PA, Mittendorf R, et al. Intake of carrots, spinach, and supplements containing vitamin A in relation to risk of breast cancer. Cancer Epidemiol Biomark Prev 1997;6:887–892.

81. Patterson RE, White E, Drist AR, et al. Vitamin supplements and risk: the epidemiologic evidence. Cancer Causes Control 1997;8:786–802.

82. Heinonen OP. Vitamin E reduces prostate cancer rates in Finnish trial: U.S. considers follow-up. J Natl Cancer Inst 1998;90:416.

83. Adlercreutz H. Western diet and Western diseases: some hormonal and biochemical mechanisms and associations. Scand J Clin Lab Invest 1990;50(suppl 201):3–23.

84. Goodman MT, Wilkens LR, Hankin JH, et al. Association of soy and fiber consumption with the risk of endometrial cancer. Am J Epidemiol 1997;146:294–306.

85. Ingram D, Sanders K, Kolybaba M, Lopez D. Case-control study of phyto-oestrogens and breast cancer. Lancet 1997;350:990–994.

86. Gammon MD, John EM, Britton JA. Recreational and occupational physical activities and risk of breast cancer. J Natl Cancer Inst 1998;90:100–117.

87. Smith-Warner SA, Spiegelman D, Yaun SS, et al. Alcohol and breast cancer in women: a pooled analysis of cohort studies. JAMA 1998;279:535–540.

88. Muti P, Trevisan M, Micheli A, et al. Alcohol consumption and total estradiol in premenopausal women. Cancer Epidemiol Biomark Prev 1998;7:189–193.

89. Swerdlow AJ, De Stavola BL, Swanwick MA, Maconochie NES. Risks of breast and testicular cancers in young adult twins in England and Wales: evidence on prenatal and genetic aetiology. Lancet 1997;350:1723–1728.

90. Yang Q, Khoury MJ, Rodriguez C, et al. Family history score as a predictor of breast cancer mortality: prospective data from the Cancer Prevention Study II, United States, 1982–1991. Am J Epidemiol 1998;147:652–659.

91. Paech K, Webb P, Kuiper GGJM, et al. Differential ligand activation of estrogen receptors Erα and Erβ at AP1 sites. Science 1997;277:1508–1510.

92. Kuiper GGJM, Gustafsson JA. The novel estrogen receptor-β subtypes: potential role in the cell- and promoter-specific actions of estrogens and anti-estrogens. FEBS Lett 1997;410:87–90.

93. Davis DL, Telang NT, Osborne MP, Bradlow HL. Medical hypothesis: bifunctional genetic-hormonal pathways to breast cancer. Environ Health Perspect 1997;105:571–576.

94. Service RF. New role for estrogen in cancer? Science 1998;279:1631–1632.

95. Ziegler RG, Rossi SC, Fears TR, et al. Quantifying estrogen metabolism: an evaluation of

the reproducibility and validity of enzyme immunoassays for 2-hydroxyestrone and 16α-hydroxyestrone in urine. Environ Health Perspectives 1997;105(3):607–614.

96. Castagnetta LA, Lo Casto M, Granata OM, et al. Estrogen content and metabolism in human breast tumor tissues and cells. In: Castagnetta L, Nenci I, Bradlow HL, eds. Basis for cancer management. New York: New York Academy of Science, 1996:314–324.

97. Telang NT, Katdare M, Bradlow HL, Osborne MP. Estradiol metabolism: an endocrine biomarker for modulation of human mammary carcinogenesis. Environ Health Perspect 1997;105:559–564.

98. Kabat GC, Chang CJ, Sparano JA, et al. Urinary estrogen metabolites and breast cancer: a case-control study. Cancer Epidemiol Biomark Prev 1997;6:505–509.

99. Meilahn EN, De Stavola B, Bradlow HL, et al. Do urinary estrogen metabolites predict breast cancer? Follow-up of the Guernsey III cohort. Br J Cancer 1998;78:1250–1255.

100. Cavalieri EL, Stack DE, Devanesan PD, et al. Molecular origin of cancer: catechol estrogen-3,4-quinones as endogenous tumor initiators. Proc Natl Acad Sci USA 1997;94:10937–10942.

101. Lavigne JA, Helzlsourer KJ, Huang HY, et al. An association between the allele coding for a low activity variant of catechol-o-methyltransferase and the risk of breast cancer. Cancer Res 1997;57:5493–5497.

102. Kuller LH, Cauley JA, Lucas L, et al. Sex steroid hormones, bone mineral density, and risk of breast cancer. Environ Health Perspect 1997;105(suppl 3):593–599.

2

The Genetics of Breast Cancer

Wendy S. Rubinstein

Physicians and poets alike have long marveled at the ability of the female breast to provide nourishment, life and comfort, sexual pleasure, and pain and death. Theories about the causes of breast health and illness have undergone a long and convoluted evolution (1). The ancient Egyptians believed that the milk from a mother who had borne a male child could be used as a sleeping potion, and for centuries, breast milk was used for medicinal purposes. We now recognize the medicinal benefits of milk to include the transmission of antibodies to the nursing infant, as well as a decreased risk of breast cancer to mothers who have nursed. Hippocrates, extrapolating from his theory that illness derived from the imbalance of the four bodily humors, believed that cessation of menses led to the inability of menstrual blood to be converted into breast milk. Ultimately, this resulted in degeneration of the blood humor into nodules, causing breast cancer in postmenopausal women. A modern explanation for the observed increased risk of breast cancer with advancing age would incite the role of the neoteric body humor estrogen and its long-term effects on the breast.

In the biotechnology era, we look to our genes to understand the etiology of disease. The seminal event in modern breast cancer genetics was the linkage of early-onset familial breast cancer to chromosome 17q21 in 1990 by Mary-Claire King and colleagues (2). This tour de force enabled the rapid identification and cloning of the 17q-linked *BRCA1* gene in 1994 (3), followed by discovery of the second breast cancer susceptibility gene, *BRCA2* within 2 years (4,5). This achievement sharply demarcates two eras: 1) a long age of primitive notions about

breast cancer etiology, followed by a period of epidemiologic insights and delineation of genetic syndromes, and 2) the explosive molecular era detailed in this book.

Epidemiologic Insights

The recognition that family history of breast cancer is a risk factor for breast cancer is well documented over the past two decades of epidemiologic literature and has led to practical models of risk assessment (6–8) (see Table 2-2). Aside from age, female gender, or specific histologic findings such as lobular carcinoma in situ (9), family history of breast cancer has the greatest magnitude of any risk factor. However, not all family histories are equivalent. Insights about genetic factors beyond simple absence or presence of a family history of breast cancer were first provided by epidemiologic studies. As seems intuitively obvious, risk increases with the number of relatives affected and closer degrees of relationship (10). Not always as obvious is the importance of paternal family history, since first-degree relatives (fathers) are rarely affected. However, having affected paternal second-degree relatives (e.g., aunt, grandmother) poses a risk similar to that of affected maternal second-degree relatives, reflecting the Mendelian inheritance of traits that show sex-dependent expression.

Bilateral breast cancer also was uncovered as a risk factor. Bilateral breast cancer due to two unique primary cancers can be difficult to distinguish from metastatic disease, that is, spread of a single primary cancer from one breast to the other. A lapse of several years between diagnoses in the absence of distant disease or the presence of unique breast cancer histologies can clarify the situation. In addition, earlier than usual age of onset of breast cancer in affected relatives, defined either by the age at diagnosis (8) or by premenopausal versus postmenopausal status, is a clear risk factor. Relative risks (RR) vary widely depending on these factors. For example, family history of a first-degree relative with postmenopausal breast cancer carries an RR of 1.5; the RR is 3.1 if the relative was premenopausal, and the RR is 8.5 to 9.0 if the relative had premenopausal bilateral breast cancer (9). The magnitude of breast cancer risk is reflective of underlying genetic etiology. Indeed, all the risk factors described above, that is, family history of the same condition, large numbers of affected relatives, close degree of relationship, bilaterality, and early age of onset, are commonly observed features in hereditary conditions (e.g., retinoblastoma). These features have been crucial for selecting families to study to identify breast cancer–predisposing genes via linkage analysis.

The genetic and epidemiologic literature contributed further insights including recognition of an association between ovarian and breast cancer (11–15), leading to a breast cancer risk model based on family history of both ovarian and breast cancer (16). A wider but not unrestricted set of cancers also emerged as female breast cancer risk factors. For example, a family history of male breast cancer was associated with an RR of 2 (17), similar to that of female breast cancer. An association between prostate cancer and female breast cancer has long been recognized (18) and has been borne out in epidemiologic studies (19–21). For some cancers, such as endometrial cancer, family history was significant in some studies (20,21) but not others (22). Similarly, family history of colon cancer has emerged as a possible risk factor in some studies (10) but not others (21). Conflicting results among epidemiologic studies may reflect sampling differences or study design. For certain cancers, such as melanoma or lung cancer, an association with breast cancer was not observed (21).

Epidemiologic studies generally do not permit conclusions about genetic versus shared environment risk within families. However, these studies parallel the recognition of discrete genetic syndromes that include specific constellations of cancer and usually are not limited to one cancer per syndrome. It is tempting to use hindsight to explain prior epidemiologic studies with currently recognized genetic mutations, such as seen in the *BRCA1* and *BRCA2* syndromes, that do suggest an increased risk of prostate cancer. However, attempts to do so would be methodologically flawed and would not take into account the fact that not all hereditary cancer syndromes have been delineated. Further, the *BRCA1* and *BRCA2* syndromes do convey an increased risk of colon cancer not always observed in the preceding studies.

A major contribution of studies exploring family history of diverse cancers was to provide evidence that different cancers may share a common etiology, which is probably at least in part genetic. Thus a complete survey of cancer family history has clinical relevance. Unfortunately, this insight has not been translated effectively into medical practice, and family history, when taken, is often restricted to the single cancer under evaluation. It seems clear that this practice ignores the risk posed by other cancers in the family and impedes the clinical recognition of hereditary cancer syndromes.

Susceptibility, Syndromology, and Environment

Contrary to information in the lay press, there is no single "breast cancer gene." A number of hereditary cancer syndromes have been delineated that pose an increased risk of breast cancer. Since these syndromes are each caused by one or more genes, the concept of a "breast cancer gene" is passé. Indeed, there are probably many more genetic susceptibility factors than hereditary cancer syndromes, such as genes that metabolize xenobiotics, genes that determine endogenous hormone metabolism, and genes that influence onset of menarche and menopause, to name a few categories. All these factors come under the rubric of *breast cancer genetics* (Fig. 2-1). The major challenge confronting modern breast cancer research is to identify these factors and merge the concepts of genetic and environmental risk (23,24).

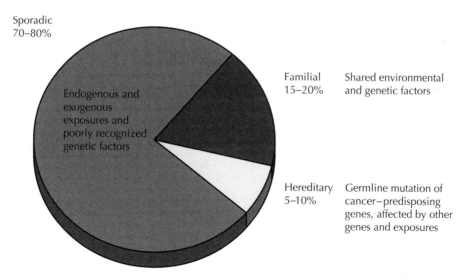

Figure 2-1. Proportion of sporadic, familial, and hereditary breast cancer.

Rather than suggest that genetic and environmental theories of carcinogenesis are competing, breast cancer genetics seeks to develop a synthetic view of breast cancer development with clear elaboration of mechanistic pathways. With this framework in mind, the known hereditary breast cancer syndromes are outlined below.

Gene-environment interactions can be studied by measuring the variation in cancer penetrance within families carrying breast cancer–predisposing genes as a function of individual exposure to carcinogens or to endogenous and exogenous hormones. Examples of such studies in *BRCA1* and *BRCA2* mutation carriers will be explored. Another approach is to dissect the roles of genes and carcinogens in population studies. For example, most epidemiologic studies have not found an association between breast cancer and smoking tobacco. However, genetic variation exists in the ability to detoxify carcinogenic aromatic amines in cigarette smoke, so gross analyses could mask an association. Ambrosone and colleagues (25) studied the relationship between genetic variation in *N*-acetyltransferase 2 (*NAT2*) gene polymorphisms indicating slow or fast acetylation phenotypes, smoking, age, and breast cancer risk in Caucasian women. For slow acetylators (i.e., those with less innate ability to detoxify carcinogens in cigarette smoke), the risk

of breast cancer in smokers increased in a dose-dependent manner. This effect was found among postmenopausal women only, perhaps because there is an intrinsic difference between pre- and postmenopausal breast cancer or because insufficient time had elapsed to see an effect in younger women. No increase in risk was detected for rapid acetylators, and neither *NAT2* genotype or smoking were independent risk factors for breast cancer. Clearly, our understanding of the interacting roles of genes and environment is in a nascent stage, but the promise of the modern paradigm is apparent.

Sporadic breast cancer is colloquially defined as occurring by chance and conceived as being due to exposure to endogenous and exogenous environmental factors, with an accumulation of genetic insults to a breast cell culminating in cancer. Genetic factors in sporadic breast cancer are poorly recognized but undoubtedly exist. With a deeper understanding of the causes of breast cancer, the term *sporadic* will evolve into more descriptive terminology. Sporadic breast cancer accounts for about 70% to 80% of breast cancer.

Familial breast cancer refers to a clustering of two or more affected blood relatives and comprises about 15% to 20% of breast cancer. Shared genetic factors and/or shared environment among family members may be etiologic. Familial breast cancer is conceived as being "possibly genetic" after known breast cancer syndromes are excluded. Unaffected relatives have an increased RR of breast cancer, which can be quantified using epidemiologic risk models (7,8) (see Table 2-2). Breast cancer is most likely familial if only two or three cases are present in the family, breast cancer age of onset is older, and there are no genetic features such as ovarian cancer. For example, three relatives with breast cancer occurring at age 60 or older most likely represents familial breast cancer. Since breast cancer is common, cases may cluster in families due to chance alone. The chance of this familial clustering being due to known breast cancer–susceptibility genes can be quantified using genetic risk assessment models and is low in this example. However, factors such as family size, ethnicity, and specific features in the medical history influence the chances of whether a genetic form of breast cancer is present. Since the chances of finding a mutation in a known breast cancer–susceptibility genes are low in this example, genetic testing does not help in clarifying risk, but genetic counseling is still valuable.

Hereditary or *genetic* breast cancer refers to breast cancer due to cancer–predisposing genes. Genetic cases comprise about 5% to 10% of all breast cancer. Most forms of hereditary breast cancer follow autosomal dominant inheritance of highly penetrant genes that cause a clustering of breast and other cancers recognizable as cancer family syndromes.

The proportion of hereditary breast cancer due to *BRCA1* and *BRCA2* is approximately 52% and 32%, respectively, as estimated by linkage studies that do not rely on the sensitivity of mutation-detection techniques (26). Other known genes account for a small fraction of hereditary cancer. Additional undiscovered genes account for most other hereditary cases (27). Models used to predict *BRCA1* and/or *BRCA2* mutation carrier status are compared and contrasted in Table 2-2.

Although a family with three cases of late-onset breast cancer is unlikely to carry a *BRCA1* or *BRCA2* mutation, a family with a single case of early-onset breast cancer (e.g., age 32) may have a mutation. A single case of breast cancer may be genetic even though it is not familial if other genetic features (such as young age at onset) are present. Population-based epidemiologic studies provide evidence that about 5% to 11% of breast cancer in women aged 40 years or younger are due to germ-line *BRCA1* mutations, with an additional contribution from *BRCA2* mutations (~3%–6%).

Although *BRCA1* and *BRCA2* have gained the spotlight of genetic testing, other breast cancer–predisposing syndromes are known and must be considered in the differential diagnosis. The contribution of Li-Fraumeni syndrome to hereditary breast cancer is uncertain. However, Li-Fraumeni syndrome is rare, and probably 1% or fewer cases of breast cancer are caused by germ-line *p53* mutations (28). Similarly, Cowden syndrome is estimated to cause 1% or fewer cases. However, many genetic syndromes including Li-Fraumeni syndrome exist in less penetrant forms. These cases may be more difficult to recognize, and without population studies, the actual genetic contribution is uncertain.

Hereditary non-polyposis colorectal cancer (HNPCC) may have breast cancer as an occasional feature. HNPCC may be the most common cancer–predisposing syndrome, occurring in about 1 in 200 individuals. Thus the contribution of HNPCC to breast cancer could be important.

Ataxia telangiectasia is an autosomal recessive condition predisposing to lymphomas and leukemias in homozygotes. Breast cancer is not a classic feature of the syndrome. However, epidemiologic studies suggest that carriers of mutations in the ataxia telangiectasia gene *ATM* (i.e., heterozygotes) may be at increased risk of breast cancer, particularly if exposed to ionizing radiation. If true, then about 8% to 18% of breast cancer may be attributable to the *ATM* gene. This controversial hypothesis is explored in detail later.

Peutz-Jeghers syndrome is a rare autosomal dominant cancer–predisposing syndrome caused by germ-line mutations in the *STK11/LKB1* gene (29,30). Peutz-Jeghers syndrome is characterized by multiple benign intestinal hamartomatous polyps and mucocutaneous pigmentation of the lips, buccal mucosa, and digits. Carriers are predisposed to benign and malignant neoplasms of the gastrointestinal tract, pancreas, testis, ovary, breast, and uterus. The RR for cancer in females has been reported as 18.5 and in males as 6.2 (31). In this study, the RR for breast and gynecologic cancers was 20.3. The condition will not be further explored here.

Hereditary Breast Cancer: Segregation Analysis and Linkage Mapping

The genetic tools of segregation analysis and linkage mapping were used successfully to provide evidence of genes predisposing to breast cancer and to determine the chromosomal location of these genes to facilitate their cloning. Mendelian inheritance theory posits that individuals receive one allele (copy) of each gene from each of their parents and that when gametes are formed, these alleles separate (i.e., segregate independently). Mating of parents with particular genotypes leads to segregation of parental alleles, leading to fixed ratios of genotypes and therefore phenotypes in offspring. Segregation analysis tests for compatibility of observed proportions of affected and unaffected offspring with Mendelian inheritance models. Thus the genetic model that best fits the family data is chosen as the model best supported by the statistical evidence.

Methods exist to aid a more complete model of inheritance than provided by simple Mendelian models. For example, reduced penetrance of a dominant gene leads to less than 50% of affected offspring in the segregation proportion, but the inheritance is Mendelian. The problem of phenocopies also must be confronted. In other words, since breast cancer incidence is high, families with genetic predisposition to breast cancer also will have members with sporadic breast cancer, confounding the analysis. Additional considerations include ascertainment bias, where the segregation proportion is influenced by nonrandom inclusion of affected individuals in the sample, and etiologic heterogeneity, where more than one genetic form of the disease as well as nongenetic causes also may exist.

Claus and colleagues (32) investigated the familial risk of breast cancer in a population-based study of 4730 histologically confirmed breast cancer patients aged 20 to 54 years and 4688 matched controls. Importantly, patients were not selected on the basis of family history,

but family history information was available from interviews with the patients and controls. Segregation analysis provided evidence for the existence of a rare breast cancer–predisposing autosomal dominant allele with a frequency of 0.0033. The risk of breast cancer to carriers compared with noncarriers was greatest for young women, but risk was increased at all ages. The cumulative lifetime risk of breast cancer for carriers was estimated as 92% versus a 10% lifetime risk for noncarriers. This study and others (33) inferred the existence of an important breast cancer–predisposing gene (or genes), laying the groundwork for the substantial efforts required to map and clone the *BRCA1* and *BRCA2* genes. In fact, the 17q-linked *BRCA1* gene first localized by Hall and colleagues (2) and subsequently cloned by Miki and colleagues (3) demonstrates a mutation frequency and penetrance similar to estimates predicted by Claus and colleagues.

A number of methods have been used to localize traits in the human genome, including linkage analysis, deletion mapping (Duchenne muscular dystrophy), chromosome aberration (retinoblastoma), and other techniques. Linkage analysis exploits the situation where segregation of traits does not occur independently; that is, two traits are co-inherited as a unit. This violation of the law of independent assortment is most readily explained if the two loci are adjacent (i.e., linked) on a chromosome. Linkage provides a high level of statistical proof that a condition has a genetic cause, but ultimate proof depends on identifying the gene, delineating the function of the gene product, and providing an explanation of the disease pathogenesis.

The probability of cosegregation of two loci depends on their genetic distance. Since analogous chromosomes in a pair undergo genetic recombination during meiosis, genetic distance can be measured by the recombination fraction. Traits on different chromosomes segregate independently, and traits far apart on the same chromosome also segregate independently, since recombination between them is highly likely. Traits adjacent to each other almost never recombine; thus the recombination fraction approaches zero (the traits are linked in the offspring exactly as in the parents). Traits close to each other, with enough distance to recombine, have a measurable recombination fraction that is proportional to their genetic distance.

Linkage analysis uses DNA markers to distinguish individual alleles on chromosome pairs. These signposts along the human genome are analyzed with respect to coinheritance of a disease trait in order to localize the trait. The log-odds (LOD) score is a summary statistic used to assess the strength of the evidence in favor of linkage at a specified genetic distance. The LOD score is the log of a ratio comparing the observed recombination fraction with that expected if the disease assorts independently of the DNA marker(s). A LOD score of 3 indicates that the odds are in favor of linkage by 1000 to 1. An LOD score of 2 indicates that the odds are in favor of linkage by 100 to 1, etc. An LOD score of 3 is conventionally accepted as sufficient evidence in favor of linkage. With this degree of certainty that a specific DNA region contains the disease gene, efforts to clone the gene (e.g., positional cloning, positional candidate gene analysis) can be targeted to this region.

An array of alleles (i.e., DNA markers) along a single chromosome, known as a *haplotype*, can distinguish individual chromosomes in a pair. In suitable families, the disease-bearing chromosome can be traced along the generations without having cloned the disease gene or clarified its function. Linkage analysis permits indirect genetic testing that can be used in genetic counseling and can guide medical management, even before a gene has been cloned. Furthermore, since current mutation-detection techniques remain unable to identify a significant proportion of mutations in known genes, linkage sometimes continues to play a role even after a gene has been cloned. In contrast to direct gene testing, linkage analysis requires the participation of multiple family members to establish phase (alignment of alleles on disease-bearing versus non-disease-bearing chromosomes).

BRCA1 and BRCA2

To set the stage for isolation of the *BRCA1* gene, it was necessary to perform genetic linkage studies to localize the gene. Once localized, another 4 years elapsed during a concerted effort to refine DNA markers and assess candidate genes. Ultimately, positional cloning was required to search through a massive DNA region for a previously unidentified gene that demonstrated mutations in affected families but not in normal control individuals. Once found, the *BRCA1* gene showed little homology with known genes. Thus, elucidating its function has been equally challenging. Delineation of the clinical syndromes and epidemiologic relevance of *BRCA1* (*http://www3.ncbi.nlm.nih.gov/Omim/searchomim .html*, OMIM No.#113705) and *BRCA2* (*http:// www3.ncbi.nlm.nih.gov/Omim/searchomim.html*, OMIM No. #600185) mutations has outpaced the understanding of gene function.

Gene Discovery

Hall and colleagues (2) performed linkage studies on 23 families with 146 cases of breast cancer. Families were selected for young age at onset of cancer, bilateral breast cancer, and male breast cancer. An LOD score of 5.98 for linkage to a genetic marker on chromosome 17, band q21, was found in families with an age at onset of less than 46 years. Strong evidence was found for linkage heterogeneity (i.e., that other breast cancer–predisposing loci exist). Other groups found linkage of hereditary breast cancer and hereditary breast-ovarian cancer in 60% to 70% of families (34,35). In a linkage study of 214 families from the Breast Cancer Linkage Consortium (BCLC), confirmatory evidence of linkage to 17q21 was found (36). The 17q locus appeared to be responsible for most hereditary breast-ovarian cancer, but only about half of hereditary breast cancer families were linked to 17q. Additional evidence that a breast cancer–predisposing gene was present in this region was provided by tumor studies in hereditary cases showing loss of the wild-type allele, consistent with involvement of a tumor-suppressor gene.

Despite these intensive linkage studies, the genetic interval containing the putative gene was large (~ 20 cM), and mutation analysis of candidate genes was not fruitful. Without information on the gene function or protein structure, positional cloning (i.e., cloning based on knowledge of genetic location only) was performed (3), implying the use of molecular brute force.

First, a genetic map of the region was refined by development of additional markers with a higher degree of polymorphism (variation). Reanalysis of genetic recombinants in families narrowed the region of interest to about 4 cM. The hunt then focused on DNA regions that were expressed as mRNA and thus were potential genes. After trial and error, a composite of cDNA sequences was constructed representing the putative *BRCA1* gene. Conceptual translation of this gene predicted a protein of 1863 amino acids. A search of known sequences in DNA databases revealed a sequence near the N-terminus homologous to zinc finger (RING finger) proteins, which bind to nucleic acids and control DNA transcription. The transcript was expressed in breast, ovary, and other tissues. Mutations were identified in five of eight kindreds. Importantly, mutations cosegregated with the *BRCA1* predisposing haplotype (people with the disease-bearing chromosome carried the mutation). Putative *BRCA1* mutations were not found in control population samples, arguing against the identification of common polymorphisms (benign variants). All families had some women with the mutation who lived to age 80 without developing cancer, consistent with studies indicating less than 100% penetrance of hereditary breast cancer (32,36).

Linkage analysis of 15 families unlinked to the *BRCA1* locus identified a second breast cancer–susceptibility locus, *BRCA2* (37), within a 6-cM interval on chromosome 13q12-q13. The associated ovarian cancer risk was smaller than noted in *BRCA1*. Linkage to *BRCA2* was shown in a family with seven male breast cancers in three generations, with tumor loss of the non-disease-associated haplotype (38). With chance favoring the prepared laboratory, further localization of *BRCA2* to a 300-kb region was fortuitously provided by analysis of a pancreatic tumor with a homozygous deletion in the putative gene region. Analysis of transcribed sequences revealed a partial gene sequence with six different mutations (4). Tavtigian and colleagues (5) reported the complete exonic structure and coding sequence of *BRCA2* and described mutations in 9 of 18 families studied, including those with male breast cancer. High levels of expression were measured in breast and thymus, with lower levels in ovary, lung, and spleen.

Ramon Gomez de la Serna wrote, "When poets speak of death, they call it the place without breasts." Fueled by a deep cultural fear of breast cancer and a gene-conscious media, *BRCA1* and *BRCA2* became two of the most famous human genes, achieving prominence in news documentaries and fictional television dramas. Although predictive genetic testing provides valuable information to families at high risk, it is worth pointing out that evidence-based knowledge of appropriate medical management and mature understanding of the ethical, legal, and social issues lagged behind the commercial availability of clinical genetic testing.

BRCA1 and BRCA2 Gene Function

There is more than one linear pathway toward the development of cancer, although early and late molecular changes may be favored in tumors. Specific tumor types, such as infiltrating ductal carcinoma, may arise through a sequence of genetic steps that could vary from one tumor to another but look identical to a pathologist's practiced eye. Breast cancer in germ-line mutation carriers may differ from sporadic cancer in its molecular progression pathway, which could have implications for survival, prognosis, and treatment.

In general, genes causing specific hereditary cancers are also involved in the genesis of sporadic tumors of the same tissue type. For example, the *Rb1* gene is causal for hereditary retinoblastoma and also is functionally lost in sporadic retinoblastomas. The *APC* gene not only causes multiple intestinal polyposis seen in familial adenomatous polyposis but also is mutated in most sporadic colorectal adenomas. For *BRCA1* and *BRCA2*, however, functional loss through gene mutation or loss of heterozygosity appears to be uncommon in sporadic breast and ovarian cancers (39–44). Rather than imply that these genes are not relevant to the pathogenesis of most breast cancers, however, it may be that functional *BRCA1* and *BRCA2* loss occurs through other mechanisms. More likely, the *BRCA* genes may comprise one component of a crucial pathway for maintenance of the normal breast epithelial cell phenotype. Thus elucidation of this pathway by studying the role that the *BRCA* genes play in normal and malignant breast tissue may lead to a clearer understanding of sporadic breast cancer and aid in the development of new therapeutic targets.

On its discovery, *BRCA1* was a large gene that bore few clues as to its function, since no genes of similar structure had yet been described. The inheritance pattern is that characteristic for a tumor-suppressor gene. Loss of heterozygosity at the *BRCA1* locus seen in breast and ovarian tumors from germ-line mutation carriers is a classic feature of a tumor-suppressor gene (39,40). The decrease in *BRCA1* mRNA levels observed during the transition from carcinoma in situ to invasive breast cancer and the accelerated growth of malignant and nonmalignant mammary cells induced by antisense *BRCA1* mRNA suggests that *BRCA1* acts as a negative regulator of mammary cell growth (45). Transfection of wild-type but not mutant *BRCA1* into breast and ovarian cell lines inhibited growth, and no inhibition was seen in non-breast/ovarian cell lines (46). The work of Thompson and colleagues (45) on the relationship between *BRCA1* expression and malignant progression is strengthened by the findings of Wilson and colleagues (47). Immunohistochemical staining showed that *BRCA1* protein was localized to nuclear foci in benign breast, invasive lobular cancers, and low-grade ductal carcinomas but was reduced or undetectable in most high-grade ductal carcinomas.

BRCA1 has an unusual gene structure with 24 exons (exons 1 and 4 are noncoding) and a very large exon 11. It is a long gene with a coding region of about 5.5 kb strewn across about 100 kb of DNA. The resulting RNA is a 7.8-kb transcript with several isoforms due to alternative splicing patterns. The N-terminal RING finger domain is evolutionarily conserved and is homologous to the mouse *BRCA1* gene. Wu and colleagues (48) performed a yeast two-hybrid screen to capture proteins that bind to the RING domain. The *BRCA1*-associated RING domain (BARD1) protein was identified in this way, and it may affect and/or regulate *BRCA1* function. The RING domain appears to be crucial because key mutations that alter amino acids in this domain

and disrupt BRCA1/BARD1 interaction cause hereditary breast/ovarian cancer. Both genes have conserved *BRCA1* C-terminal domains (BRCT) in their C-terminal regions. This motif is also found in a polypeptide that binds the *p53* tumor suppressor and *RAD9*, which mediates cell cycle arrest in response to DNA damage in yeast. A C-terminal acidic transactivation domain (49) is also highly conserved. *BRCA1* is a component of the RNA polymerase II holoenzyme (50), probably interacting via the transactivation domain, suggesting an important role in regulating the expression of downstream genes.

The *BRCA1* gene has nuclear localizing sequences in exon 11 that mediate its translocation from the cytoplasm to the nucleus (51,52) after protein translation. It is a 220-kDa protein that undergoes cell cycle–dependent phosphorylation (53–55). Aberrant subcellular localization of *BRCA1* has been hypothesized to be etiologic in breast tumorigenesis in familial and sporadic cases (56). Debate in the literature as to the size of the protein, its subcellular localization, and its possible secretion (57) may relate to differences between laboratories in antibody specificity and fixation and staining techniques (56,58,59) and splice variants (60). A comprehensive analysis by Wilson and colleagues (47) provides compelling evidence that *BRCA1* protein is a 220-kDa protein localized in discrete nuclear foci in epithelial cell lines.

BRCA1 protein is localized in the perinuclear compartment of the endoplasmic reticulum–Golgi complex and in cytoplasmic tubes that invaginate the nucleus (61), seen as nuclear dots or foci during S phase. BRCA1 associates in nuclear dots with Rad51, which mediates the repair of double-stranded DNA breaks and is involved with meiotic recombination, suggesting a role of BRCA1 in genome integrity and meiosis (62). BRCA1, Rad51, and BARD1 appear to interact in multiprotein complexes that participate in a phosphorylation-related replication checkpoint response to DNA damage (63).

BRCA2 is composed of 27 exons (exon 1 is noncoding) distributed across 70 kb of genomic DNA. Like *BRCA1*, *BRCA2* is rich in AT base pairs and has a large exon 11. The coding region is 11.2 kb long. The *BRCA2* gene encodes a protein of 3418 amino acids which, like BRCA1 protein, is highly charged. *BRCA1* and *BRCA2* gene expression is regulated by the cell cycle (64,65), and mRNA transcripts are coordinately elevated by estrogen and inhibited by tamoxifen (66). *BRCA1* and *BRCA2* in the mouse are required for embryonic cellular proliferation (67), and the homozygous null phenotype leads to lethality. *BRCA2*-deficient mouse embryos are acutely sensitive to ionizing radiation (68). In surviving *BRCA2*-deficient mice with partial gene function, spermatogenesis is halted prior to meiosis, repair of double-stranded DNA is impaired, and thymic lymphomas develop (69).

Knowledge of the biologic functions of *BRCA1* and *BRCA2* holds promise for genotype-based therapy in mutation carriers (70). Hypersensitivity of *BRCA2*-deficient cells may be a molecular Achilles' heel, whereby ionizing radiation and chemotherapeutic agents that induce double-stranded DNA breaks may be used to selectively treat mutation carriers (71). The ubiquitous roles of *BRCA1* and *BRCA2* indicated by research studies suggest that these genes play a central role in breast tumorigenesis. The differential expression found between benign mammary tissue and putative early sporadic malignancies compared with sporadic high-grade ductal carcinomas (47) suggests a direct role of *BRCA1* in sporadic breast carcinogenesis. Therefore, knowledge gained by elucidation of these molecular pathways may be exploited in the treatment of sporadic breast/ovarian cancer.

BRCA1 and BRCA2 Clinical Syndromes

Estimates of the population frequency and penetrance of *BRCA1* and *BRCA2* mutations have varied markedly among studies. Variation occurs in relation to the ethnic populations studied and methods of study group selection. Penetrance estimates of breast cancer for *BRCA1* and *BRCA2* mutation carriers were about 85% over a lifetime in a Breast Cancer Linkage Consortium study of 237 highly selected families among 9 western European and North American countries (26), confirming earlier estimates. The ovarian cancer penetrance by age 70 is 42% to 63% for *BRCA1* (72,73) and 27% for *BRCA2*(26). An ovarian cancer cluster region in *BRCA2* exon 11 may pose a higher risk than other *BRCA2* mutations (26,74).

The most characteristic feature of the *BRCA1* and *BRCA2* syndromes is an individual with cancer of the breast and ovary. Double primary cancer is the sine qua non of hereditary cancer syndromes, involving either two different organs (e.g., breast plus ovary) or paired organs (e.g., bilateral breast cancer). Because of age-dependent penetrance characteristics of *BRCA1* and *BRCA2* and survival issues, it is more common to encounter individuals who were first diagnosed with breast and then ovarian cancer. This double primary is associated with extraordinarily high pretest probabilities of *BRCA1* and *BRCA2* gene mutations, particularly when combined with young age at diagnosis, affected relatives, or Ashkenazi Jewish ancestry (75,76). Thus any individual with breast and ovarian cancer should be evaluated for hereditary breast/ovarian cancer. Absence of this feature does not argue against involvement of the *BRCA1* and *BRCA2* genes, however.

Because the *BRCA1* and *BRCA2* genes are newly discovered, longitudinal controlled studies on optimal medical management are lacking. However, studies of affected families, retrospective studies, and decision analyses have lent knowledge for the development of management guidelines based on expert opinion (77). Age-specific incidence data for breast and ovarian cancer are crucial to developing guidelines. For example, cancer development in teenage *BRCA1* and *BRCA2* carriers is almost unknown. Therefore, it is inappropriate to perform genetic testing prior to legal adulthood, when a person is able to choose whether or not to be tested and perhaps retain a full scope of life choices regarding family, relationships, and career.

The age-dependent penetrance of cancer in the *BRCA1* and *BRCA2* syndromes provides important medical management information. The risk of breast cancer rises early for *BRCA1* and is 3.6% by age 30 and 18% by age 40. For *BRCA2*, the cumulative breast cancer incidence is slightly lower: 0.6% by age 30 and 12% by age 40 (26). Therefore, the optimal benefit of prophylactic mastectomy is obtained by acting on the decision relatively soon after one is made. Similarly, recommendations to begin annual mammograms between the ages of 25 and 35 are based on data on age-specific breast cancer incidence rates.

Decision analyses of surgical prophylaxis in theoretical *BRCA* mutation carriers have provided evidence that many years of life would be added for women undergoing prophylactic mastectomy and oophorectomy in their thirties (78,79). However, when quality of life is considered, the benefit may be considerably less. Until actual *BRCA* mutation carriers are studied, prophylactic surgery remains an option, to be presented neutrally and with respect for the multiple personal issues it raises. In counseling about such decisions, it is important to draw from knowledge of the age-dependent penetrance of breast and ovarian cancer in the *BRCA1* and *BRCA2* syndromes.

The ovarian cancer risk for *BRCA2* carriers is relatively low at younger ages, that is, 0.4% cumulative risk by age 50 and 7% risk by age 60 (26). This suggests possibly marginal benefit to prophylactic oophorectomy in *BRCA2* carriers prior to the perimenopausal years. The age-dependent penetrance of *BRCA1* for ovarian cancer is less than 1% by age 40, 23% by age 50, and 30% by age 60 (72). While the ovarian cancer risk for *BRCA1* carriers is much greater than for the average woman, most cases occur after age 40 (72,80). Prophylactic oophorectomy after completion of childbearing is a surgical option available to women with mutations (77).

Male Breast Cancer

The etiology of male breast cancer is poorly understood, but some cases are attributable to genetic causes. Klinefelter syndrome (karyotype 47,XXY) is associated with about a 3% lifetime risk of male breast cancer, perhaps due to circulating endogenous estrogens. Male breast cancer in androgen-insensitivity syndrome, due to mutations in the androgen receptor gene, has been described. Both these conditions are evident on history and physical examination. A third genetic cause of male breast cancer is germ-line mutation of the *BRCA2* gene. An analysis of 237 Breast Cancer Linkage Consortium families (26) indicates that about 77% of families with male breast cancer are linked to *BRCA2* and 19% are linked to *BRCA1*. Male breast cancer has been reported in *BRCA1* families, but *BRCA2* mutations convey a higher risk of male breast cancer than do *BRCA1* mutations.

Linkage of hereditary male breast cancer to the *BRCA1* locus on chromosome 17q was originally excluded (81), but linkage was found to the *BRCA2* region on 13q (38). Several families with male breast cancer were identified as carrying *BRCA2* mutations (82–84). An Icelandic study (82) provided evidence that one particular mutation, 999del5, accounts for 40% (12/30) of male breast cancer patients in that population (complete ascertainment was likely via the Icelandic Cancer Registry). In a U.S. study (84), where a founder effect was unlikely to account for the majority of cases, 14% (7/50) of male breast cancer patients had identifiable *BRCA2* mutations. In all 3 patients of Ashkenazi Jewish descent, the same founder mutation (6174delT) was present. Eighty percent of male breast cancer patients had a family history of breast cancer, with 85% of mutation-identified patients having a positive family history. Thus ascertainment bias may have led to elevated estimates of attributable risk of *BRCA2* to male breast cancer. In a population-based study, Friedman and colleagues (85) found *BRCA2* mutations in 4% (2/54) of male breast cancer patients, one of whom had no family history of breast or ovarian cancer.

Men with germ-line *BRCA2* mutations have about a 6% lifetime risk of breast cancer (86), far less than female carriers but far more than average-risk men. Breast self-examination and awareness may lead to early detection, which would be expected to lead to improved prognosis (87).

Non-Breast/Ovarian Cancers in BRCA1 and BRCA2

Genes that are cloned following recognition that they predispose to certain cancers are usually found to cause other cancers as well. Although named for breast cancer and clearly recognized to contribute to ovarian cancer, *BRCA1* and *BRCA2* predispose to additional cancers (Table 2-1). A population-based study of three founder mutations in Ashkenazi Jews found about a fourfold increased risk of prostate cancer among older mutation carriers compared with older noncarriers (88). A study of Breast Cancer Linkage Consortium families found an increased risk of colon cancer in *BRCA1* mutation carriers (89); this finding was not duplicated in the

Table 2-1. Lifetime risk of cancer in *BRCA1* and *BRCA2* mutation carriers

Organ	Risk	Comments
Female breast	85%	Original studies on highly penetrant families
	36–56%	Ashkenazi Jewish and Icelandic studies
Ovary	20–40%	*BRCA1*
	15–20%	*BRCA2*
	16%	Ashkenazi Jewish mutations
Male breast	6%	*BRCA2*
	Low	*BRCA1*
Pancreatic cancer	7%	*BRCA2*
Extraovarian primary peritoneal carcinoma	1–2%	*BRCA1*
Colon	5–10%	
Prostate	5–10%	
Component *BRCA2* malignancies (see text)	Probably <5% each	

Ashkenazi study (88). Since prostate cancer and colon cancer are common, sporadic cases are seen frequently in families, and these cancers do not always predict carrier status. However, in a study of seven Icelandic families including two with evidence of linkage to *BRCA1*, 44% of presumed paternal carriers had a history of prostate cancer, and prostate cancer was the second most frequently observed cancer (after breast cancer) (90).

For extraovarian primary peritoneal carcinoma (EOPPC; see below), the contribution of *BRCA1* mutations to disease in the population may be substantial. Unfortunately, few published data are available on EOPPC, but one study found mutations in 3 of 17 papillary serous carcinomas of the peritoneum (91). Two patients had the Ashkenazi founder mutation 185delAG, one had an extensive family history of breast and ovarian cancer, and the other had a personal history of breast cancer. The third patient had no personal or family history of breast or ovarian cancer. Several EOPPC patients with germ-line *BRCA1* mutations have been discussed among geneticists and genetic counselors, but a large series is currently lacking. Similarly, cancer of the fallopian tube is suspected as a component *BRCA* cancer, but a case series has not been published. Mutation of *BRCA2* has been found in a family with two cases of fallopian tube cancer (92); this rare cancer may represent an infrequent but highly specific marker of germ-line *BRCA* mutation.

BRCA2 appears to predispose to a longer list of cancers than *BRCA1*. In a pedigree showing linkage to the *BRCA2* locus, Thorlacius and colleagues (38) found the following cancers in 481 members (in descending order): breast (male and female), thyroid, stomach, prostate, bladder, sarcomas, uterus, ovary, esophagus, colon, lung, kidney, and peritoneum. Grimmond and colleagues (93) found a similarly diffuse spectrum of tumors in relatives in *BRCA2*-linked families, including also melanoma and leukemia/lymphoma. Mutational analysis in cancer patients (82) in families segregating the 999del5 mutation revealed that mutation carriers developed cancer of the prostate, pancreas, ovary, colon, stomach, thyroid, cervix, and endometrium. Eleven cases of pancreatic cancer were found in mutation-positive families compared with no cases in mutation-negative families. Phelan and colleagues (83) also reported excess pancreatic cancer in families with *BRCA2* mutations, which occurred at a statistically significant younger age; available cases were shown by haplotype analysis to be obligate mutation carriers. Comparing mutation-positive with mutation-negative families, RRs of 4.2 and 2.1 were found for prostate and colon cancer, respectively. Couch and colleagues (84) corroborated findings of breast, ovarian, stomach, prostate, and colon cancer in mutation-positive families. A high RR of 7 for laryngeal cancer in *BRCA2* kindreds has been reported (86).

Little is known about the attributable risk of germ-line *BRCA2* mutations to specific cancers in the general population. A study of 41 pancreatic adenocarcinomas detected 3 (7.3%) germ-line *BRCA2* mutations (94). In another study, no *BRCA2* mutations were found among 36 pancreatic cancers analyzed, but germ-line mutations were detected in 2 of 60 hepatocellular carcinomas (95). Since the prevalence of the founder 6174delT mutation in the Ashkenazi Jewish population is 1.36%, a high attributable risk of this mutation to pancreatic cancer would be suspected. An analysis of the 6174delT mutation in an unselected series of 39 Jewish individuals with pancreatic cancer revealed 4 mutations (10%). A lifetime penetrance of 7% was estimated in mutation carriers compared with a 0.85% risk in the general population (96).

Although an increased risk of prostate cancer has been found for families with *BRCA* mutations, a study of Jewish men with prostate cancer did not detect an increased frequency of founder mutations (97). Germ-line *BRCA1* mutational analysis in 49 men with early-onset prostate cancer or a significant family history of prostate or breast cancer identified one mutation and four sequence variants of uncertain significance (98). In this study, the conclusion about whether germ-line *BRCA1* mutations contribute to prostate cancer in the general population hinges on whether the variants were pathologic or not.

Molecular evidence that *BRCA2* may be pathogenic in diverse tumors was provided by loss of heterozygosity studies and mutational analysis (42). *BRCA2* mutations were found in the following tumors: renal, lung, bladder, pancreatic, astrocytoma, and melanoma. Germ-line mutation status was not assessed for these patients but lends suspicion that these tumors may be part of the *BRCA2* phenotype.

A thorough family history of cancer is therefore required to fully assess the probability of a germ-line mutation. Available risk models do not yet employ this information, but it is clinically useful in cancer risk counseling. Screening for potentially diverse tumors, most of which probably have a low penetrance, would be problematic, and no specific recommendations have yet emerged.

Extraovarian Primary Peritoneal Carcinoma

Extraovarian primary peritoneal carcinoma (EOPPC) (99) refers to adenocarcinoma arising from the peritoneal lining of the abdomen and pelvis. The histology of EOPPC is indistinguishable from primary epithelial ovarian carcinoma, but the ovaries are uninvolved or minimally involved. Most cases are of serous histology, also called *papillary serous carcinoma of the peritoneum* (PSCP), but nonserous forms have been described. EOPPC may occur several years following bilateral oophorectomy. EOPPC is probably underdiagnosed but may comprise almost 10% of cases of serous ovarian cancer. The presentation mimics that of primary ovarian cancer, usually with ascites. Because of the extraovarian presentation, tumors are stage III or stage IV at presentation. The CA-125 tumor marker is elevated above 35 units/mL in most patients with EOPPC, as is usually seen in primary ovarian cancer. Treatment parallels that of primary ovarian cancer. Most studies show either similar or worse survival compared with primary ovarian cancer.

Although EOPPC is histologically and clinically similar to primary ovarian cancer, the two are probably separate disease entities. There may be a common embryologic origin of peritoneal epithelium and ovarian epithelium from coelomic epithelium, explaining the similarities. Another explanation is field cancerization, where an oncogenic stimulus such as carcinogen exposure places similar tissues at risk. Supporting the latter theory is the observation of multifocal disease with differences in tumor clonality, as shown by molecular markers. Another possibility is unrecognized micrometastatic disease in the ovaries (at least in some patients), manifested clinically by EOPPC. For patients with prior prophylactic oophorectomies, this could explain the occurrence of EOPPC, since pathologic examination of the resected ovaries may not have been meticulous.

EOPPC has been diagnosed in women with *BRCA1* mutations and may be part of the clinical syndrome. Because women with *BRCA1* mutations who undergo prophylactic oophorectomy are, by definition, at high risk of ovarian cancer, it is difficult to distinguish the possibility of unrecognized micrometastatic primary ovarian carcinoma manifesting as EOPPC from "true" EOPPC.

Prevalence of BRCA Mutations

Deleterious *BRCA1* mutations are present in about 1 in 345 individuals as measured by U.S. population–based studies of ovarian cancer (100). This is intermediate between estimates of 1 in 833 individuals based on families of women with incident breast cancer or ovarian cancer in England and Wales (101) and 1 in 152 individuals based on families of U.S. breast cancer cases and controls (32). *BRCA2* mutations are present in about 1 in 1136 individuals (26).

A study (102) of Ashkenazi (eastern European) Jewish DNA samples stored following genetic testing for cystic fibrosis and Tay-Sachs disease (not selected on the basis of cancer history) was performed following anonymization and informed consent (103). The 185delAG mutation was found in 0.9% (1/107) of the samples (102). The combined prevalence of three founder mutations, 185delAG and 5382insC in *BRCA1* and 6174delT in *BRCA2*, was 2.5% (104), significantly higher than in the general population. Prevalent founder mutations occur in several other populations (105), but none have been studied as thoroughly as in Jews.

Variable Penetrance of BRCA1 and BRCA2 Mutations: Modifying Factors and Treatment Implications

Common population-specific mutations may cause a high attributable risk of a certain cancer, but it is not necessarily true that these groups have a higher overall incidence of the resulting cancers. Indeed, there is no compelling epidemiologic evidence for a markedly increased incidence of breast cancer in Jews. If the cancer penetrance of common predisposing mutations is lower than average, the increase in group cancer risk may be small. A study of the three common Ashkenazi mutations in 5318 Jewish women in the Washington, D.C., area found a penetrance of 56% for breast cancer and 16% for ovarian cancer (88). A study of Jewish women with breast cancer treated at Mount Sinai Hospital in New York estimated the penetrance for *BRCA1* to be 36%

(106), about 3 times higher than the risk in the general population. These lifetime risks are much smaller than the approximately 85% risks measured in Breast Cancer Linkage Consortium studies.

The accurate use of penetrance estimates in cancer genetic counseling requires an understanding of their limitations and illustrates certain points about factors influencing penetrance. For example, lifetime cancer risk may vary among mutations. Hundreds of *BRCA1* mutations have been reported, but studies of individual mutations are limited by their rarity. Thus penetrance is generally reported in the aggregate. Certain mutations can be studied in isolation, for example, in large kindreds or in populations with prevalent mutations. Even then, penetrance may vary for those mutations when seen in other groups, since families may cosegregate other modifying genes, and ethnic groups vary with respect to other genes and cultural/environmental factors. Theoretically, for example, a 185delAG mutation may have a different penetrance between ethnic populations. In fact, there is accumulating evidence that gene-gene and gene-environment interactions play an important role in influencing penetrance for *BRCA1* and *BRCA2* carriers. It is clear that for even the simplest genetic diseases, the specific causal mutations play a restricted role in overall disease expression. For example, one specific mutation in the β-globin gene causes all cases of sickle cell disease, but clinical manifestations vary greatly among patients and are not clearly attributable to medical treatment or access to health care. Some of the other 80,000 genes in the human genome as well as environmental factors exert an effect on even the simplest gene disorders. An important implication is that genetic makeup may not equate with destiny and that medical treatments for genetic disease may be devised by applying molecular insights.

The importance of endogenous and exogenous hormone exposure in breast cancer risk has been apparent from population studies (7,107), and evidence for the existence of such gene-environment interactions is found for *BRCA1* and *BRCA2* mutation carriers. In a study of 333 *BRCA1* mutation carriers (80), the RRs of breast and ovarian cancer varied significantly according to factors such as age at menarche and parity, suggesting that endogenous hormone exposure alters the penetrance of the *BRCA1* gene. An approximately 50% reduction in breast cancer risk seen for *BRCA* mutation carriers who underwent prophylactic oophorectomy that was only partially abrogated by the use of hormone replacement therapy (108) may be related to the effect of ovarian hormones on breast tissue. Observations in these studies are consistent with in vitro evidence that *BRCA1* and *BRCA2* mRNA expression is coordinately upregulated by estrogen and decreased by tamoxifen (66).

A genetics substudy of the Breast Cancer Prevention Trial (109) will provide information on the utility of tamoxifen for breast cancer prevention in women with germ-line *BRCA1* and *BRCA2* mutations. The preceding studies would suggest that breast cancer risk in *BRCA1* and *BRCA2* carriers is modifiable by selective estrogen receptor modulators (SERMs). However, the chemopreventive effect of tamoxifen observed in the Breast Cancer Prevention Trial was on the reduction of estrogen receptor–positive tumors, and *BRCA1* carriers have a lower proportion of estrogen receptor–positive breast tumors compared with noncarriers. Therefore, the overall benefit of tamoxifen in mutation carriers, if any, is difficult to predict. Also, it is possible that an underlying propensity of *BRCA2* carriers to develop endometrial cancer will be multiplied by tamoxifen use.

With regard to hormonal modulation of ovarian cancer risk, oral contraceptive use has been associated with a markedly decreased risk in epidemiologic studies and extends to women with a family history of ovarian cancer. Women with *BRCA* mutations who used oral contraceptives for 5 years had a 50% reduction in ovarian cancer risk, and those with over 6 years of use had a 60% risk reduction (110). Thus hormonal avenues for ovarian cancer risk reduction in mutation carriers may be fruitful.

Evidence for gene-gene interactions for *BRCA* carriers also has been found. Phelan and colleagues (111) found that a rare VNTR (variable number of tandem repeats) allele of the *HRAS1* gene doubles the risk of ovarian cancer, but not breast cancer, in *BRCA1* carriers.

The MspI genetic polymorphism in the *CYP1A1* gene metabolizes estrone to 2-hydroxyestrone, which is rapidly cleared from circulation. This variant leads to decreased production of 16α-hydroxyestrone, a potent estrogen. Smoking leads to induction of *CYP1A1* and to increased 2-hydroxyestrone levels. Brunet and colleagues (112) presented preliminary evidence that *BRCA1* and *BRCA2* mutation carriers with the *CYP1A1* polymorphism who smoke are less likely to get breast cancer. This mechanism may provide an explanation for the unexpected observation that breast cancer risk was lower in *BRCA1* and *BRCA2* carriers who smoke (113). Rather than promote any possible health benefits to smoking, a more prudent approach would be to modulate estrogen-metabolizing enzyme levels in a more targeted fashion. For example, foods containing indole-3-carbinol, such as broccoli and cabbage, similarly may alter metabolism toward more favorable estrogens, an avenue that has not yet been explored (114). Also, considering the previous discussion on *NAT2* and risk of breast cancer in smokers, it is easy to conceive that it is the overall genotype that modulates cancer risk. Considering the complexity of the human genome, the effect of "beneficial" and "harmful" behaviors is difficult to predict on an individual basis.

Proportion of Breast and Ovarian Cancer Attributable to BRCA1 and BRCA2

Widespread screening of women with breast cancer is not warranted. Some further selection is required to initiate referral for cancer risk evaluation and possible genetic testing. Depending on the way study subjects are ascertained, germ-line *BRCA1* and *BRCA2* mutations contribute to a small, medium, or large amount of breast and ovarian cancer. In a population-based study of North Carolina women with breast cancer, only 3% had *BRCA1* mutations (115), arguing against the notion of population-based screening of women with breast cancer. In this study, 33% of Caucasians patients with a family history of breast and ovarian cancer had a *BRCA1* mutation, and 45% of patients with three or more cases of breast cancer and no ovarian cancer had

BRCA1 mutations. Therefore, even in this unselected population that is probably representative of the usual oncology practice setting, *BRCA1* mutations are frequent as long as further selection is done by probing the family history.

The breast cancer burden in young women attributable to *BRCA1* mutations is significant but also varies according to the setting and ascertainment method. In a population-based study of women in Washington state diagnosed with breast cancer, 6% of women under age 35 and 7% of women under age 45 with a first-degree family history of breast cancer had germ-line *BRCA1* mutations. In clinic-based studies of women with early breast cancer, 6% to 13% of non-Jewish women had *BRCA1* mutations (116). Age is a useful criterion to distinguish germ-line carriers but generally needs to be combined with other genetic indicators to achieve high pretest probabilities. Notably, however, breast cancer under age 30 carries a high risk of germ-line *BRCA* mutation even when considered alone (117). Very early breast cancer (before age 25 and possibly before age 30) should prompt an evaluation for other genetic syndromes such as Li-Fraumeni syndrome and Cowden syndrome (see below).

Among Ashkenazi Jewish women, attributable risk of breast and ovarian cancer is much greater, which relates to the higher prevalence of founder mutations. In a Boston study, 13% of Jewish women diagnosed at age 40 or younger, unselected for a family history of cancer, had the 185delAG mutation (118). A New York study identified the 185delAG mutation in 20% of Ashkenazi Jewish women with breast cancer diagnosed before age 42, all of whom had a positive family history (119). Some of the women in these studies had other mutations, not tested at the time of study. In an Israeli study of Ashkenazi Jewish women with ovarian cancer unselected for family history, one of the three founder mutations was present in 45% of patients, and a high frequency (39%) was found even with a negative or minimal family history (120). The frequency of germ-line mutations among women diagnosed with ovarian cancer in England was much lower, about 5% (121). Another Israeli study of Jewish women unselected for family history detected one of the three founder mutations in 62%

of women with ovarian cancer (122). Age at diagnosis did not predict carrier status, and family history was sometimes negative. For women with breast cancer diagnosed under age 40, 30% were mutation carriers. Remarkably, 10% of women diagnosed with breast cancer over age 40 were mutation carriers, although sporadic breast cancer incidence rates rise sharply after age 40. A higher fraction of these women probably were mutation carriers than measured in this study, since about 10% of mutations in Jews are not accounted for by the three founder mutations, and several high-risk families in the study had no identifiable mutations. Thus a higher level of suspicion must be maintained for Jewish families with an ovarian cancer diagnosis, early breast cancer, and/or any degree of family history, and risk estimates should take ethnicity into account.

BRCA1 mutations appear to be most prevalent in Russia, although population-based studies have not been done. Seventy-nine percent of families with breast/ovarian cancer had a *BRCA1* mutation, usually due to one of two founder mutations identified (105).

Given the numerous risks and benefits to genetic testing for *BRCA1* and *BRCA2* and incomplete knowledge about optimal medical management, standard of care for informed consent should include quantitative risk assessment. Several risk models exist (26,75,76,123–125) that are useful in estimating a pretest probability of a germ-line mutation, information that the patient incorporates into a decision about whether to pursue genetic testing. The models vary with respect to the elements captured in the family history, so the risk estimates vary widely. Additional information about risk models is in Chapter 4. Some experience is required to judge which estimate is the most appropriate for a specific family. The Berry-Parmigiani-Aguilar model (124,125) uses a Bayesian (posterior probability) approach, and its computerized version is called BRCAPRO. BRCAPRO was developed by David Euhus and is available in a Windows platform version called CancerGene (*http://www.swmed.edu/home_pages/cancergene/*) that also incorporates calculations for the other widely used genetic risk models. CancerGene is currently the most comprehensive and user-friendly breast cancer genetic risk assessment tool. The genetic risk assessment models are compared and contrasted in Table 2-2.

Subtle Clinical Manifestations of BRCA1 and BRCA2 Mutations

Assuming that a family history is taken, it is easy to recognize the hereditary breast/ovarian cancer syndrome in a family with multiple generations of women affected by early-onset breast and ovarian cancer. Experience shows, however, that mutations can manifest with much less striking family histories. The clinical impact

of recognizing the presence of *BRCA* mutations may be significant. For example, in a family with six cases of breast cancer but no ovarian cancer, the pretest probability of a *BRCA* mutation is high, and therefore, the risk of ovarian cancer is much higher than average. In such families, women generally are attuned to the risk of breast cancer but are not under appropriate surveillance for ovarian cancer.

Pretest probabilities of *BRCA* mutations in families with breast cancer or breast and ovarian cancer can be approximated using a variety of available tables, graphs, and computer programs

Table 2-2. Comparison of breast cancer and genetic risk assessment models

	Gail	Claus	Shattuck-Eidens	Couch	Berry BRCAPRO	Frank myriad
Model predicts	BC risk 5, 10, 20, 30-yr and lifetime risks	BC risk 10, 20, 30-yr	*BRCA1* risk only	*BRCA1* risk only	*BRCA1* and *BRCA2* risk	*BRCA1* and *BRCA2* risk
Practical limitations	See below					
Presentation type	Tables, graphs, computer program	Tables, computer, program in Cyrillic	Graphs, calculations	Tables	Computer program	Tables
Analysis type	Regression	Segregation analysis/ genetic modeling	Regression	Regression	Mendelian with Bayesian updating	Regression
Proband age	Yes	Yes	Yes	No	Yes	No
Age of BC diagnosis in proband	N/A	N/A	Yes	Yes, as part of family mean	Yes	Yes, but categorical <50 for model <40 in calculation
Age of cancer onset in relatives	No	Yes	No	Yes, as mean age	Yes	No, but only considers BC <50
Proband with BC required	N/A	N/A	Yes*	Yes*	No*	Yes*
# of family members with BC &/or OC	1st degree (max = 2)	1st, 2nd degree (max = 2)	1st, 2nd degree (min = 0, no max)	Not specified optimal⩾2	1st, 2nd degree	1st, 2nd degree (min = 1, max = 2)
Ashkenazi Jewish ancestry considered	No	No	Yes	Yes	Yes	No

*May use affected relative as "proband" for calculations, then adjust risk by relationship using Mendelian principles
BC = breast cancer; OC = ovarian cancer; N/A = not applicable.

Table 2-2 Part II. Practical Limitations

Gail model

Proband must be age 20–70 years
Overpredicts BC risk in women not having annual mammograms.
Underpredicts BC if
    There is a paternal family history of BC
    There is a second-degree family history of BC (maternal or paternal)
    Early-onset BC
    Family history of OC

Claus model

Proband must be age 20–69 years
Proband must have first- and/or second-degree female relative with BC
Underpredicts if
    Significant family history of BC (more than two relatives)
    OC

Shattuck-Eidens model

Technically not applicable for proband with BC or OC diagnosed under age 30 years
No distinction between first- and second-degree relatives
Age at onset assessed in proband only

Couch model

Family must have BC; technically not appropriate for single case (proband) of BC
No distinction between first- and second-degree relatives

Berry (*BRCAPRO*) model

Extensive family history needed — both affected and unaffected
Computerized model only
Very young-onset OC not treated as significant (age-dependent penetrance estimates used for model are
    very low below age 40)

Frank (Myriad) model

Proband* must have BC diagnosed before age 50 and first- or second-degree relative with BC diagnosed
    before age 50 or OC diagnosed at any age
No distinction between first- and second-degree relatives
Age at onset only before age 50
Does not distinguish (Ashkenazi) ethnicity

(26,75,76,123–125). The utility of risk calculations in medical decision making is illustrated in Fig. 2-2. Much more subtle family histories may occur, however, and the available methods do not take into account non-breast/ovarian cancers. Table 2-3 lists minimal features that suggest the presence of *BRCA1* or *BRCA2* mutations. The scientific literature supporting some of these features is in some cases scant but highly suggestive. The combinations listed are estimated to equate to a 10% pretest probability or greater for a germline mutation and should prompt consideration of referral for genetic counseling. Any additional features in the family history (additional cases of breast cancer, ovarian cancer, early age at diagnosis, Jewish ancestry, etc.) would increase the risk of a germ-line mutation further.

Practical Issues in BRCA1/BRCA2 Testing

The *BRCA1* and *BRCA2* genes are large, and hundreds of mutations have been found virtually all along their entirety. To detect mutations, sections of the genomic DNA sequence of coding portions of the gene and boundaries of exons and introns are first amplified using the polymerase chain reaction (PCR). Amplified DNA products are usually then either 1) directly sequenced or 2) electrophoresed on gels to detect alterations in migration patterns indicating mutations, which are then verified by DNA sequencing. The complexity of analysis means that DNA testing for *BRCA1* and *BRCA2* is expensive, currently about $2600 for DNA sequencing of both genes at a commercial laboratory.

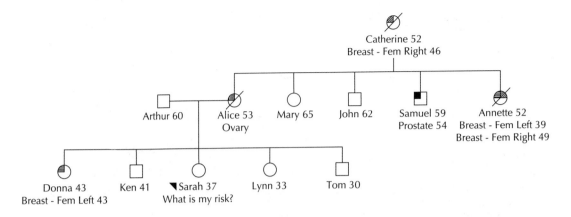

Sarah: "What is my risk?"

Quantitative risk, calculated by risk models and refined by genetic testing, guides clinical decision making for surveillance and prevention.

Risk of being *BRCA1* or *BRCA2* mutation carrier (*BRCAPRO*) = 0.46 (non-Ashkenazi family)

Breast cancer risk = carrier risk × penetrance = 0.46 × 0.83 = 38% lifetime risk of breast cancer

Similarly, lifetime ovarian cancer risk = 16%

If Donna has an identifiable *BRCA* mutation, and Sarah tests negative, Sarah's breast cancer and ovarian cancer risks are close to the population risk levels. Assuming a good breast cancer prognosis, Donna should undergo ovarian surveillance. If Sarah is positive for the familial mutation, her lifetime risk of breast and ovarian cancers is that of a known mutation carrier. If Donna tests negative, then genetic testing is uninformative in this family and surveillance/prevention is based on family history alone.

Unless she is shown to lack a known familial mutation, Lynn should be screened for breast cancer (before the usual age of 40 years) and should begin ovarian cancer surveillance. The pedigree should be probed further to discern other at-risk relatives who require screening and who may desire genetic testing.

▤ Breast - Fem Left   ▤ Ovary   ▤ Breast - Fem Right   ■ Prostate

Figure 2-2. Hereditary breast-ovarian cancer family risk calculations.

There is much clinical overlap between the *BRCA1* and *BRCA2* syndromes, and usually both genes are tested together. Once a mutation is found, then only that mutation needs to be evaluated in other family members to assess their carrier status (with some exceptions, discussed below). The cost of this analysis is about $300 to $450. In families with known mutations, genetic testing is highly sensitive and specific.

In a family without a previously identified mutation, the sensitivity of genetic testing for *BRCA1* may be as low as 63% (26). The sensitivity for *BRCA2* is probably similar. In other words, as many as one-third of families that are linked to *BRCA1* may not have detectable mutations using current technology. Laboratories that report detection rates of greater than 90% use a denominator of "detectable mutations" that are essentially limited to the coding region of the gene and intron-exon boundaries. Gene function may be altered by mutations in control regions or within introns, by DNA modification (126,127), or by large deletions (128,129) that would not be detectable by the standard methods used. Therefore, negative test results must be interpreted with great caution.

In addition, conclusions about negative test results in families highly suggestive for hereditary breast cancer are very different depending on whether or not the person tested had cancer (Table 2-4). Often, individuals without cancer are more highly motivated to seek genetic testing, but these are less than ideal candidates. The reasons are as follows: If a person without a history of cancer has a negative test result, there are several possible explanations. First, it remains possible that the family may have a *BRCA1* or

Table 2-3. Minimal features suggesting *BRCA1* and *BRCA2* mutation*

A single individual with breast and ovarian cancer (see text)

Male breast cancer in combination with
  Ashkenazi Jewish or Icelandic ancestry, or
  A family history of ovarian cancer, or
  Early-onset female breast cancer

Female breast cancer under age 30 (see text for features suggestive of LFS of Cowden syndrome)

Breast cancer in a Jewish woman under age 40

Ovarian cancer in a Jewish woman at any age

Extraovarian primary pritoneal carcinomatosis, possibly alone, or in combination with
  Ashkenazi Jewish ancestry, or
  A family history of ovarian cancer, or
  Early-onset breast cancer

Fallopian tube carcinoma in combination with
  A family history of ovarian cancer, or
  Early-onset breast cancer

Pancreatic cancer in combination with
  Ashkenazi Jewish ancestry, or
  A family history of ovarian cancer, or
  Early-onset breast cancer

A preponderance of tumors consistent with *BRCA2* mutations (see text) in combination with
  Ashkenazi Jewish ancestry, or
  A family history of ovarian cancer, or
  Early-onset breast cancer

*Any additional genetic features increase the risk of a germ-line mutation further.

Table 2-4. Various explanations of a negative *BRCA1* and *BRCA2* DNA sequencing result

A. First person tested in the family has no history of cancer and has a negative result (no mutation identified).
  1. Family has *BRCA1/2* mutation that is not detectable with DNA sequencing (e.g., promoter mutations, methylation, large deletions, intronic mutations). The test is uninformative in that particular family. The person tested might be a carrier.
  2. Family has a mutation in another gene (discovered or unknown). The "wrong gene" was tested.
  3. True negative result. Cannot be distinguished from numbers 1 and 2 above, unless a familial mutation is demonstrated in another family member.
B. First person tested in the family has a history of breast cancer and has a negative result.
  1. Number 1 as above.
  2. Number 2 as above.
  3. The person tested has sporadic cancer. A *BRCA1* or *BRCA2* mutation may be present in another family member.
C. Ideal testing situation.
  1. First person tested has cancer with genetic features (early-onset breast cancer, ovarian cancer, male breast cancer, double primary malignancy, or presumed obligate carrier based on pedigree structure).
  2. A *BRCA1* or *BRCA2* mutation is identified.
  3. Another family member (e.g., without cancer) undergoes testing for the specific familial mutation and has a negative result. This result is clearly interpretable as a true negative. Inheritance of familial predisposition to cancer is reliably excluded. (Family history from both parental lineages was considered and ethnicity taken into account when testing — see text.)

BRCA2 mutation that is not detectable with standard genetic testing. In suitable families, linkage analysis may be performed to distinguish presumed carriers from noncarriers without direct gene testing. The second explanation is that the family does not have a *BRCA1* or *BRCA2* mutation but may have a mutation in another gene (discovered or unknown) that was not tested. Until genetic testing can discriminate noncarriers with greater negative predictive value, all at-risk individuals should follow a more intensive cancer surveillance regimen based on their family of cancer, since a negative test result does not negate elevated risk. A third explanation is that a *BRCA1* or *BRCA2* mutation is present in the family but that the individual did not inherit it (true negative). This is precisely the information that people generally seek, but the problem is that a negative test result cannot be distinguished from the first or second explanation. Therefore, when testing individuals without cancer whose families do not have known mutations, a positive test result is the only reliable result. In order to learn that one has escaped the strong familial tendency to develop cancer, one must test negative for a specific, known familial mutation.

When a person with cancer is the first person tested and the result is negative, the first and second explanations remain possible. A third possibility is that the person tested had sporadic cancer (e.g., breast cancer at age 45), but the other cancers in the family may be due to *BRCA1* or *BRCA2*. This last possibility is minimized by testing individuals whose cancers have strong genetic features (e.g., young age at breast cancer diagnosis, ovarian cancer, male breast cancer, double primary cancer, or apparently obligate carrier based on the pedigree structure).

Ideally, an individual with cancer associated with strong genetic features and a high pretest probability of a mutation undergoes testing first, a mutation is identified, and other family members undergo testing for the specific familial mutation. Both sides of the family history are explored for each individual tested. If the individual is of Ashkenazi Jewish ancestry, the three Ashkenazi mutations are tested in addition to the known familial mutation. With this systematic approach to testing, a negative result is interpretable as a true negative.

In addition to positive and negative test results, a third testing outcome is a variant of unknown significance. Many polymorphisms have been detected in *BRCA1* and *BRCA2*, and new variants continue to appear. The significance of many of these is uncertain, and further understanding must await population studies or functional assays. Proper clinical interpretation is crucial. For example, inappropriate counseling that the variant was a mutation might lead to

a decision to pursue prophylactic surgery. In some cases, by testing other family members, it may be possible to show that the variant comes from the side of the family without cancer and is presumably benign. One can appreciate the consternation felt by an individual with a polymorphism when told that he or she has a DNA mutation in a gene that causes cancer, but the health consequences are not yet known. Pretest counseling and informed consent require a discussion of this third testing outcome.

Variability in the types of founder mutations based on ethnicity influences the accuracy of genetic testing. In Dutch breast cancer families, 36% of *BRCA1* mutations are due to one of three large genomic deletions (129). Large deletions are not detected by standard mutation testing methods because the normal gene gives a signal that the DNA in the deleted region is present. It is necessary to perform a Southern blot to find large genomic deletions.

For Ashkenazi Jews, the presence of three founder mutations has simplified genetic analysis and decreased the cost. Ninety percent of Jewish families with identifiable mutations have one of three common mutations, which can be tested for about $400 to $450. However, if the result is negative, there is a 10% chance that another mutation is present. Therefore, if one had a high enough suspicion to perform the initial analysis, it is prudent to perform full-length *BRCA1* and *BRCA2* sequencing. In practice, however, paying an additional $2100 to rule out a 10% chance of mutation is not appealing to many people.

Family history must be evaluated for both sides of the family for any individual receiving cancer risk assessment. When mutations are as prevalent as in Ashkenazi Jews, hereditary cancer risk may arise from both parental lineages. Therefore, even when a mutation is known on one side of the family, the founder mutations usually also require evaluation when testing additional family members.

Li-Fraumeni Syndrome

Li-Fraumeni syndrome (LFS, OMIM No. 151623, *http://www3.ncbi.nlm.nih.gov/Omim/searchomim.*

html) is a rare autosomal dominant cancer-predisposing syndrome characterized by early-onset breast cancer, sarcomas, and other cancers in children and young adults caused by germ-line mutations in the *p53* gene. (*Note*: The proper nomenclature is the *TP53* gene, but the common designation is *p53*, named for the 53-kDa protein product.) The clinical delineation of the syndrome and demonstration of its genetic cause provide a classic illustration of how cancer genetics has contributed to an understanding of tumor-suppressor genes. Linkage analysis of LFS was impractical because of its rarity and the high frequency of lethal tumors. Instead, candidate gene analysis proved a fruitful approach (130). Two important tumor-suppressor genes known in 1990 were the *Rb1* gene and the *p53* gene. The *Rb1* gene was an unlikely candidate because retinoblastomas are not a component tumor of LFS. Reasoning that the *p53* gene is inactivated in the sporadic counterparts of most component LFS tumors (i.e., sarcomas; brain, lung, and breast tumors; and leukemias) and that similar tumors were seen in transgenic mice with a mutant *p53* gene, germ-line mutation analysis of *p53* in affected families was undertaken. Analysis revealed germ-line *p53* mutations in all five families studied, and vertical transmission was shown in one family (130). An additional family with vertical transmission of a germ-line *p53* mutation was identified soon thereafter (131).

p53 Function and the Knudson Hypothesis

The *p53* gene (OMIM No. 191170, *http://www3. ncbi.nlm.nih.gov/Omim/searchomim.html*) plays a central role in normal cell growth, differentiation, and programmed cell death (apoptosis), and over half of human malignancies display *p53* mutations (132). The *p53* protein was first discovered in 1979 as a protein bound to the SV40 large-T antigen viral transforming protein and later cloned (133). In 1993, *Science Magazine* designated *p53* the "molecule of the year" (134,135). The *p53* pathway provides a cell cycle checkpoint, effecting G1 arrest in response to γ-radiation damage, ultraviolet light, or certain chemotherapeutic drugs. The result of normal *p53* function is an arrest of the cell cycle in response

to DNA-damaging agents, prevention of DNA replication in the presence of DNA damage, and an effect on DNA repair mediators. The p53 protein binds to DNA as a tetramer and functions as a transcriptional regulator of such genes as *p21* (cell cycle arrest), *mdm-2* (DNA damage response), *Bax* (apoptosis), and *GADD45* (DNA repair).

Classically, tumor-suppressor genes are recessive on the cellular level, meaning that both alleles must be inactivated for loss of tumor-suppressor function to occur. Knudson's two-hit hypothesis (136) predicts that the first hit in a germ-line mutation carrier is inherited (and present in all body cells), and the second hit is an acquired somatic event in a single cell. The likelihood that a second hit will occur during a germ-line mutation carrier's lifetime is high, since it can occur in any cell of each organ at risk. This molecular mechanism explains the early onset of cancer, multifocality and bilaterality of tumors, and frequent multiple primary malignancies seen in hereditary cancer-predisposing syndromes. An often confusing point is that the clinical predisposition is autosomal dominant, since the first hit has already occurred, but tumor-suppressor genes are recessive, requiring loss of function of both alleles to manifest cellular effects. Illustrations of the recessive nature of *p53* include the example of colorectal tumors with chromosomal deletions involving one *p53* allele and point mutations in the other allele (137).

Prevention of the second hit would have important implications if this could be achieved. If one functional allele is sufficient for tumor-suppressor function, then decreasing the chance of the second hit may be the key to cancer prevention in carriers. Indeed, *p53* function is altered by a variety of environmental agents such as viruses, cigarette smoke, alcohol, and other carcinogens, leaving open the possibility of clinical intervention in mutation carriers. The *p53* gene has been called the "gatekeeper of the genome" and illustrates a synthesis of the manifold theories of carcinogenesis, all of which can disable *p53* function.

Notwithstanding Knudson's two-hit hypothesis, certain *p53* mutations appear to abrogate the normal function of the protein product of the unmutated allele through dominant-negative or gain-of-function effects. The tetrameric configuration of *p53* and/or DNA-binding capacity may have implications that extend to the clinical realm. Dominant-negative mutations nullify the function of a normal protein like "a bad kid on the block spoiling the neighborhood (E. Hoffman)." Because *p53* is multimeric, it is easy to visualize a domino effect leading to neutralization of normal *p53* function. The implications would be that certain mutations could, in effect, cause a constitutional double hit, possibly resulting in earlier-onset tumors and a higher cancer incidence. The treatment and prevention implications for such families could be distinct from therapies useful in a classic two-hit situation. One would expect dominant-negative or gain-of-function mutations to occur in the form of missense mutations rather than inactivating mutations (including truncating mutations), since an altered protein must exist to annul the function of the normal protein. In fact, there is evidence for a highly penetrant cancer phenotype in carriers of missense mutations in the DNA-binding domain (138). Supporting the hypothesis that the increased cancer incidence and decreased age at tumor onset in these families could be due to a diminished reliance on a second hit is the finding that carriers with missense mutations in the DNA-binding domain have a decreased frequency of loss of the wild-type *p53* allele (138). Other studies, however, have not found a genotype-phenotype correlation in families with truncating versus missense mutations (139).

Clinical Features

LFS was first described following a review of medical records and death certificates on 648 children with rhabdomyosarcoma (140,141). Four families were identified in which siblings or cousins had a childhood sarcoma. Family histories were notable for a variety of tumors, including early-onset breast cancer. Three mothers of index cases developed breast cancer before age 30 years. The alternate designation, *SBLA syndrome* (142), serves to highlight the major component tumors: sarcoma, breast and brain tumors, leukemia (most commonly acute lymphocytic leukemia), laryngeal and lung cancer,

and adrenocortical carcinoma. The list of component tumors is long, also including lymphocytic or histiocytic lymphoma, melanoma, gonadal germ cell tumors, prostate carcinoma, pancreatic carcinoma, and other malignancies. The broad and variable tumor spectrum may reflect coinheritance of modifying genes that vary among individuals, families, and populations and/or environmental modifiers that also vary among exposed groups.

Hallmarks of LFS are an unusually young age of tumor onset and frequent multiple primary tumors. Bone sarcomas, soft tissue sarcomas, and brain tumors each account for about 12% of LFS tumors. Breast cancer is the most frequently observed cancer, accounting for one-quarter to one-third of all tumors, with an average age of onset of 36 years (138,143). Breast cancer in the 20s, particularly the early 20s, or in combination with such LFS features as sarcoma or adrenocortical carcinoma should prompt a consideration of LFS. One study found a single germ-line *p53* mutation among 126 consecutive patients with breast cancer onset at age 40 or younger (28). In the absence of other LFS features, the chance of a *p53* germ-line mutation is low, and germ-line *BRCA1* or *BRCA2* mutations are more likely. Adrenocortical carcinomas comprise only 3.6% of tumors in LFS, but the probability of identifying a germ-line *p53* mutation is higher when this tumor is present in the family. The average age of onset of 5 years for adrenocortical carcinoma in LFS contrasts sharply with typical onset in midadulthood for sporadic forms, providing an infrequent but useful hallmark. Childhood-onset adrenocortical carcinoma (unselected for family history of cancer) may be associated with a germ-line *p53* mutation in half of patients.

The penetrance of cancer in LFS is estimated to reach almost 50% by age 30 and over 90% by age 70. Lifetime penetrance of cancer is higher for women than for men, due to the high frequency of breast cancer in the syndrome. In a study of multiple primary cancers in 200 individuals from 24 LFS kindreds, the average risk of a second malignancy was 57% at 30 years following diagnosis of a first cancer. Younger individuals (aged 0–19) had an extraordinarily high RR of 83 for developing a second malignancy. In this study, 4% of individuals had a third primary, and 2% had four primary malignancies (144).

Like many other genetic syndromes, LFS exists in both distinct and subtle forms. Classic LFS is defined by the following stringent criteria: 1) index case with sarcoma diagnosed before age 45 years, 2) first-degree relative with LFS component cancer before age 45 years, and 3) another first- or second-degree relative with either a sarcoma diagnosed at any age or a component cancer diagnosed before age 45 years. Frebourg and colleagues (145) performed germ-line *p53* analysis in the 10 coding exons (the first of 11 exons is noncoding) in 15 LFS families meeting classic LFS criteria and identified germ-line mutations in eight families. Mutations were concentrated in exons 5 to 8, also a hotspot for somatic mutations. Additional studies have found that the most frequently mutated codons in the germ line (175,181,245,248,273, and 282) overlap with the most frequent sites of somatic mutation. However, half the families in the Frebourg study had no identifiable germ-line *p53* mutations. The detection rate of germ-line mutations may approach 70% using a stringent clinical definition for LFS and meticulous mutation-detection techniques (146) not clinically available. Possible explanations for failure to identify mutations in LFS families include incomplete gene analysis, abnormal posttranslational modification of the *p53* protein, promoter defects, or mutations in other genes in the *p53* signaling pathway, such as *p21, mdm-2,* and other genes. In a detailed molecular analysis of one LFS family meeting classic criteria, no *p53* mutation was identified, and linkage analysis provided evidence against involvement of the *p53* gene locus (147). Thus genetic heterogeneity may be a feature of LFS.

Nonetheless, individuals and families who do not meet the strict criteria for classic LFS occasionally do carry germ-line *p53* mutations. With less stringent genetic definitions, the chance of finding a germ-line *p53* mutation is diminished, but without relaxed criteria, cases are missed, and the spectrum of clinical presentation is unappreciated. About 10% to 30% of "Li-Fraumeni syndrome-like" families have germ-line *p53* mutations. Numerous criteria for LFS-like families have been advanced (139), including the following: 1) clustering of two different tumors seen in extended LFS, with any age of onset, in individuals who are first- or second-degree relatives to each other, 2) three first- or second-degree relatives with LFS-related malignancies, with at least two diagnosed under age 45, 3) one person with three primary LFS-related malignancies, or 4) proband with a childhood cancer or a sarcoma or adrenocortical carcinoma before age 45. As an example of the significance of using loosened diagnostic criteria, 4 (6.8%) of 59 children and adults with a second malignant neoplasm had germ-line *p53* mutations (148).

Genetic Counseling and Testing

Several clinical features of LFS present distinctive, challenging genetic counseling issues. One major difference between *p53* and *BRCA* testing is the issue of genetic testing in children; *p53* carriers are frequently affected in childhood, but *BRCA* carriers are not. Even testing an adult for *p53* has important ramifications for children in the family, issues that must be explored in the process of genetic counseling and informed consent.

The plethora of potential malignancies in LFS is the most impressive of any cancer-predisposing syndrome yet identified. For individuals considering genetic testing, this poses a dilemma of whether it is preferable to be confronted with the certainty of high risk after a positive genetic test result or to live with uncertainty and a modicum of hope. In truth, decision making about genetic testing is much more complex than this scenario portrays, and the choice between certainty or uncertainty also applies to other genetic tests. However, there seems to be a closer parallel of *p53* germ-line testing with Huntington disease testing than with *BRCA* testing. The penetrance of LFS approaches 100% and the penetrance of Huntington disease is 100% by late adulthood, and prevention and treatment are severely limited for both conditions. With the exception of surveillance for breast cancer, there are few medical screening options for LFS patients, leaving no recourse for early detection of major malignancies such as sarcomas, brain tumors, or leukemias or the longer list of potential cancers. For *BRCA1* and *BRCA2* mutation carriers, screening and prevention of breast and ovarian cancers are imperfect, but several viable approaches exist for both major component tumors. The use of genetic testing is higher for *BRCA1* and *BRCA2* than for *p53* testing (149), which is probably due to a complex interplay of attitudes about surveillance, family experience with cancer, perceived immediacy of risk, coping styles, and other factors.

Nancy Wexler has depicted that the plight of genetic testing for Huntington disease and the Tiresias complex has parallels to LFS as well: "It is but sorrow to be wise when wisdom profits not" (the blind seer Tiresias, confronting Oedipus the King) (150). Nonetheless, information gained by genetic testing has worth to many people at risk for Huntington disease, whether for family planning, financial planning, or a valid, albeit ill-defined, "value in knowing." Certainly, the value of potentially excluding hereditary risk of Huntington disease or LFS by genetic testing seems quite vast. Furthermore, since breast cancer is the most common malignancy in LFS, a strong argument can be made for surveillance, and thus clarification of risk may have medical benefits. The efficacy of screening mammography in women under age 50 has been debated, but the positive predictive value of mammography is increased for young women with a positive family history of breast cancer (151). Thus it seems plausible that screening mammography in young LFS carriers can have a favorable impact on morbidity and mortality, notwithstanding concerns about radiation exposure in young women with cancer-predisposing mutations. It is sobering that almost half of LFS patients whose first malignancy is breast cancer will develop a second malignancy (144), but this may reflect a higher success rate of breast cancer treatment than other cancers, even in LFS patients. Finally, the exhortation against cigarette smoking seems even more compelling for *p53* germ-line mutation carriers than for the general public because smoking causes distinctive mutations in the *p53* gene that may accelerate the development of a "second hit."

Given the significant risks and potential benefits of genetic testing for LFS and the uncertainties of medical management, recommendations for *p53* germ-line mutation testing have been put forth (152). The guidelines stress the critical role of genetic counseling in families undergoing genetic testing, given the complexities of informed consent and manifold psychosocial issues. Adequate expertise in patient selection, test interpretation, medical management, and counseling is best ensured by a multidisciplinary team of clinicians and researchers well versed with LFS. Cancer control through prevention and early detection should be pursued in affected families despite knowledge gaps about efficacy. Incomplete knowledge about LFS management underscores the importance of enrolling LFS patients in research studies. The care of patients is best advanced by efforts to enroll patients in studies to examine surveillance, chemoprevention, and exposure prevention; clarify the role of environmental carcinogens and modifying genes; refine the clinical definition of LFS and LFS-like families; assess and hone the methods of mutation analysis; and ultimately, develop genotype-specific therapies.

Hereditary Nonpolyposis Colorectal Cancer Syndrome

The hereditary nonpolyposis colorectal cancer (HNPCC) syndrome (OMIM Nos. 120435 and 120436, *http://www3.ncbi.nlm.nih.gov/Omim/search omim.html*) is one of the most common cancer-predisposing syndromes, accounting for about 6% to 13% of colon cancers (153). First described by Warthin in 1895 and published in 1913, Lynch and colleagues (154) delineated the clinical details of the syndrome, and the eponymous designation bears Lynch's name (155). Lynch syndrome I refers to families with colorectal cancer only, whereas Lynch syndrome II denotes families with extracolonic as well as colorectal malignancies. Extracolonic sites most commonly include the endometrium and ovaries, but the list of possible component tumors is long and may include breast cancer. HNPCC is caused by mutations in the mismatch repair genes, which play a crucial role in maintaining the integrity of the human genome.

Stringent diagnostic criteria devised by the International Collaborative Group on Hereditary Non-Polyposis Colorectal Cancer, termed the *Amsterdam criteria* (156), are as follows: 1) at least three individuals in the family with histologically verified colorectal cancer, one of whom is a first-degree relative of the other two, 2) at least two generations affected with colorectal cancer, and 3) at least one colorectal cancer diagnosis before the age of 50. The definition excludes the diagnosis of familial adenomatous polyposis; a few polyps may be present, but polyposis rules out HNPCC. Although rigorous criteria were essential to help define the syndrome molecularly, one failing of the Amsterdam criteria is the lack of importance afforded to the presence of extracolonic tumors, particularly endometrial cancer. Furthermore, many HNPCC colon tumors are right-sided, but the Amsterdam criteria do not take into account this characteristic feature. Many families have germ-line mutations in the genes that cause Lynch syndrome but do not meet the Amsterdam criteria. Conversely, many families that meet the Amsterdam criteria do not have detectable germ-line mutations in the mismatch repair genes. The Bethesda criteria (see below) may be useful in guiding decisions about the utility of genetic testing.

Genetic Basis

The genetic basis of HNPCC was synchronously discovered by laboratories performing genetic linkage analysis and conducting research on genetic instability in HNPCC tumors and in yeast (157–160). The mismatch repair genes are a family of genes that correct DNA mismatches and help maintain accuracy of the DNA code. When one strand in the DNA double helix does not match precisely with its partner, as would occur with a mutation, the misalignment of the two strands is recognized by the mismatch repair proteins. When the mismatch repair genes are defective, mutations accumulate throughout the genome, accelerating the progression to cancer.

Errors left unrepaired by defective mismatch repair genes result in a characteristic molecular footprint known as *microsatellite instability* (MSI). Microsatellite DNA consists of short base sequences repeated several times. For example, the DNA sequence CA might be repeated three times (CACACA) on one DNA allele and five times (CACACACACA) on the other. Because the lengths of these DNA sequences

are different, the two alleles can be distinguished on electrophoretic gels. When DNA integrity is maintained properly, microsatellite allele lengths remain constant through multiple rounds of DNA synthesis in all cells of the body. However, when the mismatch repair genes are defective, slippage of DNA at microsatellites creates different-sized alleles (e.g., CACA or CACACACA), and unrepaired genetic footprints remain behind.

The phenomenon of MSI was known from work in yeast genetics, and cloning of the human HNPCC genes was facilitated by homology with the already characterized yeast genes. Five human mismatch repair genes are known to cause HNPCC, including *MSH2, MLH1, PMS1, PMS2,* and *MSH6/GTBP*. Most cases of HNPCC with identifiable mutations are caused by *MSH2* or *MLH1*, and clinical testing is not available for the other mismatch repair genes. Lynch syndromes I and II are not distinguishable on the basis of the specific mismatch repair gene mutation present. Epigenetic modification such as DNA methylation is becoming recognized as a mechanism for silencing gene function (161). Although the end result mimics a mutation, routine methods for mutational analysis do not detect this phenomenon. In part because of epigenetic modification, the sensitivity of genetic testing for HNPCC is low. It is crucial to understand that families conforming to the Amsterdam criteria but without identifiable mismatch repair gene mutations nonetheless manifest a cancer family syndrome that requires aggressive clinical surveillance despite the negative test results.

HNPCC tumors have a high degree of microsatellite instability, and MSI has utility in the clinical diagnosis of HNPCC. Presumably, loss of mismatch repair gene function was causal in tumorigenesis and led to molecular progression of the tumor while leaving the MSI genetic footprint. The Bethesda criteria (162) allow for the use of MSI analysis of tumors to determine whether mismatch repair gene analysis is merited. If no MSI is present in a tumor, it is unlikely that the tumor was caused by an underlying mismatch repair defect. Conversely, the presence of MSI in a tumor raises the likelihood that an underlying mismatch repair defect is present.

Extracolonic Malignancies

Like some other cancer-predisposing syndromes, the list of component tumors in Lynch syndrome II is long, and there is uncertainty about whether certain tumors are part of the syndrome or are seen in families due to chance alone. Endometrial, ovarian, upper urologic, pancreatic, and gastrointestinal malignancies occur in excess in HNPCC families and are considered to be part of Lynch syndrome II. Additional tumors may be part of the syndrome, and understanding cancer risk may influence management. A variant of Lynch syndrome II called *Muir-Torre syndrome* (163) involves multiple skin tumors and may be associated with an increased risk of breast cancer (164,165), although the evidence is sparse. Mutations in *MSH2* and *MLH1* have been found in Muir-Torre kindreds, suggesting that Lynch syndrome II also could predispose to breast cancer.

One way to discern HNPCC-associated tumors is to compare the frequency of extracolonic malignancies in HNPCC families with the frequencies measured in a tumor registry for the same geographic region (166). However, methodologic flaws, such as ascertainment bias (recognition of families because of a high incidence of extracolonic malignancies that may not be part of the HNPCC syndrome) are difficult to exclude. In addition, there could be underrepresentation of specific malignancies in some families if additional interacting genes are required for cancer manifestation.

A more rigorous definition of the HNPCC tumor spectrum would rely on molecular characterization of extracolonic malignancies. Two such studies shed light on whether breast cancer is part of HNPCC. In one study, breast tumor tissue from five families was studied using molecular techniques (167). In a family with a germ-line *MLH1* mutation, a breast tumor displayed microsatellite instability. MSI is rare in breast tumors, occurring in only 0% to 20% of tumors and suggesting that a mismatch repair defect may play a role in tumorigenesis. Furthermore, this breast tumor expressed only the mutant *MLH1* allele. This finding is consistent with Knudson's hypothesis whereby the wild-type (normal) *MLH1* gene function was lost in the breast tumor, the mutant *MLH1* copy was expressed but provided inadequate function, and there was no mismatch repair capacity, leading to the MSI footprint seen. In this study, an additional four breast tumors and a metastatic breast cancer arising among four different families also showed MSI. An additional study found MSI in a breast tumor from a patient with a family history suggestive of Lynch syndrome II (168).

Thus there is some molecular evidence that breast cancer is a feature of Lynch syndrome II. However, breast cancer is not a major component tumor of the syndrome, and risk could be influenced significantly by other modifying genes. Thus far there is no compelling evidence for the routine institution of early breast cancer surveillance in HNPCC kindreds, although individualized recommendations should be influenced by the family history of breast cancer.

Ataxia-Telangiectasia

There is debate in the scientific literature about whether female mutation carriers for the autosomal recessive disorder ataxia-telangiectasia (AT, OMIM No. 208900, *http://www3.ncbi.nlm.nih.gov/Omim/searchomim.html*) are at increased risk of breast cancer. Some sources indicate that this theory is accepted dogma, but controversy still exists. Evidence in favor of the AT heterozygote hypothesis is based mainly on epidemiologic studies and is supported by biologic plausibility. The evidence for and against this hypothesis is explored below.

AT is an autosomal recessive inherited disorder characterized by progressive cerebellar ataxia, oculocutaneous telangiectasia, hypersensitivity to ionizing radiation, immunodeficiency, chromosomal instability, and a markedly increased frequency of malignancy, seen in one-third of homozygotes (169). Lymphomas, particularly of B-cell origin, and T-cell chronic lymphatic leukemia are the most common malignancies; also described are adenocarcinoma of the stomach, medulloblastoma, and glioma. Breast cancer is not usually seen in AT homozygotes; whether early death due to other causes usually precludes this presentation is unknown.

Homozygotes and heterozygotes with breast cancer have been reported in rare families with atypical AT features (170).

Fibroblasts and lymphocytes from AT patients are abnormally sensitive to induction of chromosomal breakage and killing by ionizing radiation, paralleled clinically by the radiation necrosis seen in homozygotes when given conventional treatment doses for malignancy. Exposure to ionizing radiation is a risk factor for breast cancer, as shown by studies of female survivors of the Hiroshima and Nagasaki atomic bombings and occurrence of iatrogenic radiation-induced breast cancers (e.g., breast cancer following mantle irradiation for Hodgkin's lymphoma). The AT heterozygote hypothesis is that individuals with one mutated copy of the *AT* gene (and only one normal *AT* gene) do not possess enough intrinsic ability to guard against the carcinogenic effects of radiation and thus develop cancer at a higher rate than individuals with two working copies of the *AT* gene. Based on an estimated AT homozygote frequency of 1 in 40,000 to 100,000 live births, about 1% of people are carriers of *AT* mutations (171,172). If an excess risk of breast cancer is conveyed to *AT* mutation carriers, then a significant proportion of breast cancer in the general population may be attributable to *AT* mutation carrier status. If so, then identification of these at-risk individuals and minimization of radiation exposure may have a favorable impact on the incidence of breast cancer.

The AT heterozygote theory arose out of a series of epidemiologic studies performed by Swift and colleagues. These studies assessed cancer mortality (173) and incidence in retrospective (174,175) and prospective (176) studies in blood relatives of AT homozygotes. These studies could not directly assess the mutational status of the *AT* gene because it had not yet been cloned. However, since parents are obligate *AT* mutation carriers and the relatedness of other blood relatives is quantifiable, cancer risk could be assessed in relation to the chance of carrying an abnormal *AT* allele. An RR of cancer of 6.1 in AT heterozygotes was found (175), with an estimated attributable risk of 8% to 18% for AT heterozygosity in sporadic breast cancer. It has seemed counterintuitive that such a large proportion of breast cancer would be attributable to such a rare disease as AT. However, a separate group (177) found an excess of breast cancer deaths in the mothers of AT patients, corroborating the findings of Swift's group. Swift later (176) found an RR of breast cancer of 5.1, and a case-control substudy found that women with breast cancer were more likely to have been exposed to ionizing radiation. Several methodologic objections were noted (178–182), including a "healthy spouse effect" and improper estimates of radiation exposure. Nonetheless, other groups (183,184) reported findings that upheld those of Swift's group.

The impasse encountered in the preceding epidemiologic studies became bridgeable with the cloning of the gene mutated in AT (185), called *ATM* (*AT*-mutated). Sequence homologies to an array of genes in yeast, *Drosophila*, and mammals have revealed several putative functions involved with cell cycle control, detection of DNA damage, control of telomere length, and meiotic pairing. Genetic testing of *ATM* in AT families permitted more direct probing of the AT heterozygote hypothesis. Athma and colleagues (186) performed molecular genotyping on AT patients' relatives who had breast cancer and found AT heterozygosity in 25 of 33, giving an odds ratio of 3.8. An estimated 6.6% of breast cancers were calculated to be attributable to AT heterozygosity in the United States, with a more pronounced effect in older women. In apparent contrast, FitzGerald and colleagues (187) found no evidence of increase in AT heterozygosity in young women with breast cancer. Perhaps this is reconcilable with the study of Athma and colleagues if a cumulative effect of radiation with age is important (as seen in the *NAT2*/smoking/breast cancer/age example discussed previously).

Genetic testing is not performed routinely for the clinical identification of AT heterozygotes. The possible health risks to carriers of *ATM* mutations remain to be clarified. The risk-benefit ratio of mammography has been questioned, particularly for younger women, because risk appears to be of greater magnitude. Given the naïve state of knowledge in this area, there are currently no specific health guidelines for known *ATM* carriers.

Cowden Syndrome

Cowden Syndrome (OMIM No. 158350, *http://www3.ncbi.nlm.nih.gov/Omim/searchomim.html*) is a rare autosomal dominant cancer-predisposing syndrome involving characteristic mucocutaneous lesions and cancer of the breast, thyroid, and female genitourinary tract. Named for a patient with the condition, the alternate designation is the *multiple hamartoma syndrome*. Hamartomas are benign, disorganized, hyperplastic growths that may occur in any tissue. In Cowden syndrome, hamartomas are encountered most commonly in the skin, mucous membranes, breast, and thyroid, and hamartomatous polyps of the colon and small bowel are characteristic. Multiple trichilemmomas are pathognomonic. The cobblestone-like gingival and buccal mucosa papules, verrucous skin lesions of the face and limbs, acral keratoses, and papillomatous tongue are hallmarks. Lipomas and fibromas are also typical. Penetrance of the mucocutaneous features is nearly complete by age 20.

In addition to breast hamartomas, a number of benign breast findings may occur, including ductal hyperplasia, intraductal papillomatosis, adenosis, lobular atrophy, fibroadenomas, and fibrocystic change (188), as well as nipple and areolar malformations. The risk of fibrocystic breast disease may be as high as 67%. Typical of the syndrome is the presence of a densely fibrotic hyalinized breast nodule. Ductal carcinoma in situ and invasive cancers are common, with a lifetime penetrance of 30% to 50% for breast tumors. Thyroid disease, including multinodular goiter and adenomas, is seen in 50% to 75% of individuals. There is a 3% to 10% chance of epithelial thyroid carcinoma, with papillary thyroid carcinoma being most typical. Multiple, early-onset uterine leiomyomas are characteristic, and brain tumors (i.e., meningiomas, glioblastoma multiforme) also occur. Primary neuroendocrine carcinoma of the skin, also known as *Merkel cell carcinoma* or *trabecular carcinoma*, occurs in association with Cowden syndrome. Squamous cell carcinoma, basal cell carcinoma, and malignant melanoma have been reported. Ovarian carcinoma, renal cell carcinoma, transitional cell carcinoma of the bladder, uterine carcinoma, non-small cell lung carcinoma, colorectal carcinoma, hepatocellular carcinoma, pancreatic carcinoma, and liposarcoma also have been reported.

Since the major malignancies in Cowden syndrome, breast and thyroid cancer, can be detected in early stages by surveillance, recognition of the syndrome is critical. The International Cowden Syndrome Consortium operational criteria for diagnosis are useful for weighting the pleiotropic manifestations according to major and minor criteria to make a formal diagnosis (189). The finding of a single germ-line *PTEN* mutation among 64 Cowden syndrome-like subjects who did not meet the operational diagnostic criteria provides evidence that these criteria are robust (190). Although Cowden syndrome is said to be rare, underdiagnosis is likely because of general lack of awareness of the syndrome as well as its variable expressivity and sometimes subtle manifestations (191). In addition, although inheritance is autosomal dominant, there may be lack of a family history because new mutations occur. Regardless of whether there is a family history, the risk of transmission by affected individuals is 50%; therefore, institution of cancer surveillance is crucial in at-risk relatives.

Several nonneoplastic features seen in Cowden syndrome have suggested that the gene has a crucial function during normal development. Lhermitte-Duclos disease (i.e., cerebellar ganglion cell hypertrophy, a form of hamartoma, leading to ataxia, altered gait, and seizures) and macrocephaly (megalencephaly, seen in 38%) are major diagnostic features of Cowden syndrome. Mental retardation, psychomotor developmental delay, adenoid facies, high-arched palate, thickened furrowed (scrotal) tongue, pectus excavatum, and scoliosis are some of the developmental anomalies seen. There is clinical overlap of Cowden syndrome with other dysmorphic genetic syndromes, at least one of which is allelic to *PTEN* (i.e., caused by mutations in the same gene) (192,193). Interestingly, abnormalities of all three germ cell layers (i.e., mesoderm, ectoderm, and endoderm) are seen in Cowden syndrome, suggesting disruption of a gene essential to basic development.

The gene responsible for Cowden syndrome, *PTEN* (phosphatase and tensin homologue deleted on chromosome ten), was first identified following observations of loss of heterozygosity at chromosome band 10q23 in glioblastomas and advanced prostate cancers. Repeatedly observed loss of a specific chromosomal region in tumors is a characteristic feature of a tumor-suppressor gene. Homozygous deletion mapping experiments at 10q23 in sporadic advanced prostate and breast cancers and glioblastomas narrowed the region containing the putative tumor-suppressor gene. Exon trapping and subsequent analysis of candidate genes performed in tumor cells resulted in cloning of the *PTEN* gene (194). Independently, families with Cowden syndrome were studied using linkage analysis, and the condition was shown to map to this same region. Combining the clinical features that suggested germ-line mutation of a tumor-suppressor gene with the evidence for a tumor-suppressor gene in the chromosomal region, the *PTEN* gene was analyzed in affected individuals. Liaw and colleagues (195) discovered germ-line mutations in *PTEN* in families with Cowden syndrome, and Nelen and colleagues (196) confirmed the presence of germ-line *PTEN* mutations in a large number of families and individuals with Cowden syndrome. Thus far there is no demonstration of genetic heterogeneity; i.e., all cases are consistent with mutations in *PTEN* and/or linkage to 10q23.

Tensin interacts with focal adhesions, and therefore, it is plausible that disruption of a tensin-like function in the PTEN protein could relate to metastasis and the observation of *PTEN* functional loss in advanced cancers. *PTEN* was cloned independently by Steck and colleagues (197) via analysis of sporadic glioma, prostate, kidney, and breast cancers or cell lines and named *MMAC1* (mutated in multiple advanced cancers 1). Germ-line *PTEN* mutations are not commonly observed in early-onset breast cancer. However, *PTEN* somatic loss appears to be important in the development of some common sporadic cancers, including breast, prostate, kidney, and brain cancers.

The dual-specificity tyrosine phosphatase domain is a frequent site of mutation in Cowden syndrome. The tyrosine phosphatase function antagonizes protein tyrosine kinases; loss of this function conceivably may lead to unrestricted cell growth. Experimental evidence supports a role of *PTEN* in inhibiting cell migration and integrin-mediated cell spreading. Interference with negative regulation of cell interactions with the extracellular matrix provides a plausible pathogenetic mechanism for the developmental anomalies as well as the predisposition to benign and malignant neoplasms seen in Cowden syndrome.

Eng (189) has pointed out the importance of instituting surveillance in families with mutations in this highly penetrant, autosomal dominant cancer-predisposing gene. Management depends on disease recognition using the International Cowden Syndrome Consortium operational diagnostic criteria. A team-management approach with a primary care provider, geneticist, dermatologist, neurologist, oncologist, and surgeon is optimal. The earliest documented case of breast cancer in Cowden syndrome is age 14 years, but most cases occur in the thirties and older. Physical examinations focusing on the thyroid should begin in the teen years, and self breast examination should be taught early. Annual mammography with or without breast ultrasounds should begin at age 30 or 5 years less than the youngest breast cancer diagnosed in the family, whichever is younger. Fibroadenomas may impair surveillance, cause pain and disfigurement, and require tailored surveillance strategies with the option of bilateral prophylactic mastectomy at the patient's discretion.

Modern Breast Cancer Genetics

The emerging framework of breast cancer etiology suggests numerous avenues for basic and clinical research. Most hereditary breast cancer is attributable to already discovered genes, several breast cancer risk factors have been enumerated, interactions between genes and environmental factors are emerging, there is mounting evidence that hereditary cancer risk is modifiable, nonsurgical means of decreasing risk are available, and early detection is improving. Discovery of novel genes will likely engender a redefinition of hereditary, familial, and sporadic breast cancer.

Henry Miller wrote, ''In expanding the field of knowledge, we but increase the horizon of ignorance." Many knowledge gaps exist regarding the clinical manifestations and epidemiologic significance of genetic syndromes. The use of gene status for improved early detection and prevention is rudimentary, and patients' knowledge about gene status does not always translate directly into improved surveillance behaviors. Thus far we have surmised about, more than systematically studied, the medical and economic health care impact of genetic testing. Genetic discrimination is much feared and incompletely legislated against.

Yet clinical genetic testing for hereditary breast cancer is now available. Although reviled by some as being prematurely available, the scales have tipped in the balance of clinical testing with the advent of chemoprevention, and the opportunity to rule out hereditary cancer risk cannot be overstated. Nonetheless, the embryonic state of knowledge in hereditary cancer management mandates enrollment of patients into research studies whenever possible.

As the modern era of breast cancer genetics takes shape, the cardinal aim is to serve patients as responsibly as possible while the field matures. Most practitioners are not fully conversant with the various breast cancer–predisposing syndromes, the ideal sequence of genetic testing within an appropriate family, the breadth of pre- and posttesting informed consent, the existing screening recommendations for carriers, or the full scope of detection, prevention, and treatment options for mutation carriers. Educational programs for practitioners on cancer genetics have matured (198,199) but have not yet pervaded clinical practice.

However, the services of genetic counselors experienced in cancer genetic counseling are widely available (NCI PDQ Cancer Genetics Services Directory, located at *http://cancernet.nci.nih. gov/wwwprot/genetic/genesrch.shtml*). Like other specialty referrals, genetic counselors fill a role unmatched by other practitioners. Genetic counselors can help navigate through family dynamics to test appropriate persons without coercion, aid in dissemination of genetic information within a family while respecting patient autonomy, and serve the practitioner's medicolegal need to manage hereditary risk for the family unit. Appropriate selection and interpretation of the

genetic test, up-to-date discussion of management options, and enrollment into research studies are best accomplished in consultation with genetic counselors and/or medical geneticists. This is an effective way to remain linked with the academic community and assist the efforts of the National Cancer Genetics Network (200), which aims to study mutation carriers in sufficient numbers to further the research and clinical needs of this population.

References

1. Yalom M. A History of the breast. New York: Alfred A Knopf, 1997.
2. Hall JM, Lee MK, Newman B, et al. Linkage of early-onset familial breast cancer to chromosome 17q21. Science 1990;250:1684–1689.
3. Miki Y, Swensen J, Shattuck-Eidens D, et al. A strong candidate for the breast and ovarian cancer susceptibility gene *BRCA1*. Science 1994;266:66–71.
4. Wooster R, Bignell G, Lancaster J, et al. Identification of the breast-cancer susceptibility gene *BRCA2*. Nature 1995;373:789–792.
5. Tavtigian SV, Simard J, Rommens J, et al. The complete *BRCA2*gene and mutations in chromosome 13q-linked kindred. Nature Genet 1996;12:333–337.
6. Ottman R, Pike MC, King MC, et al. Practical guide for estimating risk for familial breast cancer. Lancet 1983;2:556–558.
7. Gail MH, Brinton LA, Byar DP, et al. Projecting individualized probabilities of developing breast cancer for white females who are being examined annually. J Natl Cancer Inst 1989;81:1879–1886.
8. Claus EB, Risch N, Thompson WD. Autosomal dominant inheritance of early-onset breast cancer: implications for risk prediction. Cancer 1994;73:643–651.
9. Bilimoria MM, Morrow M. The woman at increased risk for breast cancer: evaluation and management strategies. CA 1995;45:263–278.
10. Slattery ML, Kerber R. A comprehensive evaluation of family history and breast cancer risk: the Utah population database. JAMA 1993;270:1563–1568.
11. Lynch HT, Krush AJ. Carcinoma of the breast and ovary in three families. Surg Gynecol Obstet 1971;133:644–648.
12. Go RC, King MC, Bailey-Wilson J, et al. Genetic epidemiology of breast cancer and associated cancers in high-risk families: I. Segregation analysis. J Natl Cancer Inst 1983;71:455–461.

13. Schildkraut JM, Thompson WD. Familial ovarian cancer: a population-based case control study. Am J Epidemiol 1988;128:456–466.
14. Schildkraut JM, Risch N, Thompson WD. Evaluating genetic associations among ovarian, breast, and endometrial cancer: evidence for a breast-ovarian cancer relationship. Am J Hum Genet 1989;45:521–529.
15. Thompson WD, Schildkraut JM. Familial history of gynecological cancers: relationships to the incidence of breast cancer prior to age 55. Int J Epidemiol 1991;20:595–602.
16. Claus EB, Risch Neil, Thompson WD. The calculation of breast cancer risk for women with a first degree family history of ovarian cancer. Breast Cancer Res Treat 1993;28:115–120.
17. Anderson DE, Badzioch MD. Breast cancer risks in relatives of male breast cancer patients. J Natl Cancer Inst 1992;74:1114–1117.
18. Thiessen EU. Concerning a familial association between breast cancer and both prostate and uterine malignancies. Cancer 1974; 34:1102–1107.
19. Cannon L, Bishop DT, Skolnick M, et al. Genetic epidemiology of prostate cancer in the Utah Mormon genealogy. Cancer Surv 1982;1:47–69.
20. Tulinius H, Egilsson V, Olafsdottir GH, et al. Risk of prostate, ovarian, and endometrial cancer among relatives of women with breast cancer. Br Med J 1992;305:855–857.
21. Anderson DE, Badzioch MD. Familial effects of prostate and other cancers on lifetime breast cancer risk. Breast Cancer Res Treat 1993;28:107–113.
22. Parazzini F, Negri E, LaVecchia C, et al. Family history of reproductive cancers and ovarian cancer risk: an Italian case-control study. Am J Epidemiol 1992;135:35–40.
23. Mulvihill JJ, Tulinius T. Cancer ecogenetics: studying genetic and environment interactions through epidemiology. Int J Epidemiol 1987;16:337–340.
24. Ambrosone CB, Kadlubar FF. Toward an integrated approach to molecular epidemiology. Am J Epidemiol 1997;146:912–918.
25. Ambrosone CB, Freudenheim JL, Graham S, et al. Cigarette smoking, *N*-acetyltransferase 2 genetic polymorphisms, and breast cancer risk. JAMA 1996;276:1494–1501.
26. Ford D, Easton DF, Stratton M, et al. Genetic heterogeneity and penetrance analysis of the *BRCA1* and *BRCA2* genes in breast cancer families. Am J Hum Genet 1998;62:676–689.
27. Serova OM, Mazoyer S, Puget N, et al. Mutations in *BRCA1* and *BRCA2* in breast cancer families: are there more breast cancer-susceptibility genes? Am J Hum Genet 1997;60:486–495.
28. Sidransky D, Tokino T, Helzlsouer K, et al. Inherited *p53* gene mutations in breast cancer. Cancer Res 1992;52:2984–2986.
29. Hemminki A, Markie D, Tomlinson I, et al. A serine-threonine kinase gene defective in Peutz-Jeghers syndrome. Nature 1998;391:184–187.
30. Jenne DE, Reimann H, Nezu J-I, et al. Peutz-Jeghers syndrome is caused by mutations in a novel serine threonine kinase. Nature Genet 1998;18:38–43.
31. Boardman LA, Thibodeau SN, Schaid DJ, et al. Increased risk for cancer in patients with the Peutz-Jeghers syndrome. Ann Intern Med 1998;128:896–899.
32. Claus EB, Risch N, Thompson WD. Genetic analysis of breast cancer in the Cancer and Steroid Hormone Study. Am J Hum Genet 1991;48:232–241.
33. Newman B, Austin MA, Lee M, et al. Inheritance of breast cancer: evidence for autosomal dominant transmission in high risk familes. Proc Natl Acad Sci USA 1988;85:1–5.
34. Narod SA, Feunteun J, Lynch HT, et al. Familial breast-ovarian cancer locus on chromosome 17q12-23. Lancet 1991;338:82–83.
35. Lynch HT, Watson P. Genetic counselling and hereditary breast/ovarian cancer. Lancet 1992; 339:1181. Letter.
36. Easton DF, Bishop DT, Ford D, et al. Breast Cancer Linkage Consortium. Genetic linkage analysis in familial breast and ovarian cancer: results from 214 families. Am J Hum Genet 1993;52:678–701.
37. Wooster R, Neuhausen SL, Mangion J, et al. Localization of a breast cancer susceptibility gene, *BRCA2*, to chromosome 13q12-13. Science 1994;265:2088–2090.
38. Thorlacius S, Tryggbadottir L, Olafsdottir GH, et al. Linkage to *BRCA2* region in hereditary male breast cancer. Lancet 1995;346:544–545.
39. Futreal PA, Liu Q, Shattuck-Eidens D, et al. *BRCA1* mutation in primary and ovarian carcinomas. Science 1994;266:120–122.
40. Merajver SD, Pham TM, Caduff RF, et al. Somatic mutations in the *BRCA1* gene in sporadic ovarian tumors. Nature Genet 1995;9: 439–443.
41. Miki Y, Katagiri T, Kasumi F, et al. Mutation analysis in the *BRCA2* gene in primary breast cancers. Nature Genet 1996;13:245–247.

42. Teng DH, Bogden R, Mitchell J. Low incidence of *BRCA2* mutations in breast carcinoma and other cancers. Nature Genet 1996;13:241–244.

43. Lancaster JM, Wooster R, Mangion J, et al. *BRCA2* mutations in primary breast and ovarian cancers. Nature Genet 1996;13:238–240.

44. Takahashi H, Chiu HC, Bandera CA, et al. Mutations of the *BRCA2* gene in ovarian carcinomas. Cancer Res 1996;56:2738–2741.

45. Thompson ME, Jensen RA, Obermiller PS, et al. Decreased expression of *BRCA1* accelerates growth and is often present during sporadic breast cancer progression. Nature Genet 1995;9:444–450.

46. Holt JT, Thompson ME, Szabo C, et al. Growth retardation and tumour inhibition by *BRCA1*. Nature Genet 1996;12:298–302.

47. Wilson CA, Ramos L, Villasenor MR, et al. Localization of human *BRCA1* and its loss in high-grade, non-inherited breast carcinomas. Nature Genet 1999;21:236–240.

48. Wu LC, Wang SW, Tsan JT, et al. Identification of a RING protein that can interact in vivo with *BRCA1* gene product. Nature Genet 1996;14:430–440.

49. Monteiro ANA, August A, Hanafusa H. Evidence for a transcriptional activation function of *BRCA1* C-terminal region. Proc Natl Acad Sci USA 1996;93:13595–13599.

50. Scully R, Anderson SF, Chao DM, et al. *BRCA1* is a component of the RNA polymerase II holoenzyme. Proc Natl Acad Sci USA 1997;94:5605–5610.

51. Chen CF, Li S, Chen YM, et al. The nuclear localization sequences of the *BRCA1* protein interact with the importin-alpha subunit of the nuclear transport signal receptor. J Biol Chem 1996;271:32863–32868.

52. Thakur S, Zhang HB, Peng Y, et al. Localization of *BRCA1* and a splice variant identifies the nuclear localization signal. Mol Cell Biol 1997;17:444–452.

53. Chen Y, Farmer AA, Chen C-F, et al. *BRCA1* is a 220-kDa nuclear phosphoprotein that is expressed and phosphorylated in a cell cycle-dependent manner. Cancer Res 1996;56:3168–3172.

54. Thomas JE, Smith M, Rubinfeld B, et al. Subcellular localization and analysis of apparent 180-kDa and 220-kDa proteins of the breast cancer susceptibility gene, *BRCA1*. J Biol Chem 1996;271:28630–28635.

55. Ruffner H, Verma IM. *BRCA1* is a cell cycle-regulated nuclear phosphoprotein. Proc Natl Acad Sci USA 1997;94:7138–7143.

56. Chen Y, Chen C-F, Riley DJ, et al. Aberrant subcellular localization of *BRCA1* in breast cancer. Science 1995;270:789–791.

57. Jensen RA, Thompson ME, Jetton TL, et al. *BRCA1* is secreted and exhibits properties of a granin. Nature Genet 1996;12:303–308.

58. Scully R, Ganesan S, Brown M, et al. Location of *BRCA1* in human breast and ovarian cell lines. Science 1996;272:123–125.

59. Wilson CA, Payton MN, Pekar SK, et al. *BRCA1* protein products: antibody specificity. Nature Genet 1996;13:264–265.

60. Wilson CA, Payton MN, Elliott GS, et al. Differential subcellular localization, expression and biological toxicity of *BRCA1* and the splice variant *BRCA1-δ* 11b. Oncogene 1997;14:1–16.

61. Coene E, Van Oostveldt P, Willems K, et al. *BRCA1* is localized in cytoplasmic tube-like invaginations in the nucleus. Nature Genet 1997;16:122–124.

62. Scully R, Chen J, Plug A, et al. Association of *BRCA1* with *Rad51* in mitotic and meiotic cells. Cell 1997;88:265–275.

63. Scully R, Chen J, Ochs RL, et al. Dynamic changes of *BRCA1* subnuclear location and phosphorylation state are initiated by DNA damage. Cell 1997;90:425–435.

64. Vaugh JP, Cirisano FD, Huper G, et al. Cell-cycle control of *BRCA2*. Cancer Res 1996;56:4590–4594.

65. Vaughn JP, Davis PL, Jarboe MD, et al. *BRCA1* expression is induced before DNA synthesis in both normal and tumor-derived breast cells. Cell Growth Diff 1996;7:711–715.

66. Spillman MA, Bowcock AM. *BRCA1* and *BRCA2* mRNA levels are coordinately elevated in human breast cancer cells in response to estrogen. Oncogene 1996;13:1639–1645.

67. Suzuki A. *BRCA2* is required for embryonic cellular proliferation in the mouse. Genes Dev 1997;11:1242–1252.

68. Sharan SK, Morimatsu M, Albrecht U, et al. Embryonic lethality and radiation hypersensitivity mediated by *Rad51* in mice lacking *Brca2*. Nature 1997;386:804–810.

69. Connor F, Bertwistle D, Mee PJ, et al. Tumorigenesis and a DNA repair defect in mice with a truncating *Brca2* mutation. Nature Genet 1997;17:423–430.

70. Biggs PJ, Bradley A. A step toward genotype-based therapeutic regimens for breast cancer in patients with *BRCA2* mutations? J Natl Cancer Inst 1998;90:951–953.

71. Abbott DW, Freeman ML, Holt JT. Double-strand break repair deficiency and radiation

sensitivity in *BRCA2* mutant cancer cells. J Natl Cancer Inst 1998;90:978–985.

72. Easton DF, Ford D, Bishop DT, and the Breast Cancer Linkage Consortium. Breast and ovarian cancer incidence in *BRCA1* mutation. Am J Hum Genet 1995;56:265–271.

73. Narod SA, Ford D, Devilee P, et al. An evaluation of genetic heterogeneity in 145 breast-ovarian cancer families. Am J Hum Genet 1995;56:254–264.

74. Gayther S, Mangion J, Russell P, et al. Variation of risks of breast and ovarian cancer associated with different germ-line mutations of the *BRCA2* gene. Nature Genet 1997;15:103–105.

75. Shattuck-Eidens D, Oliphant A, McClure M, et al. *BRCA1* sequence analysis in women at high risk for susceptibility mutations: risk factor analysis and implications for genetic testing. JAMA 1997;278:1242–1250.

76. Frank TS, Manley SA, Olopade OI, et al. Sequence analysis of *BRCA1* and *BRCA2*: correlation of mutations with family history and ovarian cancer risk. J Clin Oncol 1998; 16:2417–2425.

77. Burke W, Daly M, Garber J, et al. For the Cancer Genetics Studies Consortium. Recommendations for follow-up care of individuals with an inherited predisposition to cancer: II. *BRCA1* and *BRCA2*. JAMA 1997;277:997–1003.

78. Schrag D, Kuntz KM, Garber JE, et al. Decision analysis: effects of prophylactic mastectomy and oopohorectomy on life expectancy among women with *BRCA1* or *BRCA2* mutations. New Engl J Med 1997;336:1465–1471.

79. Grann VR, Panageas KS, Whang W, et al. Decision analysis of prophylactic mastectomy and oophorectomy in *BRCA1*-positive or *BRCA2*-positive patients. J Clin Oncol 1998;16:979–985.

80. Narod SA, Goldgar D, Cannon-Albright L, et al. Risk modifiers in carriers of *BRCA1* mutations. Int J Cancer 1995;64:394–398.

81. Stratton MR, Ford D, Neuhasen S, et al. Familial male breast cancer is not linked to the *BRCA1* locus on chromosome 17q. Nature Genet 1994;7:103–107.

82. Thorlacius S, Olafsdottir G, Tryggvadottir L, et al. A single *BRCA2* mutation in male and female breast cancer familites from Iceland with varied cancer phenotypes. Nature Genet 1996;13:117–119.

83. Phelan CM, Lancaster JM, Tonin P, et al. Mutation analysis of the *BRCA2* gene in 49 site-specific breast cancer families. Nature Genet 1996;12:120–122.

84. Couch FJ, Farid LM, DeShano ML, et al. *BRCA2* germ-line mutations in male breast cancer cases and breast cancer families. Nature Genet 1996;13:123–125.

85. Friedman LS, Gayther SA, Kurosaki T, et al. Mutation analysis of *BRCA1* and *BRCA2* in a male breast cancer population. Am J Hum Genet 1997;60:313–319.

86. Easton DF, Steele L, Fields P, et al. Cancer risks in two large breast cancer families linked to *BRCA2* on chromosome 13q12-13. Am J Hum Genet 1997;61:120–128.

87. Donegan WL. Cancer of the breast in men. CA 1992;41:339–354.

88. Struewing JP, Hartge P, Wacholder S, et al. The risk of cancer associated with specific mutations of *BRCA1* and *BRCA2* among Ashkenazi Jews. New Engl J Med 1997;336:1401–1408.

89. Ford D, Easton DF, Bishop DT, et al. Breast Cancer Linkage Consortium. Risks of cancer in *BRCA1* mutation carriers. Lancet 1994;343: 692–695.

90. Arason A, Barkardottir RB, Egilsson V. Linkage analysis of chromosome 17q markers and breast-ovarian cancer in Icelandic families, and possible relationship to prostate cancer. Am J Hum Genet 1993;52:711–717.

91. Bandera CA, Muto MG, Berkowitz RS, et al. Germ-line *BRCA1* mutations in women with papillary serous carcinoma of the peritoneum. Gynecol Oncol 1997;64:297. Abstract.

92. Schubert EL, Lee MK, Mefford HC, et al. *BRCA2* in American families with four or more cases of breast or ovarian cancer: recurrent and novel mutations, variable expression, penetrance, and the possibility of families whose cancer is not attributable to *BRCA1* or *BRCA2*. Am J Hum Genet 1997;60:1031–1040.

93. Grimmond SM, Palmer JM, Walters MK, et al. Confirmation of susceptibility locus on chromosome 13 in Australian breast cancer families. Hum Genet 1996;98:80–85.

94. Goggins M, Schutte M, Lu JL, et al. Germ-line *BRCA2* gene mutations in patients with apparently sporadic pancreatic carcinomas. Cancer Res 1996;56:5360–5364.

95. Katagiri T, Nakamura Y, Miki Y. Mutations in the *BRCA2* gene in hepatocellular carcinomas. Cancer Res 1996;56:4575–4577.

96. Ozcelik H, Schmocker B, DiNicola N, et al. Germ-line *BRCA2* 6174delT mutations in Ashkenazi Jewish pancreatic cancer patients. Nature Genet 1997;16:17–18.

97. Lehrer S, Fodor F, Stock RG, et al. Absence of 185delAG mutation of the *BRCA1* gene and

6174delT mutation of the *BRCA2* gene in Ashkenazi Jewish men with prostate cancer. Br J Cancer 1998;78:771–773.

98. Langston AA, Stanford JL, Wicklund KG, Thompson JD, et al. Germ-line *BRCA1* mutations in selected men with prostate cancer. Am J Hum Genet 1996;58:881–884. Letter.

99. Eltabbakh GH, Piver MS. Extraovarian primary peritoneal carcinoma. Oncology 1998;12: 813–819.

100. Whittemore AS, Gong G, Itnyre J. Prevalence and contribution of *BRCA1* mutations in breast cancer and ovarian cancer: results from three U.S. population-based case-control studies of ovarian cancer. Am J Hum Genet 1997; 60:496–504.

101. Ford D, Easton DF, Peto J. Estimates of the gene frequency of *BRCA1* and its contribution to breast and ovarian cancer incidence. Am J Hum Genet 1995;57:1457–1462.

102. Struewing JP, Abeliovich D, Peretz T, et al. The carrier frequency of the *BRCA1* 185delAG mutation is approximately 1 percent in Ashkenazi Jewish individuals. Nature Genet 1995;11: 198–200.

103. Beutler E, Burk RB, Cohen MM, et al. Genetic diseases and the Jewish community: a clarification. Congress Monthly 1998;65:3–7.

104. Tonin P, Weber B, Offit K, et al. Frequency of recurrent *BRCA1* and *BRCA2* mutations in Ashkenazi Jewish breast cancer families. Nature Genet 1996;2:1179–1183.

105. Szabo CI, King M-C. Population genetics of *BRCA1* and *BRCA2*. Am J Hum Genet 1997;60:1013–1020. Editorial.

106. Fodor FH, Weston A, Bleiweiss IJ, et al. Frequency and carrier risk associated with common *BRCA1* and *BRCA2* mutations in Ashkenazi Jewish breast cancer patients. Am J Hum Genet 1998;63:45–51.

107. Colditz GA, Willett WC, Hunter DJ, et al. Family history, age, and risk of breast cancer: prospective data from the Nurses' Health Study. JAMA 1993;270:338–343.

108. Rebbeck T, Levin A, Daly M, et al. Cancer risk reduction by prophylactic surgery in *BRCA1* and *BRCA2* mutation carriers. Am J Hum Genet 1998;63:A47.

109. Fisher B, Costantino JP, Wickerham DL, et al. Tamoxifen for prevention of breast cancer: report of the National Surgical Adjuvant Breast and Bowel Project P-1 Study. J Natl Cancer Inst 1998;90:1371–1388.

110. Narod SA, Risch H, Moslehi R, et al. Hereditary Ovarian Cancer Clinical Study Group. Oral contraceptives and the risk of hereditary ovarian cancer. New Engl J Med 1998;339:424–428.

111. Phelan CM, Rebbeck TR, Weber BL, et al. Ovarian cancer risk in *BRCA1* carriers is modified by *HRAS1* variable number of tandem repeats (VNTR) locus. Nature Genet 1996;12:309–311.

112. Brunet JS, Vesprini D, Abrahamson J, et al. Breast cancer risk in *BRCA1/BRCA2* carriers is modified by the *CYP1A1* gene. Am J Hum Genet 1998;63:A47.

113. Brunet J-S, Ghadirian P, Rebbeck TR, et al. Effect of smoking on breast cancer in carriers of mutant *BRCA1* or *BRCA2* genes. J Natl Cancer Inst 1998;90:761–766.

114. Meilahn EN, Destavola B, Allen DS, et al. Do urinary oestrogen metabolites predict breast cancer? Guernsey III cohort follow-up. Br J Cancer 1998;78:1250–1255.

115. Newman B, Mu H, Butler LM, et al. Frequency of breast cancer attributable to *BRCA1* in a population-based series of American women. JAMA 1998;279:915–921.

116. Couch FJ, Hartmann LC. *BRCA1* testing: advances and retreats. JAMA 1998;279:955–956. Editorial.

117. Shattuck-Eidens D, McClure M, Simard J, et al. A collaborative survey of 80 mutations in the *BRCA1* breast and ovarian cancer susceptibility gene. JAMA 1995;273:535–541.

118. FitzGerald MG, MacDonald DJ, Krainer M, et al. Germ-line *BRCA1* mutations in Jewish and non-Jewish women with early-onset breast cancer. New Engl J Med 1996;334:143–149.

119. Offit K, Gilewski T, McGuire P, et al. Germ-line *BRCA1* 185delAG mutations in Jewish women with breast cancer. Lancet 1996;347:1643–1645.

120. Levy-Lahad E, Catane R, Eisenberg S, et al. Recurrent *BRCA1* and *BRCA2* mutations in Ashkenazi Jews in Israel: frequency and differential penetrance in ovarian cancer and in breast-ovarian cancer families. Am J Hum Genet 1997;60:1059–1067.

121. Stratton JF, Gayther SA, Russell P, et al. Contribution of *BRCA1* mutations to ovarian cancer. New Engl J Med 1997;336:1125–1130.

122. Abeliovich D, Kaduri L, Lerer I, et al. The founder mutations 185delAG and 5382insC in *BRCA1* and 617delT in *BRCA2* appear in 60% of ovarian cancer and 30% of early-onset breast cancer patients among Ashkenazi women. Am J Hum Genet 1997;60:505–514.

123. Couch FJ, DeShano ML, Blackwood A, et al. *BRCA1* mutations in women attending clinics

that evaluate the risk of breast cancer. New Engl J Med 1997;336:1409–1415.

124. Berry DA, Parmigiani G, Sanchez J, et al. Probability of carrying a mutation of breast-ovarian cancer gene *BRCA1* based on family history. J Natl Cancer Inst 1997;89:227–238.

125. Parmigiani G, Berry DA, Aguilar O. Determining carrier probabilities for breast cancer—susceptibility genes *BRCA1* and *BRCA2*. Am J Hum Genet 1998;62:145–158.

126. Dobrovic A, Simpfendorfer D. Methylation of the *BRCA1* gene in sporadic breast cancer. Cancer Res 1997;57:3347–3350.

127. Mancini DN, Rodenhiser DI, Ainsworth PJ, et al. CpG methylation within the 5′ regulatory region of the *BRCA1* gene is tumor specific and includes a putative CREB binding site. Oncogene 1998;16:1161–1169.

128. Puget N, Stoppa-Lyonnet D, Sinilnikova OM, et al. Screening for germ-line rearrangements and regulatory mutations in *BRCA1* led to the identification of four new deletions. Cancer Res 1999;59:455–461.

129. Petrij-Bosch A, Peelen T, VanVliet M, et al. *BRCA1* genomic deletions are major founder mutations in Dutch breast cancer patients. Nature Genet 1997;17:341–345.

130. Malkin D, Li FP, Strong LC, et al. Germ line *p53* mutations in a familial syndrome of breast cancer, sarcomas, and other neoplasms. Science 1990;250:1233–1238.

131. Srivastava S, Zou ZQ, Pirollo K, et al. Germ-line transmission of a mutated *p53* gene in a cancer prone family with Li-Fraumeni syndrome. Nature 1990;348:747–749.

132. Levine AJ. *p53,* the cellular gatekeeper for growth and division. Cell 1997;88:323–331.

133. Lamb P, Crawford L. Characterization of the human *p53* gene. Mol Cell Biol 1986;6:1379–1385.

134. Culotta E, Koshland DE. *p53* sweeps through cancer research. Science 1993;262:1958–1959.

135. Harris CC. *p53:* at the crossroads of molecular carcinogenesis and risk assessment. Science 1993;262:1980–1981.

136. Knudson AG. Mutation and cancer: statistical study of retinoblastoma. Proc Natl Acad Sci USA 1971;68:820–823.

137. Baker SJ, Fearon ER, Nigro JM, et al. Chromosome 17 deletions and *p53* gene mutations in colorectal carcinomas. Science 1989;244:217.

138. Birch JM, Blair V, Kelsey AM, et al. Cancer phenotype correlates with constitutional *TP53* genotype in families with the Li-Fraumeni syndrome. Oncogene 1998;17:1061–1068.

139. Eng C, Schneider K, Fraumeni JF, et al. Third international workshop on collaborative interdisciplinary studies of *p53* and other predisposing genes in Li-Fraumeni syndrome. Cancer Epidemiol Biomark Prev 1997;6:379–383.

140. Li FP, Fraumeni JF. Soft-tissue sarcomas, breast cancer, and other neoplasms: a familial syndrome? Ann Intern Med 1969;71:747–752.

141. Li FP, Fraumeni JF. Rhabdomyosarcoma in children: an epidemiologic study and identification of a familial cancer syndrome. J Natl Cancer Inst 1969;43:1364–1373.

142. Lynch HT, Guirgis HA. Childhood cancer and the SBLA syndrome. Med Hypothesis 1979;5:515–522.

143. Kleihues P, Schauble B, zur Hausen A, et al. Tumors associated with *p53* germ-line mutations: a synopsis of 91 families. Am J Pathol 1997;150:1–13.

144. Hisada M, Garber JE, Fung CY, et al. Multiple primary cancers in families with Li-Fraumeni syndrome. J Natl Cancer Inst 1998;90:606–611.

145. Frebourg T, Barbier N, Yan Y, et al. Germ-line *p53* mutations in 15 families with Li-Fraumeni syndrome. Am J Hum Genet 1995;56:608–615.

146. Varley JM, McGown G, Thorncroft M, et al. Germ-line mutations of *TP53* in Li-Fraumeni families: an extended study of 39 families. Cancer Res 1997;57:3245–3252.

147. Evans SC, Mims B, McMasters KM, et al. Exclusion of a *p53* germ-line mutation in a classic Li-Fraumeni syndrome family. Hum Genet 1998;102:681–686.

148. Malkin D, Jolly KW, Barbier N, et al. Germline mutations of the *p53* tumor-suppressor gene in children and young adults with second malignant neoplasms. New Engl J Med 1992;326:1309–1315.

149. Patenaude AF, Schneider KA, Kieffer SA, et al. Acceptance of invitations for *p53* and *BRCA1* predisposition testing: factors influencing potential utilization of cancer genetic testing. Psycho-Oncology 1996;5:241–250.

150. Wexler N. The Tiresias complex: Huntington's disease as a paradigm of testing for late-onset disorders. FASEB J 1992;6:2820–2825.

151. Kerlikowske K, Grady D, Barclay J, et al. Positive predictive value of screening mammography by age and family history of breast cancer. JAMA 1993;270:2444–2450.

152. Li FP, Garber JE, Friend SH, et al. Recommendations on predictive testing for germ line *p53* mutations among cancer prone individuals. J Natl Cancer Inst 1992;84:1156–1160.

153. Houlston RS, Collins A, Slack J, et al. Dominant genes for colorectal cancer are not rare. Ann Hum Genet 1992;56:99–103.

154. Lynch HT, Shaw MW, Mangnuson CW. Hereditary factors in cancer: study of two large midwestern kindreds. Arch Intern Med 1966; 117:206–212.

155. Marra G, Boland CR. Hereditary nonpolyposis colorectal cancer: the syndrome, the genes, and historical perspectives. J Natl Cancer Inst 1995;87:1114–1125.

156. Vasen HFA, Mecklin JP, Khan PM, et al. The International Collaborative Group on Hereditary Non-Polyposis Colorectal Cancer (ICG-HNPCC). Dis Colon Rectum 1991;34:424–425.

157. Peltomaki P, Aaltonen LA, Sistonen P, et al. Genetic mapping of a locus predisposing to human colorectal cancer. Science 1993;260: 810–812.

158. Aaltonen LA, Peltomaki P, Leach FS, et al. Clues to the pathogenesis of familial colorectal cancer. Science 1993;260:812–816.

159. Thibodeau SN, Bren G, Schaid D. Microsatellite instability in cancer of the proximal colon. Science 1993;260:816–819.

160. Fishel R, Lescoe MK, Rao MR, et al. The human mutator gene homologue *MSH2* and its association with hereditary nonpolyposis colon cancer. Cell 1993;75:1027–1038.

161. Jones PA, Laird PW. Cancer epigenetics comes of age. Nature Genet 1999;21:163–167.

162. Rodriguez-Bigas MA, Boland CR, Hamilton SR, et al. A National Cancer Institute workshop on hereditary nonpolyposis colorectal cancer syndrome: meeting highlights and Bethesda guidelines. J Natl Cancer Inst 1997;89:1758–1759.

163. Hall NR, Williams MA, Murday VA, Newton JA, Bishop DT. Muir-Torre syndrome: a variant of the cancer family syndrome. J Med Genet 1994;31:627–631.

164. Finan MC, Connolly SM. Sebaceous gland tumors and systemic disease: a clinicopathologic analysis. Medicine 1984;63:232–242.

165. Spraul CW, Lang GE. Grossniklaus HE, Lang GK. Metastatic adenocarcinoma to the retina in a patient with Muir-Torre syndrome. Am J Ophthalmol 1995;120:248–250.

166. Benatti P, Sassatelli R, Roncucci L, et al. Tumour spectrum in hereditary nonpolyposis colorectal cancer (HNPCC) and in families with "suspected HNPCC": a population-based study in northern Italy. Int J Cancer 1993;54:371–377.

167. Risinger JI, Barrett JC, Watson P, et al. Molecular genetic evidence of the occurrence of breast cancer as an integral tumor in patients with the hereditary nonpolyposis colorectal carcinoma syndrome. Cancer 1996;77:1836–1843.

168. Bergthorsson JT, Egilsson V, Gudmundsson J, et al. Identification of a breast tumor with microsatellite instability in a potential carrier of the hereditary nonpolyposis colon cancer trait. Clin Genet 1995;47:305–310.

169. Gatti RA, Boder E, Vinters HV, et al. Ataxia-telangiectasis: an interdisciplinary approach to pathogenesis. Medicine 1991;70:99–117.

170. Stankovic T, Kidd AM, Sutcliffe A, et al. *ATM* mutations and phenotypes in ataxia-telangiectasia families in the British Isles: expression of mutant *ATM* and the risk of leukemia, lymphoma, and breast cancer. Am J Hum Genet 1998;62:234–245.

171. Swift M, Morrell D, Cromartie E, et al. The incidence and gene frequency of ataxia-telangiectasia in the United States. Am J Hum Genet 1986;39:573–583.

172. Easton DF. Cancer risk in AT heterozygotes. Int J Radiat Biol 1994;66(suppl):S177–S182.

173. Swift MR, Sholman L, Perry M, et al. Malignant neoplasms in the families of patients with ataxia-telangiectasia. Cancer Res 1976;36: 209–215.

174. Swift M, Reitnauer PJ, Morrell D, et al. Breast and other cancers in families with ataxia-telangiectasia. New Engl J Med 1987;316:1289–1294.

175. Morrell D, Chase CL, Swift M. Cancers in 44 families with ataxia-telangiectasia. Cancer Genet Cytogent 1990;50:119–123.

176. Swift M, Morrell D, Massey RB, et al. Incidence of cancer in 161 families affected by ataxia-telangiectasia. New Engl J Med 1991; 325:1831–1836.

177. Pippard EC, Hall AJ, Barker DJP, et al. Cancer in homozygotes and heterozygotes of ataxia-telangiectasia and xeroderma pigmentosum in Britain. Cancer Res 1988;48:2929–2932.

178. Kuller LH, Modan B. Risk of breast cancer in ataxia-telangiectasia. New Engl J Med 1992; 326:1357–1361. Letter.

179. Boice JD, Miller RW. Risk of breast cancer in ataxia-telangiectasia. New Engl J Med 1992; 326:1357–1361. Letter.

180. Wagner LK. Risk of breast cancer in ataxia-telangiectasia. New Engl J Med 1992;326:1357–1361. Letter.

181. Hall EJ, Geard CR, Brenner DJ. Risk of breast cancer in ataxia-telangiectasia. New Engl J Med 1992;326:1357–1361. Letter.

182. Land CE. Risk of breast cancer in ataxia-telangiectasia. New Engl J Med 1992;326:1357–1361. Letter.

183. Borresen AL, Andersen TI, Tretli S, et al. Breast cancer and other cancers in Norwegian families with ataxia-telangiectasia. Genes Chromos Cancer 1990;2:339–340.

184. Bridges BA, Arlett CF. Risk of breast cancer in ataxia-telangiectasia. New Engl J Med 1992;326:1357–1361. Letter.

185. Savitsky K, Bar-Shira A, Gilad S, et al. A single ataxia telangiectasia gene with a product similar to PI-3 kinase. Science 1995;268:1749–1753.

186. Athma P, Rappaport R, Swift M. Molecular genotyping shows that ataxia-talangiectasis heterozygotes are predisposed to breast cancer. Cancer Genet Cytogenet 1996;92:130–134.

187. Fitzgerald MG, Bean JM, Hegde SR. Heterozygous *ATM* mutations do not contribute to early onset of breast cancer. Nature Genet 1997;15:307–310.

188. Schrager CA, Schneider D, Gruener AC, et al. Clinical and pathological features of breast disease in Cowden's syndrome: an underrecognized syndrome with an increased risk of breast cancer. Hum Pathol 1998;29:47–53.

189. Eng C. Cowden syndrome. J Genet Counsel 1997;6:181–192.

190. Marsh DJ, Dahia PLM, Caron S, et al. Germline *PTEN* mutations in Cowden syndrome-like families. J Med Genet 1998;35:881–885.

191. Lynch ED, Ostermeyer EA, Lee MK, et al. Inherited mutations in *PTEN* that are associated with breast cancer, Cowden disease, and juvenile polyposis. Am J Hum Genet 1997;61:1254–1260.

192. Marsh DJ, Coulon V, Lunetta KL, et al. Mutation spectrum and genotype-phenotype analyses in Cowden disease and Bannayan-Zonana syndrome, two hamartoma syndromes with germline *PTEN*. Hum Mol Genet 1998;7:507–515.

193. DiLiberti JH. Inherited macrocephaly-hamartoma syndromes. Am J Med Genet 1998;79:284–290.

194. Li J, Yen C, Liaw D, et al. *PTEN,* a putative protein tyrosine phosphatase gene mutated in human brain, breast, and prostate cancer. Science 1997;275:1943–1947.

195. Liaw D, Marsh D, Li J, et al. Germ-line mutations of the *PTEN* gene in Cowden disease, an inherited breast and thyroid cancer syndrome. Nature Genet 1997;16:64–67.

196. Nelen MR, van Staveren WCG, Peeters EAJ, et al. Germ-line mutations in the *PTEN/MMAC1* gene in patients with Cowden disease. Hum Mol Genet 1997;6:1383–1387.

197. Steck PA, Pershouse MA, Jasser SA, et al. Identification of a candidate tumour suppressor gene, *MMAC1*, at chromosome 10q23.3 that is mutated in multiple advanced cancer. Nature Genet 1997;15:356–362.

198. Olopade OI, Offit K, Garber JE. The Task Force on Cancer Genetics Education. American Society of Clinical Oncology. Genetic testing for susceptibility to cancer. JAMA 1998;279:1612–1613. Letters.

199. Anonymous. Resource document for curriculum development in cancer genetics education. J Clin Oncol 1997;15:2157–2169.

200. Nelson N. Cancer genetics network gets under way with 5 years of funding. J Natl Cancer Inst 1997;89:10–11. News.

3

Clinical Characteristics of Genetically Determined Breast Cancer

Steven A. Narod

Family History

There is no standard definition of a hereditary breast cancer family, and it is not yet possible to clearly separate cases that are attributable to genetic mutations from nonhereditary ones on clinical grounds. Most genetics centers would consider women to be at increased risk of cancer if they have two or more relatives with early-onset breast or ovarian cancer and would offer genetic counseling accordingly. Only a minority of families of this type will be found to have a *BRCA1* or *BRCA2* mutation. Families with hereditary breast cancer are conventionally divided into two subtypes: those with the breast/ovarian cancer syndrome and those with site-specific breast cancer. The second category refers to the absence of cases of ovarian cancer and does not imply that the breast is the only site of cancer in the family. This distinction is useful at the clinical level because the presence of ovarian cancer in a family, in addition to breast cancer, increases the probability that a cancer gene mutation will be found and increases the risk of breast cancer estimated for unaffected women in the family. Women from families of both subtypes should be considered to be at increased risk for both ovarian and breast cancer. It is not possible to discriminate between the two presentations by molecular genetic studies; this is so because the major susceptibility genes, *BRCA1* and *BRCA2*, predispose to both breast and ovarian cancer. If either a *BRCA1* or *BRCA2* mutation is found, the lifetime risk of breast cancer is about 85% (1).

Families with four or more cases of breast cancer occurring below age 50 or of ovarian cancer at any age are likely to have either of the two susceptibility genes. Approximately one-third of these families present as breast/ovarian cancer families, and the remaining two-thirds are site-specific breast cancer families. Almost all families with the breast/ovarian cancer syndrome have *BRCA1* or *BRCA2* mutations; approximately 80% of these are due to *BRCA1* and 20% are due to *BRCA2* (2). Roughly equal numbers of families with site-specific breast cancer have mutations in *BRCA1* and *BRCA2* (3). However, in contrast to breast/ovarian cancer families, mutations are detected for only about one-half of families with site-specific breast cancer. The prevalence and distribution of mutations for site-specific breast cancer also vary with ethnic group. For example, Tonin and colleagues (4) found that 35 of 40 mutation-positive Ashkenazi Jewish site-specific breast cancer families carried mutations in *BRCA1* and only 5 had mutations in *BRCA2*. In contrast, the majority of the detected mutations in a group of French-Canadian families with similar clinical presentations occurred in *BRCA2* (5).

There are two hereditary breast cancer syndromes due to genes other than *BRCA1* and *BRCA2*. These syndromes are encountered rarely in clinical practice, and genetic testing for these is limited to a few centers. Cowden syndrome is the association of benign and malignant breast disease, thyroid tumors, multiple skin lesions, and colonic polyps (6). The characteristic lesion is the hamartoma. Breast cancers occur in about one-third of women with this condition. The gene for Cowden syndrome (*PTEN*) is also responsible for a proportion of families with juvenile polyposis (7).

The Li-Fraumeni syndrome is the association of early-onset breast cancer with childhood cancers of the bone, soft tissue, and adrenal cortex. The penetrance of breast cancer is about 50%. Germ-line mutations of the *p53* gene are present in the majority of families with the characteristic Li-Fraumeni phenotype but are very rare in other cancer families (8). Mutation detection should be offered to women with premenopausal breast cancer when one or more of the characteristic childhood cancers are also present. Male breast cancer is featured in families with both *BRCA1* and *BRCA2* mutations but has not been reported in the Li-Fraumeni syndrome.

Age of Onset

One of the hallmarks of hereditary breast cancer is an early age of onset. Although breast cancer at any age can be hereditary, the majority of *BRCA1*-associated breast cancers are premenopausal, and the median age of diagnosis is about 42 years. Cancer in the late twenties and early thirties is not unusual; Ford and colleagues (1) estimate the cumulative incidence of breast cancer in *BRCA1* carriers to be 4% by age 30 and 18% by age 40. *BRCA2*-associated breast cancers occur on average about 5 years later, but the lifetime risk of breast cancer is similar for the two genes (about 85%). About 10% of all breast cancers occurring below the age of 40 are hereditary.

Bilaterality

A second characteristic of hereditary breast cancer is bilaterality. Bilaterality is not in itself strongly predictive of the presence of a *BRCA1* or *BRCA2* mutation because approximately 10% of sporadic cancers are also bilateral (including both synchronous and metachronous cancers). However, the rate of contralateral breast cancer following an initial diagnosis of breast cancer is exceptionally high in *BRCA1* and *BRCA2* carriers. Robson and colleagues (9) estimate the 5-year rate of contralateral breast cancer to be 30% among

women with *BRCA1* mutations. The rate of contralateral breast cancer appears to be greater than would be expected if the cancers in the two breasts were independent. It is not clear if this excess is due to increased surveillance of the contralateral breast, the adverse effects of treatment of the initial cancer, or the selection of highly predisposed women.

Pre-Neoplastic Features

Characteristic pre-neoplastic lesions are a feature of several hereditary cancer syndromes. However, with the exception of Cowden syndrome, there does not appear to be a characteristic pre-malignant phase in the breast/ovarian cancer syndrome. Patients with Cowden syndrome are liable to a range of benign breast diseases and often will undergo multiple biopsies prior to diagnosis.

Sun and colleagues (10) reported only 4 in situ carcinomas in 36 extensive *BRCA1*-positive families. The lack of in situ cancer is particularly surprising, given that women in high-risk families are screened regularly by mammography from an early age and that the diagnosis of ductal carcinoma in situ is often made by screening mammogram. It is possible that cells with *BRCA1* mutations have the capability of early invasion. Atypical hyperplasia has not been reported to be a characteristic of breasts of women with *BRCA1* or *BRCA2* mutations. Intraductal components are also found less frequently in association with invasive breast cancer in *BRCA1* carriers than in sporadic cancers (11). These authors predicted that the rarity of in situ cancer would result in lower rates of local recurrence following surgery in *BRCA1* carriers. However, neither Verhoog and colleagues (12) nor Robson and colleagues (9) found the local recurrence rates in *BRCA1* carriers to be lower than expected.

Pathology

Hereditary breast cancers are characterized by a particular pattern of clinical features and prognostic markers that differs from sporadic cases, and it is predicted that the prognosis of hereditary breast cancer also may be different. Some characteristics of *BRCA1*-associated cancers are favorable (e.g., an increased frequency of medullary carcinomas, a decreased frequency of *erbB2* amplification), and other features are unfavorable (e.g., high mitotic grade, frequent *p53* mutations). It is therefore difficult to predict the overall influence that these secondary characteristics may have on patient relapse rates and survival. Several reports present data on the pathologic correlates of *BRCA1*-associated breast cancers (13–18). In general, the findings of high mitotic grade and a high proliferative index are consistent across all reports. Eisinger and colleagues (14) found that 81.5% of 27 *BRCA1*-associated breast cancer were of grade 3 versus 21% of registry-based control tumors ($p < 0.0001$). Marcus and colleagues (13) also found that *BRCA1*-associated cancers were of higher grade than a comparison group of tumors. In a large muliticenter study conducted by the Breast Cancer Linkage Consortium, 118 *BRCA1*-associated breast cancers and 78 *BRCA2*-associated breast cancers were compared with tumors from 547 age-matched controls (15). Both hereditary subtypes were associated with a higher grade than controls. Sixty-six percent of *BRCA1*-associated tumors were grade 3. Higher scores were found for pleomorphism, for mitotic index, and for overall grade. Eisinger and colleagues (17) found that 24 of 24 *BRCA1*-associated breast cancers were associated with a high mitotic index compared with 22 of 24 non-*BRCA1* cancers ($p = 0.0007$).

Medullary carcinoma of the breast represents only about 1% of breast cancers in the general population but is not rare in carriers of *BRCA1* mutations (12,13,15). Eisinger and colleagues (20) found that 6 (19%) of 32 cancers in *BRCA1* carriers were of medullary histology. They also found that 2 (11%) of 18 unselected breast cancers were medullary.

Molecular Features

The majority of *BRCA1*- and *BRCA2*-associated breast cancers are estrogen receptor (ER) negative (16–18,21). This is also true of the in situ components associated with invasive cancers.

Osin and colleagues (21) studied 16 patients with ductal carcinoma in situ (DCIS) associated with invasive cancers and found that two-thirds were ER negative and all were progesterone receptor (PR) negative. They concluded that ER loss is an early event in hereditary breast cancer and that these cancers are likely to be hormone resistant from their inception. They also question whether tamoxifen prophylaxis would be effective in preventing hormone-insensitive cancers.

Two groups have studied the frequency of *p53* mutations in *BRCA1*-associated breast cancers. Crook and colleagues (22) found somatic *p53* mutations in 7 of 7 *BRCA1*-associated breast tumors. Johansson and colleagues (16) found *p53* overexpression in 70% of *BRCA1*-associated breast cancers. *p53* mutations are less common in *BRCA2*-associated breast cancers and were found in only 10 (29%) of 34 *BRCA2*-assocated breast tumors in Iceland (23). This was slightly greater than the frequency in non-mutant breast cancer controls from Iceland but less frequent than in *BRCA1*-associated cancers.

Robson and colleagues (19) characterized 17 mutation-positive and 41 mutation-negative breast cancers from young Jewish women for a range of tumor markers. The *BRCA1/BRCA2* tumors were more likely to be ER negative and to be negative for ERBB2 antibody staining. No significant differences were observed for the other tumor markers, including p27, cathepsin D, epidermal growth factor receptor (EGFR), and bcl-2.

Prognosis

Because of the high frequency of high-grade, *p53*-positive, ER-negative tumors in *BRCA1* carriers, women with these cancers may be expected to have a relatively poor prognosis compared with women with nonhereditary cancer. Accurate information about prognosis is important because many *BRCA1/BRCA2* carriers opt for regular mammographic screening in lieu of prophylactic surgery. However, the value of early detection is contingent on the curability of early-stage breast cancer.

There are conflicting reports of the importance of *BRCA1* germ-line mutations on breast cancer progression. Porter and colleagues (24) studied eight Scottish breast cancer families with positive linkage to *BRCA1* and showed an 83% 5-year survival. Marcus and colleagues (13) found that *BRCA1* carriers did better than their sporadic cancer counterparts in a crude analysis (RR = 0.63), but after adjusting for age and stage, the *BRCA1* carriers did worse (RR = 1.65). Johannsen and colleagues (16) found no clear differences between *BRCA1*-associated patients and matched Swedish control patients. Verhoog and colleagues (12) also found the 5-year survival rates for *BRCA1* and sporadic patients to be equivalent. In the latter study, the data were analyzed twice, first using all 49 patients and then after exclusion of 13 probands (the woman who was first referred). After exclusion of the probands, the 5-year survival of 56% for *BRCA1* carriers was worse than that for the matched controls (71%). Robson and colleagues (18) found no differences in local and distant recurrence rates but did not measure mortality in their study.

It is difficult to estimate survival accurately for hereditary cancer patients by studying clinic records. There are several sources of selection bias in studies of this type, all of which favorably influence prognosis. This is so because these biases all result in the preferential inclusion of living women in the study cohort (selection bias or survivor bias). Several families studied for survival were those which had been ascertained initially for linkage studies. In general, linkage is informative for dominant traits such as hereditary breast cancer if there are four or more living patients with breast cancer in the family. Deceased women do not facilitate linkage studies, so families with multiple living patients will be preferentially included.

Most studies of survivorship have limited the study cohort to patients with *BRCA1*-proven breast cancer. In order to test for *BRCA1* mutation status, it is necessary to have a source of constitutional DNA. Mutation analysis is most readily done on DNA from peripheral blood. It is relatively simple to perform mutation analysis on a living patient. If the patient is deceased, it may be possible to obtain DNA from preserved tumor specimens. However, specimens may not be available in all cases. Even when a block is available, its use will be restricted to the search for a small number of known mutations. In practice, a mutation is first identified in a living affected woman, and then the same mutation is sought in the paraffin specimen. If there is no living affected women in a family, then mutation screening is not offered. For example, if a family had five members with early-onset breast cancer, all of whom were deceased, then mutation screening would not be offered. Families selected for study would then be selected for living patients.

Estimating Survival Using Archived Specimens

There are unbiased ways of estimating relative survival. The ideal study would be to follow a group of recently diagnosed incident cases of cancer prospectively and compare survivorship in mutation-positive and mutation-negative cases. An alternate method, requiring much less time, is to ascertain mutation status on an unselected sample of pathology breast specimens in a hospital tumor bank and to compare survival for women with and without mutations. Because of the frequency of recurrent *BRCA1* mutations in the Ashkenazi population, it is possible to classify Jewish women into carriers and noncarriers using tumor blocks. Foulkes and colleagues (24) analyzed survival in 187 Ashkenazi Jewish women with breast cancer ascertained at the Jewish General Hospital in Montreal, Quebec. *BRCA1*-positive cancers were more likely to be of high grade than *BRCA1*-negative cancers; 72% of the hereditary cancers were high grade versus 31% of the *BRCA1*-negative cases ($p < 0.01$). Death from breast cancer also was more common among the *BRCA1* carriers than among the controls. The 5-year breast-cancer-specific survival rate was inferior for *BRCA1* carriers than for noncarriers (70.8% versus 85.9%; $p = 0.01$). The difference was particularly striking for node-negative patients; only 58.3% of node-negative *BRCA1* carriers survived 5 years compared with 94.1% of the node-negative controls ($p = 0.0001$). Much of the difference could be attributed to the prevalence of *p53* mutations in the different groups. Among the node-negative patients, 9 of 13 *BRCA1*-positive patients were positive for *p53* versus 16 of 87 *BRCA1*-negative patients (odds ratio 9.98; $p = 0.004$). After adjustment for *p53*, *BRCA1* status was not found to be predictive of survival. Although it is often argued that *BRCA1*-associated cancers are not more aggressive than other cancers, after accounting for stage and grade, it is inappropriate to adjust for these prognostic factors if the results are to be used to help guide management decisions. A woman with a *BRCA1* mutation should be informed of the type of cancer that is most likely to develop, as well as the absolute risk of cancer, when she is counseled about different preventive options.

Screening

Women who are told that they are carriers of *BRCA1* mutations choose between prophylactic mastectomy and periodic mammographic screening. Mammographic screening is recommended routinely for high-risk women in most family cancer clinics but has not been proven to reduce mortality from breast cancer in young women (26). A recent meta-analysis of mammography trials in Sweden indicates a possible reduction of 10% to 15% associated with routine mammography in women aged 40 to 50 (27). Because the majority of *BRCA1*-associated tumors are of high grade, the risk reduction associated with mammographic screening may be less than this in the hereditary subgroup. However, the subgroup of women with a strong family history has not been studied. Because of the substantial risk of breast cancer in women aged 25 to 30 with *BRCA1* and *BRCA2* mutations, it is prudent to begin mammographic screening at age 25 and to continue annually. It is also possible that *BRCA1*-associated cancers may be more difficult to detect. In the study of Robson and colleagues (19), *BRCA1*-associated cancers were slightly larger than mutation-negative cancers (1.9 versus 1.6 cm). The difference was not significant. In two other studies there was no difference in size between *BRCA1*-positive and *BRCA1*-negative tumors (12,17).

Prevention

Tamoxifen has been shown to reduce the risk of contralateral breast cancer by 39% in women with a previous diagnosis of breast cancer (28). If the same risk reduction were obtainable for patients with hereditary breast cancer, it would be reasonable to assume that tamoxifen could prevent initial breast cancers as well. This question could be addressed either by studying the occurrence of second primary cancers in *BRCA1* carriers in relation to tamoxifen use or by identifying *BRCA1* and *BRCA2* mutation carriers among the participants of a tamoxifen prevention trial. *BRCA1*-associated breast cancers infrequently express ER. Data from the NSABP Breast Cancer Prevention Trial show no reduction in cancer incidence for ER-negative tumors. It may be that the *BRCA1* mutation reduces the requirement for estrogen to induce growth in malignant breast epithelial cells. Tamoxifen may not be effective in preventing ER-negative tumors, and it is therefore premature to consider tamoxifen therapy as a chemopreventive agent until such studies are completed.

In a recent meta-analysis it was found that current use of oral contraceptives was a significant risk factor for early-onset breast cancer (29). The magnitude of the relative risk was small, but it is not known if risk differs in the hereditary subgroup. The risk associated with oral contraceptive use appears to be limited to breast cancer in young women — of course, this is the typical age at which hereditary breast cancer presents. One small study reported an increased incidence of breast cancer in *BRCA1* carriers associated with oral contraceptive use (30). Currently, oral contraceptives are not discouraged in carriers of *BRCA1* or *BRCA2* mutations. It is of particular importance to establish the safety of oral contraceptive use in mutation carriers because of the finding that these pills reduce the incidence of ovarian cancer in both *BRCA1* and *BRCA2* carriers (30). In a second study, oral contraceptives were found to be protective against familial ovarian cancer in French-Canadians (32).

Early menopause, whether natural or surgically induced, offers some protection against breast cancer. It has not yet been determined to what extent oophorectomy diminishes the risk of hereditary breast cancer, if at all. Surgical menopause is also associated with increased risks of cardiovascular disease and osteoporosis (33). These risks may be diminished by estrogen replacement therapy, but the safety of postmenopausal estrogen replacement in women who are at high risk for cancer is a matter of debate. There is probably a modest increase in breast cancer risk for women taking prolonged hormone replacement (34), and many physicians are reluctant to offer estrogen to women who are known to carry *BRCA1* mutations. It is hoped that new drugs such as raloxifene will be useful in preventing both osteoporosis and breast cancer. Prospective studies of antiestrogens and hormone replacement therapy, alone or in combination, in *BRCA1* and *BRCA2* carriers will allow these critical clinical questions to be answered.

References

1. Ford D, Easton DF, Stratton M, et al. Genetic heterogeneity and penetrance analysis of the *BRCA2* genes in breast cancer families. Am J Hum Genet 1998;62:676–679.
2. Narod SA, Ford D, Devilee P, et al. An evaluation of genetic heterogeneity in 145 breast-ovarian cancer families. Am J Hum Genet 1995;56:254–256.
3. Serova OM, Mazoyer S, Puget N, et al. Mutations in *BRCA1* and *BRCA2* in breast cancer families: are there more breast cancer susceptibility genes? Am J Hum Genet 1997;60:486–495.
4. Tonin P, Weber B, Offit K, et al. Frequency of recurrent *BRCA1* and *BRCA2* mutations in Ashkenazi Jewish breast cancer families. Nature Med 1996;2:1179–1183.
5. Tonin PN, Mes-Masson A-M, Futreal A, et al. Founder *BRCA1* and *BRCA2* mutations in French-Canadian breast and ovarian cancer families. Am J Hum Genet 1998;63:1341–1351.
6. Lloyd KM, Dennis M. Cowden's disease: a possible new symptom complex with multiple system involvement. Ann Intern Med 1963;58:136–142.
7. Olschwang S, Serova-Sinilnikova O, Lenoir GM, Thomas G. *PTEN* germ-line mutations in juvenile polyposis coli. Nature Genet 1998;18:12–13.
8. Malkin D, Li FP, Strong LC, et al. Germ-line *p53* mutations in a familial syndrome of breast cancer, sarcomas and other neoplasms. Science 1990;250:1233–1238.
9. Robson M, Gilewsli T, Haas B, et al. *BRCA*-associated breast cancer in young women. J Clin Oncol 1998;16:1642–1649.
10. Sun CC, Lenoir GM, Lynch H, Narod SA. In situ breast cancer and *BRCA1*. Lancet 1996;348:408.
11. Jacquemier J, Eisinger F, Guinebretiere J-M, et al. Intraductal component and *BRCA1*-associated breast cancer. Lancet 1996;348:1098.
12. Verhoog LC, Brekelmans CTM, Synaeve C, et al. Survival and tumor characteristics of breast-cancer patients with germ-line mutations of *BRCA1*. Lancet 1998;351:316–321.
13. Marcus JN, Watson P, Page DL, et al. Hereditary breast cancer, pathobiology, prognoisis, *BRCA1* and *BRCA2* gene linkage. Cancer 1996;77:697–709.
14. Eisinger F, Stoppa-Lyonnet D, Longy M, et al. Germ-line mutation at *BRCA1* affects the histo-prognostic grade in hereditary breast cancer. Cancer Res 1996;56:471–474.
15. Lakhani SR, Easton DF, Stratton MR, et al. Pathology of familial breast cancer: differences between breast cancers in carriers of *BRCA1* or *BRCA2* mutations and sporadic cases. Lancet 1997;349:1505–1510.
16. Johannson OT, Idvall I, Anderson C, et al. Tumor biological features of *BRCA1*-induced breast and ovarian cancer. Eur J Cancer 1997;33:362–371.
17. Eisinger F, Jacquemeir J, Guinebretiere J-M, et al. *p53* involvement in *BRCA1*-associated breast cancer. Lancet 1997;350:1101.
18. Karp SE, Tonin PN, Begin LR, et al. Influence of *BRCA1* mutations on nuclear grade and estrogen receptor status in breast cancers in Ashkenazi Jewish women. Cancer 1997;80:435–441.
19. Robson M, Rajan P, Rosen PP, et al. *BRCA*-associated breast cancer: absence of a characteristic immunophenotype. Cancer Res 1998;58:1839–1842.
20. Eisinger F, Jacquemier J, Charpin C, et al. Mutations at *BRCA1*: the medullary breast carcinoma revisited. Cancer Res 1998;58:1588–1592.
21. Osin P, Crook T, Powles T, et al. Hormone status of in situ cancer in *BRCA1* and *BRCA2* mutation carriers. Lancet 1998;351:1487.
22. Crook T, Crossland S, Crompton M, et al. *p53* mutations in *BRCA1*-associated familial breast cancer. Lancet 1997;350:638–639.
23. Gretarsdottir S, Thorlacius S, Valgardsdottir R, et al. *BRCA2* and *p53* mutations in primary breast cancer in relation to genetic instability. Cancer Res 1998;58:859–862.
24. Porter DE, Cohen BB, Wallace MR, et al. Breast cancer incidence, penetrance and survival in probable carriers of *BRCA1* mutation in families linked to *BRCA1* on chromosome 17q12-21. Br J Surg 1994;81:1512–1515.
25. Foulkes WD, Wong N, Brunet JS, et al. Germline *BRCA1* mutation is an adverse prognostic factor in Ashkenazi Jewish women with breast cancer. Clin Cancer Res 1997;3:2465–2469.

26. Miller AB, Baines CJ, To T, Wall C. Canadian National Breast Screening Study: 1. Breast cancer detection and death rates among women aged 40–49 years. Can Med Assoc J 1992;147: 1459–1476.

27. Nystrom L, Wall S, Rutqvist L, et al. Update of the overview of the Swedish randomized trials on breast cancer screening with mammography. In: NIH consensus development conference. Washington: NIH Press, 1997.

28. Early Breast Cancer Trialists Collaborative Group. Systematic treatment of early breast cancer by hormonal, cytotoxic or immune therapy. Lancet 1992;339:1–5,71–78.

29. Collaborative Group on Hormonal Factors in Breast Cancer. Breast cancer and hormonal contraceptives: collaborative reanalysis of individual data on 53,297 women with breast cancer and 111,239 women without breast cancer from 54 epidemiological studies. Lancet 1996;347:1713–1727.

30. Ursin G, Henderson BE, Haile RW, et al. Does oral contraceptive use increase the risk of breast cancer in women with *BRCA1/BRCA2* mutations more than in other women? Cancer Res 1997;57:3678–3681.

31. Narod SA, Risch H, Moslehi R, et al. Oral contraceptives and the risk of hereditary ovarian cancer. New Engl J Med 1998;339:424–428.

32. Godard B, Foulkes WD, Provencher D, et al. Risk factors for familial and sporadic ovarian cancer among French-Canadians: a case-control study. Am J. Obstet Gynecol 1998;179:403–410.

33. Stampfer MJ, Colditz GA, Willet WC, et al. Postmenopausal estrogen therapy and cardiovascular disease: ten-year follow-up from the Nurses Health Study. New Engl J Med 1989; 321:293–297.

34. Steinberg K, Thacker S, Smith S, et al. A meta-analysis of the effect of estrogen replacement therapy on the risk of breast cancer. JAMA 1991;265:1985–1990.

4

Quantitative Breast Cancer Risk Assessment

Suzanne O'Neill

What Is Quantitative Risk, and Why Calculate It?

Risk is usually defined as the probability that a harmful event will occur. *Risk assessment* is the process of identifying the factors that contribute to that probability. Simply identifying these factors allows us to predict risk in a *qualitative* way, whereas measuring the precise contribution of each piece and any interactions between them allows us to assess risk in a *quantitative* way. This is a central focus of modern epidemiology. The progress made in the last few decades in identifying the epidemiologic parameters of breast cancer has led to an ability to quantify breast cancer risk in some individuals with ever-increasing precision. In contrast to some other cancers, such as lung cancer, breast cancer epidemiology has experienced greater advances in quantifying genetic risk factors than environmental risk factors. Identification of genetic predisposition through mutation carrier testing may be considered the most sophisticated quantitative risk-assessment tool to date. There is much we do not know, and to say that we can assess risk with the precision achieved in the diagnostic arena would be untrue. However, the field of quantitative risk assessment has been developed to the extent that its application is ready to move from theoretical research into clinical practice.

Quantitative breast cancer risk assessment is important on several levels. First, on an individual level, many women want a more precise estimate of their personal breast cancer risk than the generic 1 in 9. Many women either know or suspect that features of their personal history may have an impact on their risk. A tailored assessment may help to guide decisions about medical interventions, lifestyle modifications, and future plans. For many, accurate information leads to a sense of control over otherwise random events. Similarly, an accurate assessment of individual risk informs the physician or clinical provider. It provides a starting point for determining what medical interventions may be needed, what preventive strategies may be undertaken, and on the most basic level, what one should be looking for in a patient and her family members. On the population level, quantification of risk permits research to be done in the most effective manner. Investigations can be targeted to populations likely to derive the most benefit. Finally, identification of at-risk populations drives the formation of public health policy and facilitates the most efficient and effective distribution of health care resources.

This chapter is organized according to the hierarchy of epidemiologic investigation. The most basic quantification of risk is the population incidence data. The often-quoted 1 in 9 (when lifetime is considered up to age 85) or 1 in 8 (with lifetime considered beyond 95 years) breast cancer risk figures are derived from incidence tables formulated through the national SEER (Surveillance, Epidemiology, and End Results) Registry. Basic incidence tables allowed the identification of increasing age as the most significant predictor of risk, with most cases of breast cancer occurring after the age of 50 years. Some of the tools and statistical methods of breast cancer epidemiology are reviewed in order to foster critical appraisal of the models presented in later sections.

Breast cancer risk identification based on four large population-based studies is reviewed. Two quantitative models derived from these studies, the Gail (1) and the Claus (2) models, are discussed and their application demonstrated. Population studies revealed that the second largest risk factor for breast cancer was family history. Thus the field of breast cancer genetic epidemiology was born, and the rapid and extensive progress in this discipline highlighted by the discovery of breast cancer–predisposing genes led to the development of four new models to predict mutation carrier status (and by extension, breast cancer risk in this subpopulation) (3–6). The theoretical basis of these models, along with methods of application, are discussed.

Finally, although not the focus of this chapter, some of the psychosocial dynamics of breast cancer risk assessment, including who should perform and communicate risk to patients, are mentioned. Breast cancer risk assessment is perhaps a prototype for the future of patient profiling in the age of genomic medicine. The methodologies developed in this area may set precedents for quantitative risk assessment for many other common multifactorial disorders.

Epidemiologic Risk

Quantification of the risk of developing disease is a central feature of epidemiology. Incidence rates and exposures or risk factors are systematically tallied in an effort to assign causality and effect prevention at the population level. Breast cancer is a common disease, the most common cancer found among women and the second major cause of cancer death. It is estimated that 176,300 new cases of breast cancer will be diagnosed in 1999 and that about 1300 new cases of breast cancer will be diagnosed in men (7). Therefore, the preliminary search for causality or risk factors for breast cancer must be population-based. Once risk factors are elucidated, subpopulations of individuals with unique risks can be defined

and stratified and individual risk more precisely quantified. One of the basic premises of statistical epidemiology is the fact that statistically derived risk probabilities only apply for the population that provided the original data. We often consider statistics based on large population studies to be widely applicable, but we must understand the study population characteristics in order to be aware of the limitations. On a large scale, a comparison of cancer incidence figures from different countries illustrates this principle (8) (Table 4-1). In the context of breast cancer risk assessment, particularly for the high-familial-risk subpopulations, knowledge of the features of the underlying study population is crucial.

The Tools of Epidemiology

Traditionally, epidemiologic investigation is sparked by case reports, spurred on by collection of case series, and formalized in cross-sectional and prospective population studies. The two major types of population studies, the cohort study and the case-control study, have provided the framework for the development of statistical methods of inferring risk.

Cohort Studies and the Relative Risk

The relative risk (or risk ratio) is derived from cohort studies of populations matched as closely as possible for all factors except a particular exposure. These types of studies are generally prospective; that is, subjects are followed over a period of years, and incidence of the disease of interest is monitored in both exposed and unexposed groups. Retrospective cohort studies are possible if the exposure can be precisely and definitively measured.

Relative risk is a measure of the strength of the association between an exposure and a disease, with a relative risk of 3 or greater generally indicating a strong association. It is calculated as

Relative risk (RR)
$$= \frac{\text{incidence of disease in exposed group}}{\text{incidence of disease in unexposed group}}$$

This mathematical formula is often represented by use of a 2 × 2 table where

Table 4-1. Cumulative breast cancer risk for female gene carriers, nongene carriers, and total population for the United States, Germany, and Japan by age groups[a]

Age (yrs)	Gene Carriers[b]	United States			Germany		Japan	
		Nongene Carriers[b]	Total[c]	Total[d] (SEER Data Registries, Whites)	Nongene carriers[c]	Total[d] (Sarland Cancer Registry)	Nongene Carriers[c]	Total[d] (Osaka Cancer Registry)
29	0.0167	0.0002	0.0003	0.0004	0.0003	0.0004	0.0002	0.00025
39	0.1444	0.0027	0.0036	0.0051	0.0039	0.0044	0.0018	0.0023
49	0.3758	0.0138	0.0162	0.0205	0.0150	0.0162	0.0066	0.0078
59	0.5477	0.0275	0.0309	0.0443	0.0300	0.0317	0.0121	0.0139
69	0.6743	0.0497	0.0538	0.0785	0.0501	0.0522	0.0181	0.0203
79	0.9452	0.0798	0.0855	0.1173	0.0710	0.0739	0.0228	0.0258

[a]Calculations are based on a gene frequency of 0.0033.
[b]From Easton et al. (1993).
[c]Calculated from Eq. (1).
[d]From Parkin et al. (1992).
Source: Adapted from Becher H, Chang Claude J. Estimating disease risks given family history. Genet Epidemiol 1996;13:229–242. By permission of Wiley-Liss, Inc., a subsidiary of John Wiley & Sons, Inc.

a = number of exposed subjects with disease
b = number of exposed subjects without disease
c = number of unexposed subjects with disease
d = number of unexposed subjects without disease
$a/a + b$ = incidence rate in exposed group
$c/c + d$ = incidence rate in unexposed group

and

$$\text{Relative risk (RR)} = \frac{a/(a+b)}{c/(c+d)}$$

While cohort studies are the most direct and unbiased, they involve a considerable amount of time and are expensive to conduct. Relatively large numbers of subjects are usually required, and a cohort study may not be feasible if the disease of interest is rare. Breast cancer risk data have been provided by four large cohort studies in the United States over the past 30 years, the Breast Cancer Detection and Demonstration Project (BCDDP), the Cancer and Steroid Hormone (CASH) Study, the Nurses Health Study (NHS), and the Breast Cancer Prevention Trial (BCPT).

Case-Control Studies and the Odds Ratio

The most common epidemiologic studies are case-control studies. These studies begin with a group that has the disease or outcome of interest (cases) and a matched control group with no disease (controls). Exposure levels are then ascertained in each group and the odds ratio derived. Case-control studies are retrospective, since they begin with a population that already has the disease. Therefore, they are relatively inexpensive, less time-consuming, and more suitable for rare diseases than cohort studies. However, they are often subject to ascertainment or selection biases and biases in exposure recall and measurement.

It is important to recognize that the odds ratio is only an approximation of the relative risk and is derived indirectly. The odds ratio estimate also relies on two assumptions: 1) that the frequency of the disease in the population is small and 2) that the study cases and controls are representative of the cases and non-cases in the population. However, it should be noted that the odds ratio does not depend on the prevalence of the exposure in the population.

$$\text{Odds ratio (OR)} = \frac{\text{exposure ratio in cases}}{\text{exposure ratio in controls}}$$

$$\text{OR} = \frac{(a/c)}{(b/d)} = \frac{ad}{bc}$$

Relative Risk versus Odds Ratio

The terms *relative risk* and *odds ratio* are often used interchangeably in the medical literature, although their derivations and meanings are different. Relative risk is the "gold standard" of exposure/disease association. A relative risk denotes the probability that a given exposure will result in disease relative to the unexposed condition. For example, a woman who has had two biopsies before age 50 has a relative risk of developing breast cancer of approximately 3. Thus she is three times more likely to develop breast cancer than a woman who has had no biopsies before age 50.

The odds ratio is an indirect approximation of the relative risk. It denotes the probability that a person with a disease was exposed to the risk factor in question. Using the preceding example, an odds ratio of 3 would indicate that women with breast cancer were three times more likely to have had two or more biopsies before age 50 than women without breast cancer. The odds ratio approximates the relative risk only when the incidence of the outcome in the study population is low (<10%). The more frequent the outcome, the more the odds ratio will either overestimate or underestimate the relative risk. Several correction methods are used to adjust the odds ratio so that it more closely approximates the relative risk (9).

Relative Risk versus Absolute Risk

While relative risk is the statistic of choice in epidemiologic terms, *absolute risk* is far more useful in a clinical setting. The magnitude of a relative risk is expressed in relation to the control group used in the study, which may or may not reflect the population at large or the population used for other studies. Conversion of a relative risk to an absolute risk provides a defined risk over a specific time interval, such as a 5% chance of developing breast cancer over the next 10 years. This allows a patient to conceptualize the risk more concretely and to compare the risk with the likelihood of other adverse outcomes.

It is important to note that one cannot simply multiply the relative risk due to a specific exposure by the population incidence rate. While this is sometimes possible if disease incidence is very small, this is not the case for breast cancer (10). Breast cancer incidence rates change with age and mortality from other causes. Thus it is necessary to incorporate age-dependent corrections in estimating absolute cumulative risks for breast cancer. These corrections are

described in the section on the Gail model below. Similarly, one cannot add or multiply relative risks obtained in different studies because the reference (control) group is not the same.

Logistic Regression

Logistic regression is a method for calculating the odds ratio while simultaneously adjusting for a number of variables. For each variable, a *weight* (known as the *covariate coefficient*) is calculated corresponding to its influence on the outcome. In the context of the models discussed in this chapter, outcome may be either probability of developing breast cancer or probability of carrying a *BRCA* mutation. The form of the logistic equation is

$$\log[p/(1-p)] = \alpha + \beta_1 \text{ factor}_1 + \beta_2 \text{ factor}_2 + \beta_3 \text{ factor}_3 + \cdots + \beta_x \text{ factor}_x$$

where $\log[p/(1-p)]$ = logarithm of the odds
p = probability of the outcome
α = y intercept
β_x = the coefficients or weights
factor = risk factor or covariate

In practice, each variable is tested for significance separately and then retested for significance in the overall model equation, either by sequential addition (stepwise forward regression) or sequential omission (stepwise backward regression).

Logistic regression is exquisitely sensitive to a given data set, which in the case of the following studies is the relevant study population. Thus known risk factors such as bilaterality, age at menarche, or Ashkenazi Jewish descent may be statistically relevant in one study population and not in another.

Bayesian Analysis

Bayesian analysis is a tool often used by geneticists to modify the Mendelian risks associated with disease transmission. It is particularly well suited to reducing risk estimates when an individual has not yet exhibited some of the traits expected if she or he had indeed inherited a familial genetic disease. Bayesian analysis is often used in breast cancer risk assessment to modify the probability that a mutation was inherited by an individual who has reached an advanced age without developing disease. It also can be used to modify risk given new information such as genetic testing results.

Bayes' rule states that

$$p(A|B) = \frac{p(A \text{ and } B)}{p(B)}$$

where

$p(A|B)$ = probability of A given that B has occurred (conditional probability)
$p(A \text{ and } B)$ = probability of A and B occurring together (joint probability)
$p(A)$ = probability of A occurring
$p(B)$ = probability of B occurring

Deriving the probability rules for two mutually exclusive events, such as carrying a mutation or not carrying a mutation, the equation becomes

$$p(A|B) = \frac{[p(B|A)p(A)]}{[p(B|A)p(A) + p(B|\text{not}A)p(\text{not}A)]}$$

As an example, in a family in which a *BRCA1* mutation is assumed or has been identified, a theoretical estimation can be made of the probability that a woman in the direct line of descent carries that mutation given the fact that she has lived to

an advanced age without developing disease. If direct testing is not possible, this could provide at least a rough estimation that she carries the mutation (and can pass it on to her children).

Consider a family in which a 60-year-old unaffected woman has a sister with an identified *BRCA1* mutation. Her prior probability of having the same mutation as her sister is 50% or 0.5 [$p(C)$]. Her prior probability of not being a mutation carrier is also 50% [$p(NC)$]. Her conditional probability of being unaffected at age 60 if she is a mutation carrier [$p(U|C)$] can be estimated from *BRCA1* carrier penetrance data. Her conditional probability of being unaffected at age 60 if she is a not a mutation carrier [$p(U|NC)$] depends on the age-specific cumulative incidence rate. The posterior probability that this woman is a mutation carrier, given the fact that she is unaffected at age 60, is then

$$p(C|U) = \frac{p(U|C)p(C)}{p(U|C)p(C) + p(U|NC)p(NC)}$$
$$p(C|U) = \frac{(1 - 0.77)(0.5)}{(1 - 0.77)(0.5) + (1 - 0.04)(0.05)} = 23\%$$

Note that the actual data values used in this calculation are uncertain. There are varying estimates of the penetrance values for *BRCA* mutations. For the purposes of illustration, *BRCA1* penetrance and the cumulative incidence for noncarriers were derived from Table 4-2

Table 4-2. Cumulative risk of breast cancer for the general population, *BRCA1* heterozygotes in families with multiple cases of breast and ovarian cancer, and individuals in the Ashkenazi Jewish population analyzed for specific *BRCA* mutations

Age	General Population	*BRCA1* Heterozygotes in High-Risk Families	*BRCA2* Heterozygotes in Selected Families	*BRCA* Heterozygotes in General Population (Ashkenazi Jews)
40	0.005	0.16	0.14	0.14
45	0.01	0.42		0.30
50	0.02	0.59	0.32	0.33
55	0.03	0.72		0.46
60	0.04	0.77	0.53	0.53
65	0.06	0.80		0.56
70	0.07	0.82	0.67	0.58
75	0.09	0.84		0.63
80	0.10	0.86	0.77	0.61

Sources: Data from Easton et al., 1993; Ries et al., 1990; cited in King et al., 1993; Fig. 1B in Streuwing et al., 1997; Shubert et al., 1997. Adapted from Offit K. Clinical Cancer Genetics: Risk Counseling and Management. New York: Wiley-Liss, 1998:77. By permission of Wiley-Liss, Inc., a subsidiary of John Wiley & Sons, Inc.

(11). The BRCAPRO mutation carrier risk model is based on a sophisticated recursion of this type of Bayesian adjustment.

Offit (11) provides an illustration of the use of Bayesian analysis to determine the chance that an unaffected woman who has had genetic testing and received a negative result could in fact be a mutation carrier (Table 4-3). In his example, an Ashkenazi Jewish woman has tested negative for the three common founder mutations but wants to know her chances of being a carrier of another mutation. Again, this analysis depends on the prevalence of other mutations in this population, and the evidence is still tentative. He uses data from a study by Tonin and colleagues (12) (Table 4-4) that

estimate that approximately 90% of Ashkenazi Jewish families with two or more cases of both breast and ovarian cancer harbor one of the three founder mutations. While this woman's risk of carrying a mutation is reduced from 50% to 9%, full mutation sequencing may be able to clarify her risk more precisely.

It is important to recognize that Bayesian analysis depends not only on accurate estimates of the probability of particular "conditioning events" such as receiving a negative test result but also on the general framework of the original question that establishes the prior probability. Thus, in the preceding example, the analysis might be different if the woman had been affected (her "real" prior probability of being a gene carrier may be higher) or if an affected family member had been tested and found to carry a founder mutation (the conditional probabilities would then be based on the sensitivity and specificity of the mutation assay).

Table 4-3. Bayesian analysis of mutation carrier probability for an unaffected Ashkenazi Jewish woman who has tested negative for three common founder mutations but has an extensive family history of breast and ovarian cancer

	Being a Gene Carrier	Not Being a Gene Carrier
Prior probability	0.5	0.5
Conditional probability	0.10	1.0
Joint probability	0.05	0.5
Posterior probability	0.09	0.91

Source: Adapted from Offit K. Clinical Cancer Genetics: Risk Counseling and Management. New York: Wiley-Liss, 1998:238. By permission of Wiley-Liss, Inc., a subsidiary of John Wiley & Sons, Inc.

Modeling Breast Cancer Risk in the General Population

Population Studies

There have been four major prospective population studies that have tracked the incidence of breast cancer along with data on possible risk factors such as family history, reproductive factors, and medical, lifestyle, and environmental

Table 4-4. Frequency of *BRCA1* and *BRCA2* mutations in Jewish breast cancer families

	Mutation (%)			
	Total Families	185delAG	5382insC	6174delT	Any (%)
---	---	---	---	---	---
Site-specific breast cancer (no ovarian cancer)					
2 breast cancers	48	10	2	0	12 (25.0%)
3 breast cancers	43	7	3	1	11 (25.6%)
4+ breast cancers	47	11	2	4	17 (36.1%)
Total	138	28	7	5	40 (29.0%)
Breast/ovarian cancer syndrome					
2+ breast, 1 ovarian	54	22	9	4	35 (64.8%)
2+ breast, 2+ ovarian	28	21	4	0	25 (89.3%)
Total	82	43	13	4	60 (73.2%)

Source: Adapted from Tonin P, Weber B, Offit K, et al. Frequency of recurrent *BRCA1* and *BRCA2* mutations in Ashkenazi Jewish breast cancer families. Nature Med 1996;2(11):1179–1183.

Table 4-5. Features of the four major population studies investigating risk factors for breast cancer

Feature	BCDDP	CASH Study	NHS	BCPT
Study design	Nested case-control study from a multicenter screening program of 284,780 women	Nested population-based case-control study in 8 SEER regions (validation based on 83% of women for whom risk factor data were available)	Self-administered questionnaire follow-up study of 115,172 nurses	Multicenter, randomized, controled clinical trial of women at increased risk for breast cancer (validation based on 5969 women without a history of lobular carcinoma in situ in the placebo group)
No. of incident breast cancer cases[a]	2852	4715	2396	204
Race	White	White	Mainly white	White
Age, yrs[b]	31–81	20–54	29–61	35–79
Calendar period of follow-up[c]	1973–1980	1980–1982	1976–1988	1992–1998
Frequency of mammography	Annual	Rare	Rare before 1983	Annual
Risk model	Original Gail	Claus		NCI Gail

[a]Includes all in situ and invasive cancers. For the validation of model 2 by use of BCPT data, 49 in situ cases were excluded.
[b]Age at diagnosis for BCDDP and CASH. Age at baseline for NHS and BCPT.
[c]Period for the CASH case-control study was the period that the cases were diagnosed.
Source: Adapted from Costantino JP, Gail MH, Pee D, et al. Validation studies for models projecting the risk of invasive and total breast cancer incidence. J Natl Cancer Inst 1999;91(18):1541–1548. By permission of the National Cancer Institute.

exposure histories. Although much data have emerged, the only risk factors (other than age) with effects large enough to be incorporated in predictive models have been family history, ages at menarche and first childbirth, and breast biopsy history. Table 4-5 summarizes features of the four studies.

BCDDP

The Breast Cancer Detection Demonstration Project (BCDDP) was undertaken between 1973 and 1975. Two hundred and eighty thousand primarily Caucasian women recruited as volunteers in 28 national centers were offered screening mammography on an annual basis, and the incidence of breast cancer (both in situ and invasive) during this time period was tabulated (13). A nested case-control study was done to develop a relative-risk model using compilations of risk factors of 2852 Caucasian women who developed breast cancer and 3146 controls (1). It should be noted

that this population was almost entirely Caucasian, and by definition, all were undergoing screening mammography. Risk factors that had been confirmed in other studies were sufficiently represented in this cohort; these showed strong association with breast cancer and were included in a model that came to be known as the *Gail model*.

For the study population, these risk factors were age at menarche, age at first live birth, number of previous breast biopsies, number of first-degree relatives with breast cancer, and age of the individual. Individuals diagnosed with benign breast disease at biopsy during the original BCDDP study were followed through 1986, and an association was seen between the finding of atypical hyperplasia and subsequent development of breast cancer (14). Therefore, an additional risk factor—atypical hyperplasia demonstrated on biopsy—was later incorporated into Gail's original model.

CASH

The Cancer and Steroid Hormone (CASH) Study was a population-based, case-control study conducted by the Centers for Disease Control (15,16). This multicenter study enrolled 4730 patients, aged 20 to 54 years, with histologically confirmed in situ or invasive breast cancer years during the years 1980–1982. There were 493 cases of epithelial ovarian cancer. Controls (4688) were matched on geographic location and age within 5-year increments. Patients and controls were interviewed to obtain family history of breast cancer in first- and second-degree relatives. Only information on first-degree relatives (mothers and sisters) was used to derive the Claus model, since cancer incidence in second-degree relatives was underreported relative to the SEER data gathered in the mid-1970s (17). Nonwhites were excluded because of small numbers, and daughters also were excluded for the same reason (presumably, many were not old enough to develop breast cancer). Family history of male breast cancer was not obtained, although menstrual and pregnancy history, oral contraceptive use, and a wide variety of exposure covariates were enumerated.

Using segregation analysis, Claus and colleagues (16) found that the breast cancer incidence and transmission in this population best fit a major locus model, with autosomal dominant inheritance of a rare allele coexisting with a high frequency of non-familial cases. Previous epidemiologic studies had indicated a two- to threefold increase in breast cancer risk in women whose mothers or sisters had breast cancer. It also had been shown that early-onset breast cancer is strongly associated with a positive family history of breast cancer. Claus's model confirmed these findings.

NHS

The Nurses Health Study, based in Boston, is a prospective cohort study following 117,988 women aged 30 to 55 years at enrollment in 1976. Biennial data collection has permitted examination of various risk factors such as family history and dietary and lifestyle patterns (18). While no quantitative models have been postulated based on these data, the Gail model was validated using this data set (19). It should be noted that the incidence of breast cancer in

members of this cohort who had two or more affected first-degree relatives was lower than in other studies (20).

BCPT

The Breast Cancer Prevention Trial was a prospective, randomized, controlled clinical trial designed to assess the efficacy of tamoxifen as a preventive for invasive breast cancer in women at increased risk (21). To be eligible for the BCPT, a woman had to be 60 years old or between 35 and 59 years old with a projected 5-year risk of invasive breast cancer of at least 1.66% (the risk of a 60-year-old). A modified Gail risk model was produced for use in the trial (called *NCI Gail* in this chapter), and the women in the placebo arm of the trial provided a population in which to validate both this new model and the original Gail model. The placebo study population consisted of 5969 white women between the ages of 35 and 79 who were followed for an average of 48.4 months.

Gail Model

Study Population

The original Gail model of breast cancer risk assessment is based on data gathered during the BCDDP study. The modified NCI Gail model is discussed separately.

Risk Factors

Five risk parameters were identified, and relative-risk coefficients were calculated for each using logistic regression. Table 4-6 lists these risk factors and their associated relative risks. A composite relative risk is obtained by multiplication of the number associated with each relative-risk factor. The risk factors included in the model may be said to represent three distinct domains: hormonal or reproductive history (age at menarche, age at first live birth), medical history (number of breast biopsies, atypical hyperplasia as a pathologic finding), and family history (number of affected first-degree relatives). A woman's age is incorporated both as an adjustment for relative risk due to biopsy and in the overall calculation of age-specific absolute interval risks. *Absolute risk*, defined as the probability of developing breast cancer over a specified time interval, is computed using a

Table 4-6. NCI Gail risk model: Risk factor coefficients and absolute risk tables

Risk Factor Category	Relative Risk Factor	Baseline 5-Year Risk, %		
		Age, yrs	Black	Not Black
A. Age at menarche, yrs				
≥14	1.00	20–24	0.014	0.012
12–13	1.10	25–29	0.050	0.049
<12	1.21	30–34	0.120	0.134
B. No. of breast biopsies		35–39	0.224	0.278
Age at counseling, <50 years old		40–44	0.310	0.450
0	1.00	45–49	0.355	0.584
1	1.70	50–54	0.416	0.703
2	2.88	55–59	0.511	0.859
Age at counseling, ≥50 years old		60–64	0.562	1.018
0	1.00	65–69	0.586	1.116
1	1.27	70–74	0.646	1.157
≥2	1.62	75–79	0.713	1.140
		80–84	0.659	1.006

C. Age at first live birth, yrs	No. of first-degree relatives with breast cancer	
<20	0	1.00
	1	2.61
	≥2	6.80
20–24	0	1.24
	1	2.68
	≥2	5.78
25–29 or nulliparous	0	1.55
	1	2.76
	≥2	4.91
≥30	0	1.93
	1	2.83
	≥2	4.17
D. Atypical hyperplasia (AT)		
No biopsies		1.00
At least one biopsy and no AT found in any biopsy specimen		0.93
No AT found and hyperplasia status unknown for at least one biopsy specimen		1.00
AT found in at least one biopsy specimen		1.82

Note: To compute overall relative risk, multiply four component relative risks from categories A, B, C, and D. For example, a 42-year-old white nulliparous woman who began menstruating at age 12 years, who has no affected first-degree relatives, and who has had one previous breast biopsy with specimens interpreted as benign and no evidence of atypical hyperplasia has an overall relative risk of $1.10 \times 1.70 \times 1.55 \times 0.93 = 2.70$. From the data on 5-year baseline risk, her projected 5-year risk of invasive breast cancer is $2.70 \times 0.450 = 1.2\%$.

Source: Adapted from Gail MH, Costantino JP, Bryant J, et al. Weighing the risks and benefits of tamoxifen treatment for preventing breast cancer. J Natl Cancer Inst 1999;91(21):1829–1846. By permission of the National Cancer Institute.

baseline proportional hazards estimation derived from the BCDDP population.

Risk Calculation

The Gail model is used to calculate absolute interval risks for both invasive and in situ breast cancer. Clinical calculation of the Gail absolute risks has undergone technical evolution. Originally, a method of linear interpolation using manual multiplication and lookup tables was necessary (1); then a graphic method that was far more practical in the clinical setting was developed (22). Simplest of all is a DOS-based computer program called *RISK* (designed by Benichou) that calculates the absolute risk for any time interval (from age 20 to age 80) as a point estimate with associated confidence intervals (23). This program is distributed by the author (Benichou) to any interested parties.

Strengths and Limitations

The Gail model is perhaps the most widely known and used quantitative risk-assessment tool and is the only one to be statistically validated in several large study populations. As stated earlier, it encompasses several risk domains, and its use may be justified in assessing a preliminary risk in the general population. It is extremely important, however, to understand its limitations in women who have a positive family history of breast cancer. It considers only first-degree female relatives (mothers and sisters) and thus cannot include any paternal history. It does not consider age of breast cancer diagnosis in female relatives and thus cannot distinguish between possible hereditary and sporadic occurrences of breast cancer. In addition, the model was based on white women in active screening regimens (annual mammography) and is less accurate in assessing risk in other groups.

Validation Studies

A valid model should be able to predict the number of incident cases over a defined interval based on the enumerated risk factors of the study population. There are two components involved in the production of a final Gail risk value — the relative-risk component (which depends on the risk factors being considered) and the absolute-risk component (which depends on the baseline incidence of disease in the whole study population). Validation studies have looked at the performance of both components, with most discrepancies found to be due to the underlying population differences. With certain restrictions, the Gail model has been validated in studies undertaken by Bondy and colleagues (24), Spiegelman and colleagues (19), and Costantino and colleagues (25).

The study of Bondy and colleagues (24) followed 1981 women with a family history of breast cancer identified through the American Cancer

Society 1987 Texas Breast Screening Project. Thirty-nine cases of breast cancer occurred in this cohort during the 5 years of the study. In general, the expected number of cases predicted by the model was in agreement with the observed number of cases, although none of the risk factors alone proved statistically significant in this population. The model did overpredict risk in younger women and underpredict risk in older women. While the relative-risk portion of the model "performed reasonably well," incidence rates compiled from the SEER databases from both 1979 and 1983–1987 provided better estimates than the BCDDP rates for absolute risk.

The study by Spiegelman and colleagues (19) was designed to test the applicability of the Gail model to a large population independent of the model. The Nurses Health Study data used in the Spiegelman study were obtained from 115,172 women followed over a 12-year period (18). A comparison of observed breast cancer cases (2396) with expected cases derived from the Gail model (3196) again indicated overprediction of risk, particularly in younger women. While overprediction was estimated to be about 30% in most risk categories, twofold increases were seen among premenopausal women, women with two or more first-degree relatives with breast cancer, and women whose age at first birth was below 20 years. As in the other validation studies, this overprediction could not be explained totally by nonadherence to yearly mammography, although overall the model worked best for Gail's suggested population. While acknowledging limitations of the model for special cases, such as evidence for genetic linkage through molecular studies or recent immigration from a geographically "low risk" area, Gail maintains that the model is sound when used in a population that undergoes annual screening. This, of course, would not include young women who do not have regular mammography screenings (26). In addition, the incidence of breast cancer in the members of the NHS cohort who had two or more affected first-degree relatives was lower than in other studies (20).

The third formal validation of the Gail model was done using data from the placebo arm of the Breast Cancer Prevention Trial (21). It was possible to investigate the validity of both the original Gail model and the revised NCI Gail model in this population. The overall expected-to-observed (E/O) ratio using the original Gail model was 0.84 (CI = 0.73–0.97), although there was greater underestimation of risk for women over 60 years old. It also underestimated risk for women in the lowest quintile of risk. The modified NCI Gail model had a similar profile. The overall E/O ratio was 1.03 (CI = 0.88–1.21), although there was no underprediction in the over-60 age group. However, the modified model underpredicts risk by 30% for those in the lowest quintile of projected risk (expected-to-observed ratio = 0.70; 95% CI = 0.47–1.11) and overpredicts risk by 21% for those in the highest quintile (expected-to-observed ratio = 1.21; 95% CI = 0.92–1.64). Although the NCI Gail model is able to calculate risk for African-American women, no independent validation was possible because only 1.7% of the BCPT participants were African-American.

NCI Gail Model

While the modified model uses the same relative-risk factors as the original, the composite age-specific incidence rates used to determine the absolute risks were changed in three ways. The new rates are based on invasive breast cancer incidence only (the original model included in situ cancers), the age-specific rates are derived from the SEER Registry national incidence rates instead of the composite rates from the BCDDP, and age-specific composite SEER rates for African-American women were added.

Risk Calculation

Five-year risk of invasive breast cancer can be approximated manually by use of Table 4-6. Relative-risk factors are multiplied as in the original model, and absolute 5-year risk can be obtained by multiplying the relative risk by the value in the "Baseline 5-Year Risk" column (on the right) corresponding to present age and race. Recently, the National Cancer Institute released a Windows-based Breast Cancer Risk Assessment Tool based on the NCI Gail model (27). It calculates 5-year risks and a lifetime risk (calculated up to age 90) after entry of risk factor data and provides information about risk factors. It is available through the NCI's Cancer

Information Service (telephone: 800-4-Cancer, or Web site: *http://cancerTrials.nci.nih.gov*). A hand-held risk calculator that provides 5-year and lifetime risks is also available from Zeneca Pharmaceuticals. Computer-generated risks are slightly more accurate than those which are calculated manually because they include factors for competing mortality. Risk for development of in situ breast cancer may be approximated by multiplying the projected 5-year risk by 0.53 for women 49 years of age or younger and by 0.31 for women 50 years of age or older.

Strengths and Limitations

The strengths and limitations of the NCI Gail model are similar to those of the original model. The Costantino validation also revealed a possible cohort effect in that number of biopsies is not as predictive of risk in younger women as it was in the original BCDDP population. This may reflect the increasing number of biopsies performed in younger women since the advent of needle-biopsy procedures and increased mammographic screening. This model is the first to include risk estimations specifically applicable to black women. Although the computerized model seems to indicate that there is a separate calculation for Asian women, in actuality, the same rate tables are used as for white women. It is likely that the rates of invasive breast cancer predicted for white women overestimate the correct rates for Hispanic women, since the age-adjusted ratio comparing breast cancer rates of Hispanic women with those of non-Hispanic white women in the United States is 0.60. There are few data on the prevalence of breast cancer risk factors among Hispanic women; therefore, the model could not be modified to include this group.

While not precisely a limitation, one feature of the NCI Gail model that deserves attention is its ubiquitous availability in the form of marketed computer programs. The national distribution of both the NCI Gail computer program and the hand-held risk calculators may mislead both practitioners and the public into a sense of false security regarding breast cancer risk assessment. It is important to note that almost 55% of breast cancer develops in the absence of any known risk factors (28) and that the model is not appropriate for many women with a family history of breast cancer. On the other hand, the widespread availability of the tool may foster the practice of routine risk assessment and evaluation in a variety of clinical settings, increasing referral to both comprehensive risk-assessment specialists and entry into clinical trials. Because the NCI Gail model risk was used as a criterion for choosing the study population, it may be the best tool to use for establishing risk levels in potential candidates for tamoxifen therapy. The NCI recently published a preliminary set of decision-making tools to assist women and their physicians in exploring the risk-benefit ratio of tamoxifen use (29). Since the side effects of tamoxifen therapy are potentially serious, including an increased risk of endometrial cancer, pulmonary embolism, and deep vein thrombosis, it is imperative that accurate models for decision making be developed.

Claus Model

Study Population
The Claus model is based on data from the CASH study.

Risk Factors
Risk factors include history of breast cancer in female first- and second-degree relatives and age of onset. Paternal lineage can be included, since breast cancer history in paternal aunts and grandmothers is incorporated. Tables provide predicted cumulative probabilities (up to age 79) for occurrence of breast cancer when various combinations of first- and second-degree relatives are affected.

Risk Calculation
The patient must provide a family history of breast cancer diagnoses (including age of onset) in her mother, sisters, grandmothers, and paternal and maternal aunts, although the model can only provide risks based on a maximum of two relatives. Seven look-up tables are available for various combination pairs of relatives. These tables provide the cumulative risks for discrete patient age levels. Risks are higher for first-degree history than for second-degree history and for two relatives in a direct line of descent rather than on opposite sides of the family. Absolute risk is calculated over defined time intervals such as the next 10 or 20 years by applying the following formula to any two cumulative risk probabilities. The following calculation also subtracts the portion of risk that is abolished by achieving a given age without developing breast cancer.

Absolute interval risk

$$= \frac{[\text{cumulative risk (2)} - \text{cumulative risk (1)}]}{[1 - \text{cumulative risk (1)}]}$$

For example, consider a 45-year-old patient who has a mother who had breast cancer at age 35 and a maternal aunt with breast cancer onset at age 50. Using the table for an affected mother and maternal aunt (Table 4-7), one would find the cumulative risk at age 49 (age intervals are "up to" the age indicated) for the relative age

Table 4-7. Predicted cumulative probability of breast cancer for a woman who has mother and maternal aunt affected with breast cancer, by age of onset of the affected relatives

Proband Age (yrs)	Age of Onset of Mother		30–39			
	Age of Onset of Maternal Aunt (yrs)					
	20–29	30–39	40–49	50–59	60–69	70–79
29	0.018	0.017	0.016	0.014	0.011	0.009
39	0.061	0.058	0.053	0.046	0.039	0.031
49	0.147	0.139	0.128	0.112	0.094	0.076
59	0.262	0.249	0.229	0.203	0.172	0.140
69	0.367	0.350	0.323	0.287	0.246	0.204
79	0.433	0.414	0.383	0.343	0.296	0.248

Source: Adapted from Claus EB, Risch N, Thompson WD. Autosomal dominant inheritance of early-onset breast cancer: implications for risk prediction. Cancer 1994;73(3):643–651. By permission of Wiley-Liss, Inc., a subsidiary of John Wiley & Sons, Inc.

combination of 30 to 39 years and 50 to 59 years. Risk up to age 49 is 0.112. To determine the patient's absolute risk over the next 20 years, one looks up the cumulative risk at 69 years (0.287) and substitutes these risk values into the absolute interval risk formula:

20-year interval risk

$$= \frac{(\text{cumulative risk at } 69 - \text{cumulative risk at } 49)}{(1 - \text{cumulative risk at } 49)}$$

$$= (0.287 - 0.112)/(1 - 0.112)$$

$$= 0.175/0.888 = 19.7\%$$

Strengths and Limitations

While the Claus tables are only useful for a small subset of women (those with a family history of breast cancer), they may be more accurate than the Gail model for this cohort. Nearly one-third of women with breast cancer have one or more first-degree relatives with the disease, although it is estimated that only 4% to 9% of those women with breast cancer truly have hereditary breast cancer described by an autosomal dominant model (30). The inclusion of information concerning second-degree relatives is particularly important if vertical transmission of an autosomal dominant trait with variable penetrance is assumed. Paternal inheritance can only be considered if second-degree relatives are included.

The probabilities in the look-up tables are model-derived rather than empirically based. Model-derived risks allow for extrapolation of risk estimates to other cases beyond those found in the original study, although an obvious limitation of this model is its restriction to inclusion of history of a maximum of two relatives. Bilaterality was omitted from the models because it did not seem to increase risk in the CASH population. Although the presence of ovarian cancer in relatives has been shown to increase breast cancer risk, this parameter is not included in the original Claus model. Claus later developed additional look-up tables to estimate the risk of breast cancer based on first-degree family history of ovarian cancer (31). However, additional analysis indicated that most of the breast cancer risk involved with ovarian cancer history was a result of being a *BRCA* mutation carrier. Claus calculated that 92% of the case subjects and 95% of

the control subjects probably were not mutation carriers (32). Still, 25% of noncarriers reported a family history of breast cancer.

Although Claus has examined the model in the CASH population, and observed versus expected cases showed good fit, the model tends to underestimate risks for relatives of patients with very early onset (20–29 years) because of the small number of cases that fit this profile. An included error analysis, recalculating risk numbers with parameters raised or lowered by twice the standard error, resulted in maximum errors of 10% of the risk probabilities. The Claus model has not been validated in independent studies.

Calculating Breast Cancer Risk in the General Population

The development of standards for breast cancer risk assessment in the general population is an urgent problem. A more educated and media-driven populace demands expert advice, advanced but expensive surveillance tools require targeted use, and clinical trials are most effective in risk-prone subpopulations (33). In the past, the only tools that were available were general tables of odds ratios, lists of factors that might individually increase risk by small increments. These tables, while still useful to provide a composite qualitative sense of individual risk, have been supplemented by risk models that are able to combine certain risk factors and provide a finite estimate of the absolute risk of developing disease over defined time intervals. Still, questions remain: How will we use these models? Where will we use them? When will we use them? How will we incorporate additional risk factors, such as environmental exposures, that are not included in the models? These questions are beyond the scope of this chapter, as is the matter of qualitative interpretation of risk, although they are addressed, in part, in the chapters that consider specific options for the management of women with increased risk.

The Gail model, in either the original or the NCI version, is a validated tool that has been shown to predict breast cancer risk reasonably well on the population level. It is known to overpredict risk in younger women and in women not involved in annual screening mammography regimens. It tends to underpredict risk in post-menopausal women. It may underpredict risk in women with a family history of breast or ovarian cancer. As such, it should never be used in the absence of some method to elicit family history of cancer. The Claus model is a simple tool that can incorporate a limited maternal and paternal family history of breast cancer. Still, because it does not incorporate some of the features of hereditary syndromes, it is not sufficient to quantify risk to individuals in that risk group.

It is recognized that clinical practice is time-limited and task-intensive; thus risk-assessment tools must be developed that can easily and quickly stratify women at different risk levels. It may be suggested that the optimal way to preliminarily screen women for breast cancer risk would be to use both the Gail and Claus models together. Integrated computer programs have been developed that can perform both operations simultaneously. In practice, most unaffected women will have no family history of breast cancer. A calculated Claus risk could act as a "flag" to explore the family history further. A woman without any Claus risk factors (no affected first- or second-degree relatives) would be unlikely to have a significant measurable *BRCA* mutation risk, unless there were a family history of ovarian or other rare cancers. Any woman who has two or more affected relatives should be assessed further using modeling specific to hereditary breast cancer.

The pedigree in Figure 4-1 demonstrates the case of a woman at possibly significant risk who would not be identified by the Gail model at all and whose risk would be underestimated by the Claus model. At 42 years old, this unaffected woman, with age of menarche of 12, first live birth at age 22, a paternal aunt with breast cancer, and no biopsy history, would have a 10-year Gail risk of 1.9% (5-year NCI Gail risk of 0.6%) and a 10-year Claus risk of 2.5%. Her risk actually may

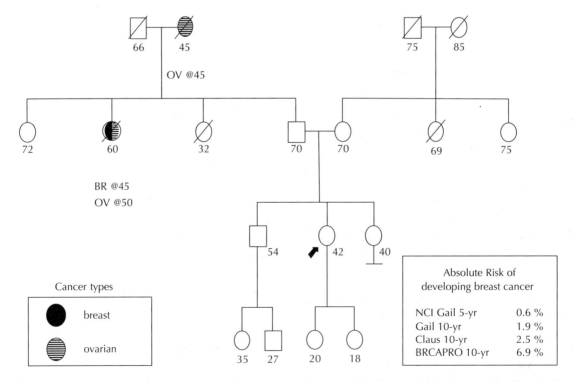

Figure 4-1. Pedigree 1. Patient is a 42-year-old woman with no personal history of cancer. Her first live birth was at age 22, her first menstrual period was at age 12, and she has had no biopsies. She has no first-degree relatives with breast cancer, although her paternal aunt and paternal grandmother were affected. Breast cancer risk probabilities, as calculated by different statistical models, are provided.

be far greater, as will be shown in the section covering mutation modeling.

There are two additional caveats to keep in mind when using the Gail model clinically. First, it is primarily age-dependent and adjusts for competing mortality. Thus a woman in her forties with a 10-year risk of 5.8% has a 20-year risk of 10.9%. The 20-year risk is not double that of the 10-year risk. Similarly, if a woman with the same risk factors presented at 50 years of age, her 10-year risk would be 5.5%. The message here is that one cannot simply add up the interval risks; one must recalculate the Gail risks periodically, particularly if any of the risk factors have changed (such as development of breast cancer in a relative or a new biopsy procedure). Another problem is defining the term *biopsy* and the pathologic finding of *atypical hyperplasia*. In practice, some women do not clearly know if they have had a breast biopsy or, more precisely, what was found when the biopsy was obtained. With the increased use of needle-biopsy procedures, many women do not distinguish between needle aspirations of a cyst and a diagnostic core biopsy. In fact, if pathologic studies are performed on the cyst aspirate, clinical distinctions may blur. Most women have not heard of the term *atypical hyperplasia*, and patient responses on this factor may be unreliable.

Modeling *BRCA1* and *BRCA2* Mutation Carrier Risk in Individuals with a Positive Family History

Pedigree Analysis

Genetic counselors traditionally derive risk estimates for disease using Mendelian principles based on individual pedigree analysis. Patterns of disease occurrence in a family may provide evidence of autosomal dominant, autosomal recessive, or X-linked transmission. Familial clustering in the absence of a specific pattern may lead one to suspect multifactorial origins of disease, that is, a combination of genetic and environmental factors. *Segregation analysis* is a statistical method of examining large or multiple pedigrees in order to determine the most likely mode of transmission of a particular trait or disease. Modification of Mendelian risk for variable penetrance

by Bayesian analysis or estimation of risk for multifactorial disorders is done using empirical data, although these data are often limited, particularly in the case of rare diseases.

Pedigree analysis is an irreplaceable tool in quantifying risk for those with a family history of breast cancer and cannot be supplanted by any of the models devised to date. All the models described below (with the exception of BRCAPRO, which requires a pedigree for input) can miss important features of hereditary breast cancer. A three-generation pedigree, including the patient (the proband), all siblings, and parental and grandparental generations, is a minimum requirement. In addition, inquiries should be made about children, nieces, and nephews. Not only can these descendants occasionally develop early-onset cancers, but motivation for risk assessment and possible genetic testing is strongly influenced by concern for the risk to offspring.

A complete pedigree is used not only to establish possible transmission of the most common highly penetrant genes but also may identify unusual or related cancers that would lead to suspicion of rarer cancer syndromes such as Cowden's disease or Li-Fraumeni syndrome.

Linkage Analysis

While segregation analysis is used to establish the transmission pattern of a genetic disease (i.e., autosomal dominant, autosomal recessive, X-linked), *linkage analysis* is a method of pinpointing the location of the responsible gene(s). Genetic "markers" with known genomic locations are traced throughout a pedigree in order to establish an association between those markers and disease occurrence. Genetic markers are particular DNA sequences that may be within genes but more commonly are close-by sequences that happen to be polymorphic; that is, they vary among individuals to such a degree that there is a high probability of finding unique versions of these sequences in different family members. These markers are generally VNTRs (variable number of tandem repeats) or STRs (short tandem repeats) and, more recently, ESTs (expressed sequence tags) and SNPs (single-nucleotide polymorphisms). The Human Genome Project has identified the chromosomal location of thousands of these markers, with more identified each day (34). Cotransmission of particular versions of these marker sequences and the disease phenotype can establish the chromosomal "address" of a disease-causing gene.

Linkage analysis depends on the availability of large, multigenerational, highly affected families with living members available for testing. Statistical methods have been devised that allow us to combine the information from many smaller families, resulting in what is known as the *LOD score*, or *logarithm of the odds of linkage* (for a further discussion, see Chap. 2).

The Breast Cancer Linkage Consortium (BCLC) is a worldwide cooperative network now encompassing approximately 100 centers sharing data on over 700 breast cancer families from Europe, Canada, and the United States. Founded in 1989 in Lyon, France, its linkage analysis studies in families with multiple cases of breast cancer were instrumental in locating the two known predisposition genes, *BRCA1* and *BRCA2* (see *http://ruly70.medfac.leidenuniv.nl/~devilee/BC-LC/history.htm#start*). The most widely quoted estimates of the prevalence, penetrance, and resulting cumulative cancer risks conferred by the breast cancer genes *BRCA1* and *BRCA2* come from BCLC studies. The original data on 214 breast cancer families, including 57 breast/ovarian cancer families, estimated the cumulative *BRCA1*-associated breast cancer risk to be 59% by age 50 and 82% by age 70 (35). Later estimates were based on 33 families in whom development of second cancers in individuals already affected with breast cancer were used to postulate an estimated cumulative risk of cancer in gene carriers. The estimates of an 87% penetrance of breast cancer and 44% of ovarian cancer by age 70 are widely quoted today, although subsequent studies in less affected families have shown much lower penetrances (36–40). BCLC analysis estimates that *BRCA2* mutations confer a 84% risk for breast cancer and a 27% risk for ovarian cancer by age 70 (41).

The BCLC linkage estimates of attributable risk are occasionally used in cancer risk assessment, and penetrance and prevalence estimates are incorporated into one of the mutation-probability models (BRCAPRO), although the confidence limits are wide. For instance, given a family with four cases of breast cancer onset under 60 years of age and no ovarian cancer, tables from Ford and colleagues (1998) would indicate a probability of 28% (95% CI = 0.11–0.50) that the family carried a mutation linked to *BRCA1* (41). This is not the probability of finding such a mutation by sequence analysis. In fact, mutation identification by testing was calculated to have only 63% (95% CI = 51–77) sensitivity when using presumed linkage as a reference.

While the knowledge gained through the collaborative efforts of the BCLC has built the foundation of breast cancer genetic epidemiology, in general, linkage analysis provides preliminary estimates for prevalence and penetrance that are best used only until more accurate empirical data can be collected. It must be emphasized that these estimates are based on a limited number of families preselected for very high penetrance. In addition, the penetrance estimates are not entirely empirical, since they are derived from highly theoretical computational methods used in linkage analysis such as maximization of LOD scores over varying values of the penetrance function. These methods rely on a variety of simplistic assumptions that may or may not reflect true conditions at the population level. Ongoing direct genetic testing in the huge family repository collected by the BCLC will provide more reliable estimates.

Logistic Regression Models of Mutation-Carrier Probability

Immediately following the successful cloning of the *BRCA1* gene (42) and the *BRCA2* gene (43), genetic testing of individuals with suggestive family histories began. Initially, testing was performed under research-only protocols, facilitating the collection of individual and family data. This permitted empirically based statistical analysis of the prevalence of mutations (both deleterious and ambiguous), the disease penetrance of mutations (causing breast, ovarian, and other cancers), and familial patterns of disease that might predict the presence of a mutation. Commercial testing for both mutations is now available, and additional data are being collected systematically.

Three models have been developed that predict mutation-carrier probabilities based on logistic regression of the risk parameters found to be significant in their respective study populations. As those of us who use the following models clinically know, the probability that a given patient carries a *BRCA* mutation is estimated differently by each of the following models. Two of the models, Shattuck-Eidens and Couch, only calculate the probability of carrying a *BRCA1* mutation. Ashkenazi Jewish descent is not included in the Frank model. The Couch model only includes age of breast cancer diagnosis as a composite family average. Whether a particular risk factor is included and how it is quantified (as a categorical yes or no or as a continuous value) has implications for the applicability of the model to an individual patient. While the three study populations probably included a limited number of third-degree relatives, inclusion of these relatives in risk calculations is uncertain. In addition to the small numbers involved, accuracy of patient-reported diagnoses for more distant relatives can be questionable (44,45).

The Couch Model

The *BRCA* mutation-risk data available before 1997 were based on the highly penetrant families who had been ascertained for linkage research. The first study to examine the mutation frequency in a more typical clinical population was that of Couch and colleagues (3) at the University of Pennsylvania.

Study Population. While this study technically included 263 unrelated women affected with breast cancer, the final model was based on only the 169 women who were referred to the breast cancer risk clinics at the University of Pennsylvania because of a positive family history. Although these women all had at least some family history (ranging from 1 to 11 breast cancer cases per family; mean, 4 cases), they had been excluded from previous linkage-analysis studies because the numbers of affected relatives available for testing were insufficient. *BRCA1* mutations were identified in 16% (27/169) of the affected women.

Risk Factors. There are no individual risk factors included for the proband. Risk is derived from the average age of onset of all breast cancers in the family. Family risk factors include the types of cancer found in the family, that is, breast cancer cases only, breast and ovarian cancer cases, or breast and ovarian cancer in a single individual. Ashkenazi Jewish descent is also considered.

Risk Calculation. Tables derived from all permutations of the logistic regression equation are provided (Table 4-8). The applicable family risk is found by obtaining the average age at diagnosis of all breast cancers and referring to the category that describes the types of cancers found in the family. There are separate tables for non-Ashkenazi and Ashkenazi women. If the proband is unaffected, the risk is calculated for the nearest affected relative and adjusted by Mendelian extrapolation. For instance, in the case of pedigree 2 Figure 4-2, where the Ashkenazi Jewish proband is unaffected, but her mother had breast cancer at age 45, her maternal aunt had breast cancer at age 50, and her maternal grandmother had breast cancer at age 80, her risk would be computed as 50% of the family risk. The family risk would be based on an average age at diagnosis of 58 and found in Table 4-8 under the heading "Ashkenazi Jewish Families with Breast Cancer Only." The family risk is 8.4%, but since the proband is unaffected, her risk is based on her nearest affected relative (her mother) and would be one-half of 8.4%, or 4.2%.

Strengths and Limitations. The Couch model predicts risk probability for *BRCA1* only; thus it will underestimate the risk of being a mutation carrier because risk due to *BRCA2* is not included. It assumes that all affected individuals are mutation carriers and, as a strictly empirical model, does not distinguish familial relationships. The greatest limitation of the model is the need to average the ages at breast cancer diagnosis. The presence of a relative with breast cancer onset in her 80s (perhaps a sporadic "phenocopy") will dilute the effect of having another relative with onset in her 30s. The mean number of cancers per family in this study was four, and only 4 of 169 families had only one case of breast cancer. Therefore, the "average age" computation is probably not

Table 4-8. Probability of detecting a *BRCA1* mutation in families with a history of breast or ovarian cancer (Couch model)

Average Age at Diagnosis of Breast Cancer (yrs)	Predicted Percent Probability (95% CI)	Average Age at Diagnosis of Breast Cancer (yrs)	Predicted Percent Probability (95% CI)
Families with Breast Cancer Only		**Ashkenazi Jewish Families with Breast Cancer Only**	
<35	17.4 (6.5–38.8)	<35	47.9
35–39	11.7 (5.1–24.6)	35–39	36.7 (12.8–69.6)
40–44	7.7 (3.6–15.6)	40–44	26.8 (9.7–55.3)
45–49	5.0 (2.3–10.8)	45–49	18.7 (6.8–42.0)
50–54	3.2 (1.2–8.1)	50–54	12.7 (4.3–31.8)
55–59	2.1 (0.6–6.5)	55–59	8.4 (2.5–24.8)
>59	1.3 (0.3–5.5)	>59	5.5 (1.3–20.0)
Families with Breast and Ovarian Cancer		**Ashkenazi Jewish Families with Breast and Ovarian Cancer**	
<35	55.0 (27.2–80.0)	<35	84.3
35–39	43.5 (22.4–67.2)	35–39	77.1 (40.1–94.4)
40–44	32.7 (17.0–53.5)	40–44	67.9
45–49	23.4 (11.4–42.1)	45–49	57.2 (24.9–84.3)
50–54	16.2 (6.7–34.2)	50–54	45.7
55–59	10.8 (3.5–28.8)	55–59	34.7 (10.8–70.0)
>59	7.1 (1.7–24.8)	>59	25.1
Families with Breast and Ovarian Cancer in a Single Member		**Ashkenazi Jewish Families with Breast and Ovarian Cancer in a Single Member**	
<35	77	<35	93.6
35–39	67.8 (37.1–88.3)	35–39	90.2
40–44	57.1 (28.4–81.7)	40–44	85.3
45–49	54.5	45–49	78.5
50–54	34.6 (12.1–67.0)	50–54	69.8
55–59	25.0	55–59	59.3
>59	17.3	>59	47.8
Families with Breast and Ovarian Cancer and One Member with Both Breast and Ovarian Cancer		**Ashkenazi Jewish Families with Breast and Ovarian Cancer and One Member with Both Breast and Ovarian Cancer**	
<35	96.6	<35	98.8
35–39	92.4 (72.0–98.3)	35–39	96.8
40–44	88.5 (63.4–97.2)	40–44	98.1
45–49	82.9 (52.0–95.6)	45–49	95.5
50–54	75.4	50–54	93.0
55–59	65.9	55–59	89.4
>59	54.9	>59	81.3

Source: Adapted from Couch FJ, DeShano ML, Blackwood MA, et al. *BRCA1* mutations in women attending clinics that evaluate the risk of breast cancer. New Engl J Med 1997; 336 (20):1409–1415. Copyright © 1997 Massachusetts Medical Society. All rights reserved. Adapted with permission.

valid for less than two affected individuals and would be most accurate for families with three or more affected individuals. The underlying data set was relatively small, with only 27 identified mutations, and confidence intervals are wide for many categories. The table, however, is very simple to use and easy to refer to in a clinical setting.

The Shattuck-Eidens Model

With the cloning and development of commercially available molecular mutation analyses for

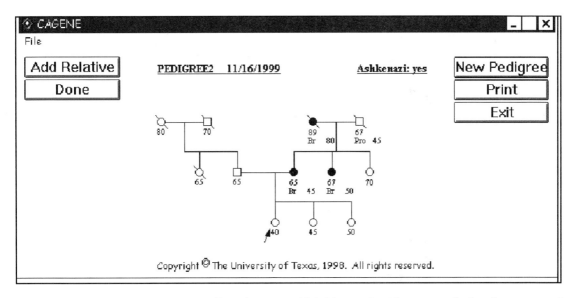

Figure 4-2. Pedigree 2. Patient is an unaffected 40-year-old Ashkenazi Jewish woman who has three maternal relatives affected with breast cancer. The probability that she is a *BRCA* mutation carrier varies according to which risk model is used to calculate carrier risk. Pedigree drawn using CancerGene software. (Reproduced with permission from David Euhus.)

BRCA1 and *BRCA2* genes, development of risk-assessment models capable of predicting probability of mutation-carrier status became a priority. Myriad Genetics, Inc., sponsored the development of two models based on clinical populations of women likely to contain mutation carriers. The Shattuck-Eidens (SE) model (4) predicts the probability of carrying a mutation in *BRCA1*, and the Frank model (5) predicts the probability of carrying a mutation in either *BRCA1* or *BRCA2*. These models, as derived, are only applicable to women already diagnosed with cancer. However, mutation-carrier probabilities can be extrapolated from affected relatives using Mendelian principles.

Study Population. The SE model is based on a logistic regression analysis of a multi-institution population ascertained through 20 familial risk clinics across the United States and Europe. Probands (798) were selected because they were members of putative high-risk families. A high-risk family was defined as having multiple cases of breast cancer, members with an early age of onset of breast cancer, or members with ovarian cancer. None of the families had known linkage to *BRCA1*, and only one proband per family

was selected. The model was based on a subset of 593 affected women (with either breast or ovarian cancer). Full-sequence mutation analysis was performed for each proband, resulting in a total mutation frequency of 12.8%, with higher frequencies noted in probands from families with ovarian cancer or of Ashkenazi Jewish descent.

Risk Factors. Risk factors included in the final model are based on characteristics of both the proband and her family. For the proband, the risk factors are breast or ovarian cancer status including age at onset and Ashkenazi Jewish heritage. For the family, factors include breast or ovarian cancer status but not age at onset or degree of relatedness. Cancer status for both the proband and family members are categorized according to the presence of breast cancer alone, ovarian cancer alone, or both cancers in the same individual. Bilaterality is also considered for the proband.

Risk Calculation. Graphs are provided in the paper for estimates of risk when none or only one family member is affected. One finds the graph that fits the family situation (i.e., no affected relatives, one relative with breast cancer, one

Table 4-9. Shattuck-Eidens model *BRCA1* mutation carrier risks (%)

		Non-Ashkenazi Proband Diagnosis					Ashkenazi Proband Diagnosis				
	Proband Age at Diagnosis	Unilateral Breast Cancer	Bilateral Breast Cancer	Ovarian Cancer with No Breast Cancer	Unilateral Breast Cancer with Ovarian Cancer	Bilateral Breast Cancer with Ovarian Cancer	Unilateral Breast Cancer	Bilateral Breast Cancer	Ovarian Cancer with No Breast Cancer	Unilateral Breast Cancer with Ovarian Cancer	Bilateral Breast Cancer with Ovarian Cancer
No affected relatives	30	8%	25%	33%	42%	50%	27%	57%	67%	75%	80%
	40	4%	13%	18%	25%	31%	14%	38%	47%	57%	65%
	50	2%	6%	9%	13%	17%	7%	21%	29%	38%	45%
	60	1%	3%	4%	6%	8%	3%	11%	15%	21%	27%
	70	0%	1%	2%	3%	4%	1%	5%	8%	11%	14%
One relative with breast cancer	30	11%	31%	40%	50%	57%	34%	65%	73%	80%	85%
	40	5%	17%	23%	31%	38%	19%	45%	55%	65%	71%
	50	2%	8%	12%	17%	21%	9%	27%	35%	45%	53%
	60	1%	4%	6%	8%	11%	4%	14%	20%	27%	33%
	70	1%	2%	3%	4%	5%	2%	7%	10%	14%	18%
One relative with ovarian cancer	30	21%	49%	58%	68%	74%	52%	80%	85%	90%	92%
	40	11%	30%	39%	49%	56%	33%	64%	72%	79%	84%
	50	5%	16%	22%	30%	37%	18%	44%	54%	63%	70%
	60	2%	8%	11%	16%	21%	9%	26%	34%	44%	51%
	70	1%	4%	5%	8%	10%	4%	14%	19%	26%	32%
One relative with breast and ovarian cancer	30	33%	64%	72%	80%	84%	67%	88%	91%	94%	96%
	40	18%	44%	54%	64%	70%	47%	76%	83%	88%	91%
	50	9%	26%	35%	44%	52%	29%	59%	68%	76%	81%
	60	4%	14%	19%	26%	33%	15%	40%	49%	59%	66%
	70	2%	7%	10%	14%	18%	8%	23%	30%	39%	47%

Source: Data derived from logistic regression equation of Shattuck-Eidens et al. JAMA 1997;278:15.

relative with ovarian cancer, or one relative with breast and ovarian cancer) and estimates the *BRCA1* risk from the point on the curve corresponding to the proband's age at onset and type(s) of cancer(s). The same information can be expressed in tabular form for those who prefer this format (Table 4-9). If more than one relative is affected, risk can be derived using the provided regression equation. The logistic regression equation (as well as the derived graphs and tables) is not considered accurate for women diagnosed before age 30.

To calculate *BRCA1* carrier probability for the proband's affected mother in pedigree 2 (see Fig. 4-2), the graphs cannot be used because she has more than one affected relative (her own mother and her sister). Risk probability must be derived by using the regression equation. The risk factors used in the equation would be proband age at diagnosis of 45, Ashkenazi descent, unilateral breast and no ovarian cancer, and two relatives with breast cancer only, resulting in a computed *BRCA1* risk of 17.2%. The probability based on Mendelian inheritance that the unaffected 40-year-old daughter is a *BRCA1* carrier is half of that, or 8.6%.

Strengths and Limitations. The SE model calculates risk for *BRCA1* only, thus underestimating the probability of being a mutation carrier. While the graphs provided are easy to use, they are only applicable for probands with either no or one affected relative. If more than one affected relative is present in the family, the risk probability can be calculated from the regression equation, but this may not be convenient in the clinical setting. Neither age at onset nor bilateral breast cancer is considered in affected relatives. A strength of the model is its inclusion of ovarian cancer diagnosis in the proband. However, age at ovarian cancer diagnosis in the proband is multiplied by the same substantial coefficient that is used for breast cancer diagnosis. It is uncertain if ovarian cancer has the same early-onset tendency as breast cancer in mutation carriers.

The Frank Model
Study Population. The Frank model is based on an analysis of 223 women who all developed breast cancer before age 50. Subjects were drawn from familial risk clinics in the United States and were selected because of a high-risk family history, with all having at least one relative with breast cancer diagnosed before age 50 or at least one relative with ovarian cancer. Subjects with known linkage to or identified *BRCA1* or *BRCA2* mutations were excluded. Thirty-nine percent of subjects had identified mutations, 26% in *BRCA1* and 13% in *BRCA2*. Forty-nine percent of the families had a history of ovarian cancer, and 20% were Ashkenazi Jewish.

Risk Factors. Although risk probability is derived from logistic regression, the risk factors considered in this model are all discrete (i.e., present or absent). Risk factors for the proband include a breast cancer diagnosis under age 50 (which is required for the model to be used), a breast cancer diagnosis under age 40 (which is only counted if there is an additional relative with breast cancer diagnosed before age 50), and the presence of bilateral breast or ovarian cancer. In most cases, the contribution of family history is limited to one relative with breast cancer diagnosed under age 50 or one relative with ovarian cancer at any age, and one of these conditions must be met in order for the model to apply. The model can include history for two relatives (one with ovarian cancer and one with breast cancer before age 50) only if the proband has a breast cancer onset under age 40.

Risk Calculation. No calculations are required for risk assessment because a chart is provided that lists risks for each constellation of risk factors (Table 4-10). Although male breast cancer was included in the logistic regression equation from which the risk figures are derived, it was not included as a category in the chart because there were too few cases. Technically, a Frank model risk could not be derived for the family in pedigree 2 because there are not two breast cancer cases with onset below age 50.

Strengths and Limitations. The Frank chart is extremely simple to use in the clinical setting (laminated reference charts are available from Myriad Genetics, Inc.). However, its applicability is limited to families with at least two early-onset breast cancer cases or an ovarian

Table 4-10. Modeled probabilities of women with breast cancer under 50 years of age carrying a mutation in *BRCA1* or *BRCA2* (Frank model)

Relative with Breast Cancer <50 Yrs	Relative with Ovarian Cancer	Proband: Bilateral Breast Cancer or Ovarian Cancer	Proband: Breast Cancer <40 Yrs	Probability of Mutation in *BRCA1* (%)	Probability of Mutation in *BRCA2* (%)	Probability of Mutation in *BRCA1* or *BRCA2* (%)
+				10.1	14.5	25
+			+	28.2	11.6	40
+		+		41.5	9.5	51
+		+	+	71.1	4.7	76
	+			22.9	12.5	35
	+		+	22.9	12.5	35
	+	+		65.0	5.7	71
	+	+	+	65.0	5.7	71
+	+			22.9	12.5	35
+	+		+	50.9	7.9	59
+	+	+		65.0	5.7	71
+	+	+	+	86.7	2.2	89

Source: Adapted from Frank TS, Manley SA, Olopade OI, et al. Sequence analysis of *BRCA1* and *BRCA2*: correlation of mutations with family history and ovarian cancer risk. J Clin Oncol 1998;16(7):2417–2425.

case. It is often mistakenly assumed that this model can be used when a proband has ovarian cancer only, since the complete study population did include women with ovarian cancer. These cases, however, were eliminated from the final model. The only possible proband is a woman who has breast cancer before age 50, and onset below age 40 is only considered under certain conditions. Bilateral cancer is not included for relatives. Ashkenazi descent is not included, and since 20% of the study population was Ashkenazi Jewish, the risk estimates for non-Ashkenazi women may be inflated.

Bayesian Model

BRCAPRO: The Berry-Aguilar-Parmigiani Model

Berry and colleagues (46) devised a mathematical model using Bayesian principles to estimate the probability of carrying a *BRCA1* mutation, and the model was later revised to include *BRCA2* (6). Age at onset in the affected relatives and current ages of the unaffected relatives are important components of this model. History of both breast and ovarian cancer is considered. The model is based on Mendelian principles but depends on known mutation frequencies and penetrance estimates. Because of this dependence, the model can be modified as these estimates become more precise. Theoretically, it can incorporate multiple genes as they are discovered, variable frequencies of mutant alleles among different ethnic populations, and other risk factors such as associated cancers.

The model is computationally intensive and must be done by computer. BRCAPRO is a software program authored by Donald Berry, Giovanni Parmigiani, Ed Iversen, and Omar Aquilar from the Institute of Statistics and Decision Sciences at Duke University and is available at *http://www.stat.duke.edu/~gp/brcapro.html*. The stand-alone program is not widely used, but BRCAPRO is included in the software program CancerGene, an integrated computer program by David Euhus from the University of Texas Southwestern Medical Center (*http://www.swmed.edu/home_pages/cancergene/*). CancerGene constructs a pedigree based on family history input, computes breast cancer risk based on the Claus and Gail models, and computes mutation-carrier risks for the Couch model (referred to as U.Penn), the Shattuck-Eidens model (referred to as Myriad I), the Frank model (referred to as Myriad II), and the Berry-Parmigiani model (referred to as BRCAPRO). It also estimates absolute breast and ovarian cancer risk based on the BRCAPRO mutation probability and published mutation penetrance estimates. CancerGene has additional features, including a glossary of familial cancer syndromes and the ability to save family data to a relational database.

Study Population

Since the BRCAPRO model is based on Bayesian updating of individual pedigree configurations, there is no study population involved per se. However, BRCA mutation incidence and breast and ovarian cancer penetrance rates are derived from BCLC data. *BRCA1* breast and ovarian penetrance is derived from the Easton and colleagues 1995 study (47), and *BRCA2* penetrance is derived from the Easton and colleagues 1997 study (48). Prevalence rates for *BRCA1* and *BRCA2* are derived from the Ford and Easton 1995 study (49) and the Andersen 1996 study (50), respectively. Rates for non-carriers are based on SEER data (adjusted to subtract out estimated *BRCA* carrier cases).

Risk Factors

Risk factors include breast and ovarian cancer in the proband and all first- and second-degree relatives (including males) with age at onset and breast bilaterality included. Present age or age at death is also included to account for development (or nondevelopment) of second cancers. Age is included for all unaffected relatives. The model also can include *BRCA1* or *BRCA2* mutation testing results, with adjustments possible for varying sensitivity and specificity. It incorporates Ashkenazi Jewish ancestry.

Risk Calculation

Risk is calculated as a posterior probability of carrying a mutation given family history. The prior probability of carrying a mutation is based on mutation frequency in the population, and conditional probabilities are based on the likelihood of the family members being mutation carriers based on their age, their cancer status, and their position in the pedigree. Bayesian updating is based on "the probability of the genetic status of the offspring, given that of the parents; the probability of the genetic status of the parents, given their offspring; and the probability of disease outcome given genetic

status" (6). An uncertainty correction is applied for the penetrance and prevalence rates.

BRCAPRO has two underlying components: the computation program (BRCA.exe) and the rate tables. There are presently two different rate tables containing prevalence and penetrance data for non-Ashkenazi and Ashkenazi individuals. The *CancerGene* computer interface itself consists of a series of input screens for collection of family history data. Relatives (and their input data) are added according to their relationship to the proband, and risks are calculated for the proband directly. The proband may be affected or unaffected. In practice, if a proband is unaffected, it is sometimes necessary to use another member of the family as a "surrogate proband" to capture informative family members because the input options only extend to second-degree relatives. In these cases, Mendelian principles are used to extrapolate the original proband's risk. The BRCAPRO *BRCA1* mutation risk for the proband in pedigree 2 is 7.4%. However, the combined risk for *BRCA1* and *BRCA2* is 28%, substantially higher than the risks calculated by previous models.

Strengths and Limitations

If one looks at Figure 4-3, it becomes obvious that the BRCAPRO model includes the most comprehensive enumeration of family history. It is based on Mendelian inheritance and Bayesian analysis rather than on empirical data from a possibly unique subpopulation. The present limitations of the model, however, are its indirect dependence on just such a data set. As stated earlier, the BCLC estimations of prevalence and penetrance of the *BRCA1* and *BRCA2* genes are based on highly affected families with many cases of both breast and ovarian cancer. The most serious limitation in this model is caused by the lack of early-onset ovarian cancer cases in BCLC data set, which results in calculation of a low probability of mutation in either *BRCA1* or *BRCA2* when age at onset of ovarian cancer is below 40 years.

Another limitation is the restriction to second-degree relatives when entering family history. The use of a "surrogate proband" will eliminate the automatic Bayesian updating based on the age of an unaffected proband, although this calculation can be done manually.

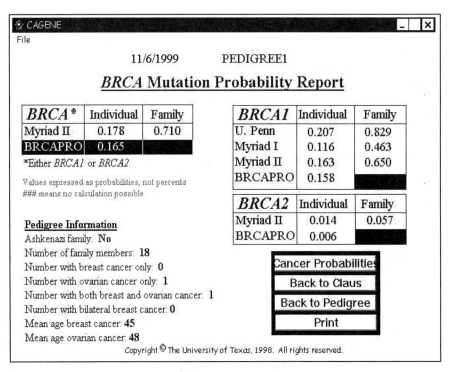

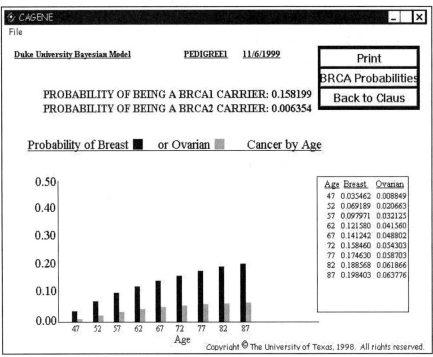

Figure 4-4. CancerGene *BRCA* mutation probability output screens. Risks are calculated separately using each of four risk models, U.Penn (Couch et al.), Myriad I (Shattuck-Eidens et al.), Myriad II (Frank et al.), and BRCAPRO (Berry et al.). BRCAPRO mutation carrier probability is multiplied by age-dependent breast and ovarian cancer penetrance rates to estimate absolute cancer risk over time. These output screens are based on the proband in pedigree 1. (Reproduced with permission from David Euhus.)

estimate than the Couch model, since it directly includes the age at breast cancer onset of a single individual. The Frank (Myriad II) model predicts a family risk of 65% for *BRCA1* and 5.7% for *BRCA2* (and a 17.8% combined risk for the proband). It captures breast cancer onset under age 50, the ovarian cancer in the same individual, and ovarian cancer in the paternal grandmother. It might be noted that a diagnosis age under 40 years in the aunt would not have conferred any higher risk, but overall, this model fits this type of pedigree configuration quite well. In this case, BRCAPRO may be slightly underestimating risk due to the presence of the ovarian cancer in the grandmother with a relatively early onset. However, it is also including the fact that the proband and her sister have lived into their 40s without developing cancer and one paternal aunt has lived to 72 without developing cancer. It estimates a combined *BRCA1* and *BRCA2* probability for the proband of 16.5%. All the models predict similar risks in this case and provide a reasonable basis for testing.

Next, consider the same pedigree with the line of transmission reversed; that is, the affected relatives become a maternal aunt with breast cancer at age 45 and ovarian cancer at age 50 and a maternal grandmother with ovarian cancer at age 45. The mutation probabilities for all the logistic regression models remain the same, since none are based on type or degree of familial relationship. The BRCAPRO model, however, predicts a combined risk of only 5.1% because it considers the fact that the mother (through whom the mutation would have had to pass in order for the proband to be at risk) has lived until age 70 without developing cancer. Such updating was not possible in the former configuration because penetrance in males is low in the case of breast cancer and nonexistent in the case of ovarian cancer. In this case, the BRCAPRO model would best approximate the actual risk.

Again consider pedigree 1 if the 35-year-old niece of the proband developed ovarian cancer. The Couch and Frank models would calculate the same risk because they are categorical. The Shattuck-Eidens model–derived risk for the family would rise to 64% if based on the paternal aunt and 83% if based on the niece,

although the validity of including third-degree relationships for any of the logistic regression models is uncertain. BRCAPRO, however, uses the proband as the reference, and all the affected relatives are second degree for her. The joint mutation probability calculated is now 22% not only because of the additional ovarian cancer but also because a line of genetic transmission is more firmly established.

Who Should Do Breast Cancer Risk Assessment

Just as there are different levels and different methods of risk assessment for different purposes, the providers of these assessments may vary according to the circumstances involved. Risk assessment for the purpose of entry into a clinical trial is a different endeavor than individual risk assessment for consideration of genetic testing. While a computerized screening risk assessment may be acceptable for flagging patients in need of further evaluation, a comprehensive risk assessment for a woman with a strong family history should be done by a professional trained in cancer genetics. As demonstrated in the preceding examples, there are subtleties in all the currently available risk models that require expert interpretation. In addition, complete pedigree analysis may identify unusual cancer syndromes. Hoskins and colleagues (56) suggest a stratification of individuals into moderate-risk (for whom the Gail and Claus risks may best apply and who may be managed by a primary care provider) and high-risk groups (who should have comprehensive risk assessment by trained specialists). In addition to risk assessment, many other services are provided in cancer risk counseling (57) (Table 4-11). Basic guidelines for referral may be found in Table 4-12, and cancer risk counseling professionals are actively developing standardized referral guidelines and strategies. Both the National Cancer Institute and the National Society of Genetic Counselors maintain Web-based directories of cancer genetic professionals available for referral and consultation (see *http://cancernet.nci.nih.gov/genesrch.shtml* and *http://www.nsgc.org/Resource_link.html*).

Table 4-11. Components of familial cancer risk counseling

Screening	Family history screening questionnaires
	Tumor markers
	Tumor registries
Brief risk assessement, interventions, and triage	History and documentation
	Genetic education
	Health promotion
	Supportive psychosocial counseling
	Referral
Comprehensive cancer risk assessment and counseling	Full pedigree analysis
	Genetic syndrome diagnosis
	Risk calculation and communication
	Genetic susceptibility testing
	DNA banking
	Psychosocial evaluation and counseling
	Customized medical surveillance
	Referral to and coordination with research studies

Source: Adapted from Peters JA, Stopfer JE. Role of the genetic counselor in familial cancer. Oncology (Huntington) 1996;10(2):159–166, 175. With permission of PRR, Inc., Melville, NY.

Table 4-12. General features of hereditary cancer syndromes

Cancer in two or more close relatives
Bilateral cancer in paired organs
Multiple primary tumors in same individual
Earlier-than-usual onset of disease
Specific constellation of tumors that comprise a
  known cancer syndrome

Source: Adapted from Peters JA, Stopfer JE. Role of the genetic counselor in familial cancer. Oncology (Huntington) 1996;10(2):159–166, 175. With permission of PRR, Inc., Melville, NY.

Although individual physicians trained in risk assessment may wish to provide this service, many others may not have the time, expertise, or inclination to perform comprehensive risk assessment and counseling. In one recent study, almost one-third of physicians misinterpreted the results of genetic testing (58). There also may be liability issues relating to failure to recognize and warn patients of genetic predisposition (59,60). Recommending bodies such as the American Society of Human Genetics and the American Society of Clinical Oncology agree that genetic testing should not be done in the absence of sufficient pre- and posttest counseling, including informed consent.

How Should Cancer Risk Be Communicated

The personal perception of risk and the effective communication of objective risk are becoming established fields of inquiry. A growing body of research that bridges psychological, health behavior, and cognitive processing is emerging. It is clear that the computation of an "objective" risk is only one component of the clinical interaction. Possible changes in health behaviors are important but are not the only outcomes that should be measured. In all the flurry surrounding genetic testing and risk assessment, it is perhaps easy to forget that there are some individuals who would just rather "not know." A comprehensive review of the current issues involved in risk perception and communication is available in a recent JNCI monograph entitled, *Cancer Risk Communication: What We Know and What We Need to Learn* (61).

Future of Breast Cancer Risk Assessment

Breast cancer risk assessment has developed to the point that it is feasible to institute preliminary risk screening for every woman in the primary care, obstetrics and gynecologic, or mammography clinical setting. Risk models will improve as we gather more information about risk in the general population. We need refined prevalence/penetrance estimates for mutation carriers that will only be available as more people are tested, and we must develop approaches for collecting these data. The National Cancer Institute recently announced the formation of the Cancer Genetics Network, which will develop a national database to analyze the links between genetics and cancer. Penetrance may depend on specific mutations, and other major genes may be involved. There are a number of families who have strong family histories and yet have not shown linkage or tested positive for *BRCA1* and *BRCA2*. The search for a putative *BRCA3* gene is ongoing.

Claus has shown that there is a proportion of risk due to family history that is not attributable to major high-penetrance genes (32). There may be modifying genes that have significant environmental interactions in subpopulations. Rebbeck uses the term *polygenes* to refer to common gene variants with small effects, such as the variable alleles of the P450 cytochrome and *N*-acetyltransferase genes involved in metabolic activation and detoxification of carcinogens. Although their effect may be small, the prevalence of these allelic variants may make their population attributable risk high (62).

How will we find all these genes, and how will we integrate vast amounts risk information? The emerging chip genotyping technologies may make it easy to test for panels of genes known to have a relationship to particular common disorders. We will need enhanced informatics capabilities to do risk assessment in the future. Many genes with different quantities of effect and cross-interactions will necessitate computationally intensive algorithms for analysis.

A new paradigm of standardized risk evaluation could center medical care on prevention, and presymptomatic intervention and personal interaction with health care providers could be more individually focused.

References

1. Gail MH, Brinton LA, Byar DP, et al. Projecting individualized probabilities of developing breast cancer for white females who are being examined annually. J Natl Cancer Inst 1989;81(24):1879–1886.
2. Claus EB, Risch N, Thompson WD. Autosomal dominant inheritance of early-onset breast cancer: implications for risk prediction. Cancer 1994;73(3):643–651.
3. Couch FJ, DeShano ML, Blackwood MA, et al. *BRCA1* mutations in women attending clinics that evaluate the risk of breast cancer. New Engl J Med 1997;336(20):1409–1415.
4. Shattuck-Eidens D, Oliphant A, McClure M, et al. *BRCA1* sequence analysis in women at high risk for susceptibility mutations: risk factor analysis and implications for genetic testing. JAMA 1997;278(15):1242–1250.
5. Frank TS, Manley SA, Olopade OI, et al. Sequence analysis of *BRCA1* and *BRCA2*: correlation of mutations with family history and ovarian cancer risk. J Clin Oncol 1998;16(7):2417–2425.
6. Parmigiani G, Berry D, Aguilar O. Determining carrier probabilities for breast cancer-susceptibility genes *BRCA1* and *BRCA2*. Am J Hum Genet 1998;62(1):145–158.
7. American Cancer Society. Breast cancer facts and figures, 1999. Available at *http://www.cancer.org/statistics/cff99/selectedcancers.html#breast*.
8. Becher H, Chang-Claude J. Estimating disease risks for individuals with a given family history in different populations with an application to breast cancer. Genet Epidemiol 1996;13(3):229–242.
9. Zhang J, Yu KF. What's the relative risk? A method of correcting the odds ratio in cohort studies of common outcomes. JAMA 1998;280(19):1690–1691.
10. Dupont WD, Plummer WD Jr. Understanding the relationship between relative and absolute risk. Cancer 1996;77:2193–2199.
11. Offit K. Clinical cancer genetics: Risk counseling and management. New York: Wiley-Liss, 1998.
12. Tonin P, Weber B, Offit K, et al. Frequency of recurrent *BRCA1* and *BRCA2* mutations in Ashkenazi Jewish breast cancer families. Nature Med 1996;2(11):1179–1183.
13. Baker LH. Breast cancer detection demonstration project: five-year summary report. CA 1982;32(4):194–225.
14. Carter CL, Corle DK, Micozzi MS, et al. A prospective study of the development of breast

cancer in 16,692 women with benign breast disease. Am J Epidemiol 1988;128(3):467–477.

15. Wingo PA, Ory HW, Glusman, et al. The evaluation of the data collection process for a multicenter, population-based case-control design. Am J Epidemiol 1988;128:206–217.

16. Claus EB, Risch N, Thompson WD. Genetic analysis of breast cancer in the cancer and steroid hormone study. Am J Hum Genet 1991;48(2):232–242.

17. Young JL, Percy CL, Asire AJ. Surveillance, epidemiology, and end results: incidence and mortality data, 1973–1977. National Institutes of Health publication no 81-2330. Bethesda, MD: Department of Health and Human Services, 1981.

18. Colditz GA. Epidemiology of breast cancer: findings from the Nurses' Health Study. Cancer 1993;71(suppl 4):1480–1489.

19. Spiegelman D, Colditz GA, Hunter D, Hertzmark E. Validation of the Gail et al. model for predicting individual breast cancer risk. J Natl Cancer Inst 1994;86(8):600–607.

20. Kelsey JL, Gammon MD. The epidemiology of breast cancer. CA 1991;41(3):146–165.

21. Fisher B, Costantino JP, Wickerham DL, et al. Tamoxifen for prevention of breast cancer: report of the National Surgical Adjuvant Breast and Bowel Project P-1 Study. J Natl Cancer Inst 1998;90(18):1371–1388.

22. Benichou J, Gail MH, Mulvihill JJ. Graphs to estimate an individualized risk of breast cancer. J Clin Oncol 1996;14(1):103–110.

23. Benichou J. A computer program for estimating individualized probabilities of breast cancer [published erratum appears in Comput Biomed Res 1994;27(1):81]. Comput Biomed Res 1993;26(4):373–382.

24. Bondy ML, Lustbader ED, Halabi S, et al. Validation of a breast cancer risk assessment model in women with a positive family history. J Natl Cancer Inst 1994;86(8):620–625.

25. Costantino JP, Gail MH, Pee D, et al. Validation studies for models projecting the risk of invasive and total breast cancer incidence. J Natl Cancer Inst 1999;91(18):1541–1548.

26. Gail MH, Benichou J. Validation studies on a model for breast cancer risk [published erratum appears in J Natl Cancer Inst 1994;86(10):803]. J Natl Cancer Inst 1994;86(8):573–575.

27. National Cancer Institute. Breast Cancer Risk Assessment Tool for Health Care Providers. Bethesda, MD: Office of Cancer Communication, National Cancer Institute, 1998. Windows computer program.

28. Madigan MP, Ziegler RG, Benichou J, et al. Proportion of breast cancer cases in the United States explained by well-established risk factors. J Natl Cancer Inst 1995;87:1681–1685.

29. Gail MH, Costantino JP, Bryant J, et al. Weighing the risks and benefits of tamoxifen treatment for preventing breast cancer. J Natl Cancer Inst 1999;91(21):1829–1846.

30. Lynch HT, Lynch J, Conway T, et al. Hereditary breast cancer and family cancer syndromes. World J Surg 1994;18(1):21–31.

31. Claus EB, Risch N, Thompson WD. The calculation of breast cancer risk for women with a first-degree family history of ovarian cancer. Breast Cancer Res Treat 1993;28(2):115–120.

32. Claus EB, Schildkraut J, Iversen ESJ, et al. Effect of BRCA1 and BRCA2 on the association between breast cancer risk and family history. J Natl Cancer Inst 1998;90(23):1824–1829.

33. Vogel VG. High-risk populations as targets for breast cancer prevention trials. Prev Med 1991;20(1):86–100.

34. Hoffee PA. Quick look genetics USMLE step 1: A visually oriented review. Madison, CT: Fence Creek Publishing, 1999.

35. Easton DF, Bishop DT, Ford D, Crockford GP. Genetic linkage analysis in familial breast and ovarian cancer: results from 214 families. The Breast Cancer Linkage Consortium. Am J Hum Genet 1993;52(4):678–701.

36. Ford D, Easton DF, Bishop DT, et al. Risks of cancer in BRCA1-mutation carriers. Breast Cancer Linkage Consortium. Lancet 1994;343(8899):692–695.

37. Struewing JP, Hartge P, Wacholder S, et al. The risk of cancer associated with specific mutations of BRCA1 and BRCA2 among Ashkenazi Jews. New Engl J Med 1997;336(20):1401–1408.

38. Newman B, Mu H, Butler LM, et al. Frequency of breast cancer attributable to BRCA1 in a population-based series of American women. JAMA 1998;279(12):915–921.

39. Schubert EL, Lee MK, Mefford HC, et al. BRCA2 in American families with four or more cases of breast or ovarian cancer: recurrent and novel mutations, variable expression, penetrance, and the possibility of families whose cancer is not attributable to BRCA1 or BRCA2. Am J Hum Genet 1997;60(5):1031–1040.

40. Serova OM, Mazoyer S, Puget N, et al. Mutations in BRCA1 and BRCA2 in breast cancer families: are there more breast cancer-susceptibility genes? Am J Hum Genet 1997;60(3):486–495.

41. Ford D, Easton DF, Stratton M, et al. Genetic heterogeneity and penetrance analysis of the

BRCA1 and *BRCA2* genes in breast cancer families. The Breast Cancer Linkage Consortium. Am J Hum Genet 1998;62(3):676–689.

42. Miki Y, Swensen J, Shattuck-Eidens D. A strong candidate for the breast and ovarian cancer susceptibility gene *BRCA1*. Science 1994;266:66–71.

43. Wooster R, Bignell G, Lancaster J, et al. Identification of the breast cancer susceptibility gene *BRCA2* [published erratum appears in Nature 1996;379(6567):749]. Nature 1995;378(6559): 789–792.

44. Parent ME, Ghadirian P, Lacroix A, Perret C. The reliability of recollections of family history: implications for the medical provider. J Cancer Educ 1997;12(2):114–120.

45. Love RR, Evans AM, Josten DM. The accuracy of patient reports of a family history of cancer. J Chron Dis 1985;38(4):289–293.

46. Berry DA, Parmigiani G, Sanchez J, et al. Probability of carrying a mutation of breast-ovarian cancer gene *BRCA1* based on family history . J Natl Cancer Inst 1997;89(3):227–238.

47. Easton DF, Ford D, Bishop DT. Breast and ovarian cancer incidence in *BRCA1*-mutation carriers. Breast Cancer Linkage Consortium. Am J Hum Genet 1995;56(1):265–271.

48. Easton DF, Steele L, Fields P, et al. Cancer risks in two large breast cancer families linked to *BRCA2* on chromosome 13q12-13. Am J Hum Genet 1997;61(1):120–128.

49. Ford D, Easton D. The genetics of breast and ovarian cancer. Br J Cancer 1995;72:805–812.

50. Andersen TI. Genetic heterogeneity in breast cancer susceptibility. Acta Oncol 1996;35(4): 407–410.

51. Biesecker BB, Boehnke M, Calzone K, et al. Genetic counseling for families with inherited susceptibility to breast and ovarian cancer [published erratum appears in JAMA 1993;270(7): 832]. JAMA 1993;269(15):1970–1974.

52. Hopwood P. Psychological issues in cancer genetics: current research and future priorities. Patient Educ Couns 1997;32(1–2):19–31.

53. Kash KM. Psychosocial and ethical implications of defining genetic risk for cancers. Ann N Y Acad Sci 1995;768:41–52.

54. Lerman C, Croyle RT. Emotional and behavioral responses to genetic testing for susceptibility to cancer. Oncology (Huntingt) 1996;10(2): 191–195, 199.

55. Statement of the American Society for Clinical Oncology: genetic testing for cancer susceptibility. J Clin Oncol 1996;14:1730–1736.

56. Hoskins KF, Stopfer JE, Calzone KA, et al. Assessment and counseling for women with a family history of breast cancer: a guide for clinicians. JAMA 1995;273(7):577–585.

57. Peters JA, Stopfer JE. Role of the genetic counselor in familial cancer. Oncology (Huntingt) 1996;10(2):159–166, 175.

58. Giardiello FM. Genetic testing in hereditary colorectal cancer. JAMA 1997;278:1278–1281.

59. Severin M. Genetic susceptibility for specific cancers. Cancer 1999;86(8):1744–1749.

60. Severin MJ. Hereditary cancer litigation: a status report. Oncology (Huntingt) 1996;10(2):211–214.

61. National Cancer Institute. Cancer risk communication: what we know and what we need to learn. NCI Monogr 1999;XX:25

62. Rebbeck TR. Inherited genetic predisposition in breast cancer: a population-based perspective. Cancer 1999;86(suppl 8):1673–1681.

5

Clinical Characteristics of Genetically Determined Ovarian Cancer

Patricia A. Shaw, Michael T. Deavers, and Gordon B. Mills

Ovarian cancer is the fifth most common cancer in women and is the most common cause of death from gynecologic malignancies. The observation of familial clustering of ovarian cancer, often in association with breast cancer or with bowel and endometrial cancer, indicated that a subgroup of patients with ovarian cancer likely carried germ-line genetic mutations predisposing to the development of ovarian cancer. Over the last decade it has become clear that germ-line inheritance of a number of different genetic mutations predispose to the development of ovarian cancer, often in association with other forms of cancer.

Predisposition to Sex Cord–Stromal Tumors

A number of inherited disorders predispose to sex cord–stromal neoplasia. Peutz-Jegher syndrome is an autosomal dominant disorder associated with diverse types of ovarian tumors, which are, however, usually benign sex cord–stromal tumors. A rare tumor, sex cord tumor with annular tubules, occurs with an increased frequency in this syndrome. Women with the autosomal dominant basal cell nevus syndrome (Gorlin syndrome) develop ovarian fibromas, a form of sex cord–stromal tumors. Despite predisposing to sex cord–stromal tumors, neither Peutz-Jegher nor Gorlin syndrome, however, appears to increase the risk of the more common epithelial types of ovarian cancer.

Predisposition to Epithelial Ovarian Cancer

Risk factors for the development of epithelial ovarian cancer include nulliparity, early menarche, late menopause, and a family history of ovarian or breast cancer. Multiparity and oral contraceptive use are associated with a diminished risk. The spectrum of predisposing factors has led to the theory that "incessant ovulation" is critical to the development of epithelial ovarian cancer. Ovulation may lead to repeated injury and repair of the ovarian surface epithelium (OSE), the presumed cell of origin for the majority of epithelial ovarian cancers. This injury or repair process may result in the proliferation of the surface epithelium, leading to the accumulation of somatic mutations in genes contributing to the development of ovarian cancer. Indeed, frequent ovulation is associated with an increased incidence of mutations in *p53* in subsequent ovarian cancers (1). The incidence of ovarian cancer is higher in the United States and other industrialized countries than elsewhere in the world, suggesting a role for as yet unidentified environmental or dietary factors. The spectrum of mutations observed in *p53* in ovarian cancer more closely reflects those which would be expected to accumulate from random mutation than those which would be expected if a specific toxin or toxins such as those contained in cigarette smoke were a causal factor.

Women with a family history of epithelial ovarian cancer are three to four times more likely to develop epithelial ovarian cancer compared with the general population. To what extent this reflects an inherited abnormality in specific cancer-predisposition genes, environmental or lifestyle factors, or clustering of cases remains to be fully determined. However, it is clear that a significant proportion of the risk is due to a germ-line inheritance of abnormalities in cancer-predisposition genes. Germ-line cancer-predisposition genes can be divided into those which are relatively rare and demonstrate a high penetrance and those which are relatively common but demonstrate a low penetrance. The rare, high-penetrance cancer-predisposition genes responsible for a hereditary predisposition to ovarian cancer are being identified and characterized rapidly. However, the potential spectrum of relatively common, low-penetrance genes that likely predispose to the development of ovarian cancer have proven recalcitrant to analysis. Further, whether this family of genes contributes directly to the development of ovarian cancer or modifies the activity of the rare, high-penetrance ovarian cancer–predisposition genes requires further evaluation.

At least 5% to 10% of epithelial ovarian carcinoma cases result from the inheritance of specific abnormalities in rare, highly penetrant cancer-predisposition genes (2–4). Epidemiologic and, more recently, genetic evidence has indicated that there are at least two hereditary epithelial ovarian cancer syndromes: hereditary breast/ovarian cancer (HBOC) syndrome and hereditary non-polyposis colorectal cancer (HNPCC) syndrome.

Hereditary Breast/Ovarian Cancer Syndrome

The hereditary breast/ovarian cancer (HBOC) syndrome, which accounts for at least 75% of all hereditary ovarian cancer cases, is characterized by an increased frequency of ovarian and breast cancers in family members (4–9). In many high-risk families, both breast and ovarian cancer can be documented in the same individual. The HBOC syndrome appears to be a consequence of inherited mutations in two different genes, *BRCA1* on chromosome 17q21 and *BRCA2* on chromosome 13q12-13, with mutations in *BRCA1*

being the more prevalent. Families with abnormalities in *BRCA2* may demonstrate an increased frequency of male breast cancer and, potentially, pancreatic cancer. Mutations in *BRCA1* and *BRCA2* are relatively rare, afflicting approximately 1 in 500 individuals. However, due to founder mutations in *BRCA1* and *BRCA2*, the HBOC syndrome is observed more frequently in individuals of Ashkenazi Jewish descent. A third syndrome, site-specific ovarian cancer syndrome, has been proposed because studies have identified families with multiple cases of ovarian cancer in the absence of breast or bowel cancer. Identification of subsequent cases of breast cancer in some of the potential site-specific ovarian cancer families on follow-up called into question the existence of this syndrome as a separate entity. Further, genetic linkage analysis of these families indicated that most of these families are linked to *BRCA1*, and thus their cancers are likely due to inherited mutations in *BRCA1* (10). A recent study (11) reported 8 cases of ovarian cancer in one Ashkenazi Jewish family without an identified case of breast cancer. The 8 patients all carried a 185delAG mutation in *BRCA1*, one of the so-called "founder" mutations of *BRCA1* in Jewish women. It is likely, therefore, that site-specific ovarian cancer is a variant of HBOC syndrome rather than a separate syndrome. The modifying effects that determine the relative spectrum of breast and ovarian cancer in a family have not been fully characterized but could represent specific mutations in *BRCA1* or *BRCA2*. Alternatively, this may reflect modifying effects of other genes. While there remains a possibility that other high-penetrance cancer-predisposition genes account for a small proportion (10%) of the predisposition to breast and ovarian cancer, mutations of these aberrant genes, if they exist, are rare.

The incidence of ovarian cancer is significantly lower than for breast cancer in carriers of abnormalities in *BRCA1* and, particularly, *BRCA2*. Early studies of high-risk families indicated that the penetrance of both *BRCA1* and *BRCA2* for breast and ovarian cancer was high. These studies may have been biased as a result of analysis of the high-risk families used to identify *BRCA1* and *BRCA2*. Indeed, original consortium analyses suggested that the risk of a carrier of an abnormality in *BRCA1* developing ovarian cancer was as high as 30% by age 60 and 63% by age 70 (12,13). More recent analysis suggests that the risk is likely to be much lower, peaking at between 30% and 50% (14). The estimated likelihood of developing ovarian cancer for carriers of an abnormality in *BRCA2* is approximately 0.4% by age 50, 7% to 10% by age 60, and 18% to 27% by age 70 (15,16). Mutations in *BRCA1* seem to impart a much greater risk of developing ovarian cancer than do mutations in *BRCA2*.

The clinical expression of *BRCA1* and *BRCA2* mutations varies from family to family potentially due to different degrees of penetrance related to the specific mutation present. However, the effects also can differ within families, suggesting the influence of other genes on the *BRCA1* and *BRCA2* phenotype or possibly of environmental or hormonal effects. Epidemiologic studies originally suggested that there may be two groups of *BRCA1* mutation carriers: one group in which there is a high penetrance of ovarian cancer with an incidence of 84% by age 70 and a second group in which there is a lower penetrance with a risk of ovarian cancer of 32% by age 70 (12). Whether this distinction will be confirmed by analysis based on specific mutations in *BRCA1* or *BRCA2* remains to be determined. While mutations in both *BRCA1* and *BRCA2* are dispersed throughout the genes, some studies have suggested that the location of the mutation may influence the risk of developing ovarian cancer. In these studies, mutations within the 3′ end of the *BRCA1* gene were associated with a lower risk of ovarian cancer than mutations in the other two-thirds of the gene (17,18). This association has not been confirmed in subsequent studies. A high proportion of carriers of mutations in *BRCA2* who develop ovarian cancer have mutations clustered in the middle third of exon 11 bordered by nucleotides 3035 and 6629, an area that has been designated as the *ovarian cancer cluster region* (15). A more recent study exhibited similar findings but with wide confidence intervals (16). The data suggest that the penetrance of the *BRCA1* and *BRCA2* hereditary ovarian cancer–predisposition genes is modified by a number of factors, including the specific genetic lesion.

The risk of developing ovarian cancer appears to be increased when carriers of abnormalities in *BRCA1* also carry rare alleles of the *HRAS1* variable number of tandem repeats (VNTR) polymorphism (19). This may represent a relatively common, low-penetrance cancer-predisposing gene.

Narod and colleagues (20) reported that the risk of developing ovarian cancer in women with mutations in *BRCA1* is influenced by reproductive factors. The incidence of ovarian cancer decreased with increasing age at last childbirth and increased with increasing parity. This latter observation is in contrast to that observed in the general population. Recent evidence suggests that oral contraceptive use, a protective factor in the general population, also decreases the risk of ovarian cancer in both *BRCA1* and *BRCA2* carriers. A case-control study of 207 women with hereditary ovarian cancer carrying a pathogenic mutation in either *BRCA1* or *BRCA2* and 161 sister control women demonstrated that oral contraceptive therapy protected against ovarian cancer, with an odds ratio of 0.5 for carriers of *BRCA1* mutations and an odds ratio of 0.4 for carriers of *BRCA2* mutations (21). This finding demonstrates that the penetrance of mutations in *BRCA1* and *BRCA2* is altered by the hormonal or ovulatory environment and provides a "proof of principle" for chemoprevention of ovarian cancer in high-risk patients. However, the effect of oral contraceptive use on the risk of breast cancer in *BRCA1* carriers must be clarified. Indeed, in one study, oral contraceptive use was associated with an increased risk of breast cancer in Ashkenazi Jewish carriers of mutations in *BRCA1* and *BRCA2* (22).

BRCA1 and *BRCA2* Mutations in Sporadic Ovarian Cancers

Cancer-predisposition genes (such as *p53*) demonstrate a high frequency of somatic mutations in sporadic tumors. Thus an understanding of the function of cancer-predisposition genes is expected to contribute to an improved comprehension of the molecular events in sporadic tumors. Sporadic ovarian cancers exhibit a high frequency of loss of heterozygosity

(LOH) at chromosome 17q21 leading to the expectation that *BRCA1* mutations also would be frequent in nonfamilial cases of ovarian cancer. However, somatic mutations in sporadic, nonfamilial cases of ovarian cancer are rare. This suggests that the frequent allele loss at chromosome 17q21 in ovarian cancer is not entirely due to *BRCA1* mutations but indicates the involvement of another tumor-suppressor gene(s). Testing for *BRCA1* mutations in tumor samples from unselected, sporadic cases of ovarian cancer in three separate studies found *BRCA1* mutations in only 4% of the cases. Matsushima found 4 germ-line mutations but no somatic mutations in 76 apparently sporadic Japanese ovarian cancer patients (23). Takahashi found *BRCA1* mutations in 7 of 115 unselected ovarian tumor tissues, all of which were present in the germ-lines of patients who had germ-line mutations and with significant family histories (24). Stratton and colleagues found probable germ-line mutations in 13 of 374 women who were diagnosed with ovarian carcinoma before age 70 (25). These authors reported a laboratory sensitivity of 70% and therefore estimated the incidence of *BRCA1* germ-line mutations in ovarian cancer to be approximately 5% in a heterogeneous population, a figure that corresponds well to the prevalence of mutations estimated by Ford and colleagues (13). Although the patients of Ford and colleagues were not selected for family history, 9 of 12 women with truncating mutations had a family history of breast and/or ovarian cancer. Recent publications identified germ-line mutations in approximately 8% to 10% of unselected ovarian cancers (26,27).

Prevalence of Mutations in *BRCA1* and *BRCA2*

The distribution and prevalence of mutations differ among ethnic groups, with specific "founder" mutations being seen in particular populations (28–33). A 2804delAA *BRCA1* mutation has not been reported outside the Netherlands (34). Nine families in Iceland have been found to have the same *BRCA2* mutation (35). The French-Canadian population also has been shown to express common founder mutations, including the *BRCA1* C4446T and the *BRCA2* 8765delAG mutations (35a). The carrier rate for abnormalities in *BRCA1* and *BRCA2* in the Ashkenazi Jewish population is probably over 2%, 5 to 10 times higher than that of other populations in North America and Europe (30,32,33). There are three important founder mutations that predispose to ovarian cancer in Ashkenazi Jewish women: two in *BRCA1* (185delAG and 5382insC) (30,31) and one in *BRCA2* (6174delT) (36). The *BRCA2* mutation (6174delT) is particularly prevalent among carriers, present in 1.3% of all Ashkenazi Jewish women (32,33). In the Jewish population, a significant proportion of all cases of ovarian cancer are associated with mutations in *BRCA1* or *BRCA2*. Indeed, the 185delAG mutation may account for 35% to 40% of early-onset ovarian cancers (under age 50 years) in Jewish women (13,37).

Ovarian Cancer in the Hereditary Nonpolyposis Colorectal Cancer Syndrome

The hereditary nonpolyposis colorectal cancer (HNPCC) syndrome, also known as Lynch syndrome II, is characterized by a family history of bowel cancer in the absence of polyps, endometrial cancer, and a number of other cancers, including epithelial ovarian cancer, other gastrointestinal cancers, and cancers of the upper urologic tract (38). A number of different criteria have been used to identify families with a likelihood of carrying abnormalities in the DNA mismatch repair genes predisposing to HNPCC. As compared with the original Amsterdam criteria, which failed to identify a significant proportion of high-risk families, the current National Institutes of Health (NIH) criteria of a family history of three or more first-degree relatives with colorectal and/or endometrial cancer, with at least two of the cancers occurring at an age of less than 50 years (38), appears more suited to the identification of high-risk families. Colon tumors arising in HNPCC syndrome patients are associated with genetic mutations in genes that control DNA mismatch recognition and repair, with more than 90% of all mutations occurring in either *hMSH2* or *hMLH1*. In colorectal tumors of patients with the HNPCC syndrome, microsatellite instability occurs as a consequence of inherited mutations in the DNA mismatch repair genes. Strikingly, microsatellite instability is also frequent in sporadic bowel cancers, suggesting a similar etiology for sporadic and HNPCC-related bowel cancers.

A small percentage (3%–15%) (5,39) of hereditary ovarian cancers are a component of the HNPCC syndrome. The risk of ovarian cancer in HNPCC family members is three to four times that in the general population, with a lifetime risk of approximately 5%. In contrast to colonic tumors, microsatellite instability is relatively uncommon in both hereditary and sporadic ovarian cancers and occurs with equal frequency in hereditary and sporadic ovarian cancers (40). Mutations of *hMSH2* and *hMLH1* were found rarely in ovarian cancers, even when microsatellite instability was observed. Further, the patterns of microsatellite instability, when present, appear to be different from those in bowel cancers (40). Taken together, the role that mutations in the DNA mismatch genes play in both hereditary and sporadic ovarian cancers is unclear, and further, when ovarian cancers occur as part of the HNPCC syndrome, a different mutation in the mismatch repair genes may be responsible as compared with families where ovarian cancer is not part of the HNPCC syndrome.

Age at Onset

The presence of a germ-line mutation in a cancer-susceptibility gene may affect the relative importance of cofactors in the initiation and promotion of the cancer and influence the sensitivity to carcinogens, possibly accelerating the carcinogenesis. Since a minimum of five separate genetic mutations are required in a single cell for the development of most common cancers, patients with an inherited germ-line abnormality may require fewer somatic mutations for the development of a cancer. Mutations in DNA mismatch repair genes and possibly in *BRCA1* and *BRCA2* may contribute directly to genetic instability. These factors could contribute to patients carrying germ-line mutations developing cancers at a younger age than that observed for those with sporadic cancers.

For example, in patients with HNPCC syndrome, colon cancer patients present at a mean age of 44 years and those with endometrial cancer at 40 years, both significantly younger than the age at onset in unselected populations (38). Breast cancer presents at an earlier age in patients with abnormalities in *BRCA1* and *BRCA2* than in sporadic breast cancer patients (mean, 42.8 versus 62.9 years) (41). Similarly, the age at onset for *BRCA1*-associated ovarian cancers appears to be earlier than for sporadic cancers, although the evidence for the difference in age at presentation between hereditary ovarian cancer and sporadic ovarian cancer is not as clear-cut as it is for breast cancer. Reports from the Gilda Radner Familial Ovarian Cancer Registry have shown that if there are at least two cases of ovarian cancer in first-degree relatives, ovarian cancer presents at a younger age than in the general population (42,43), with a mean age at diagnosis of 54.4 years in patients with two affected first-degree relatives and 52.1 years in patients with three or more affected first-degree relatives as compared with 60.8 years in the control group. Other studies of familial clusters have shown similar findings.

In patients with only one first-degree relative with ovarian cancer, no difference in age at onset was detected (44,45). However, Bewtra and colleagues (5) reported, the mean age at diagnosis of HOBC (defined in his report as families with two or more cases of breast/ovarian cancer) to be 50 years compared with 59 years in the control group. Two families with apparent site-specific ovarian cancer had a mean age at diagnosis of 56 years. In support of a contention that early ovarian cancers are more likely to be due to an effect of a germ-line mutation, when unaffected women have one first-degree relative with ovarian cancer, the likelihood of eventually developing ovarian or breast cancer is greater with a younger age at onset of the affected relative (45,46). Even women with only one first-degree relative with ovarian cancer diagnosed at a young age may be at increased risk (46). Thus presentation of ovarian cancer at a younger age appears to be more likely in hereditary ovarian cancer. When a germ-line mutation of *BRCA1* is documented in an individual patient, there does appear to be an unequivocal earlier age at onset regardless of family history, with the average age of diagnosis reported as 48 to 53 years (25,34,47,48). In a population-based study, Risch and colleagues (27) reported an average age at diagnosis for *BRCA1*-associated ovarian carcinomas of 50.2 years compared with 56.2 years in patients with no detected mutations.

The age at onset in patients with mutations in other ovarian cancer–predisposition genes has only been assessed in a small number of patients. Ovarian cancers also appear to present at an earlier age in patients with inherited abnormalities in the HNPCC-predisposition genes, since the seven patients assessed had a mean age of 41 years (5). In contrast, mutations in *BRCA2* have not been associated with an earlier onset of ovarian cancer, and evidence suggests that unlike most hereditary cancers, such cancers occur at a later age. In the study by Risch and colleagues (27), the average age at onset for patients with *BRCA2* mutations was 59.9 years.

If age at diagnosis of ovarian cancer in an affected relative was before 45 years, the relative risk of developing ovarian cancer is 14.2 (45). In contrast, a proband with only one first-degree relative affected after age 45 has a relative risk of between 2.8 to 4.3 for developing ovarian cancer. Once again, these observations are compatible with ovarian cancer occurring at an earlier age in patients with germ-line abnormalities in *BRCA1* or *BRCA2*.

Histology

Overview

The majority of ovarian cancers are epithelial tumors, presumably derived from the ovarian surface epithelium, epithelial inclusions, or cysts. However, there is both epidemiologic and genetic evidence that at least some endometrioid and clear cell ovarian cancers may arise in endometriotic implants on the ovary (49). Serous carcinomas account for approximately 50% of sporadic epithelial ovarian carcinomas, endometrioid 20% to 25%, clear cell 5% to 10%, and mucinous 5% to 10%. Less common histologic types include transitional cell carcinomas, carcinosarcomas, and undifferentiated carcinomas. These rare types account for 5% to 15% of all primary ovarian cancers. Epithelial ovarian tumors are further categorized as benign, borderline, or invasive. Serous,

endometrioid, clear cell, and mucinous carcinomas all have benign and borderline counterparts. Borderline (tumors of low malignant potential, atypically proliferating tumors) ovarian tumors are most commonly of serous type, followed by mucinous and, rarely, endometrioid or clear cell histology. Borderline tumors show cellular proliferation combined with cytologic features of low-grade malignancy but no evidence of stromal invasion. The distinction between mucinous borderline tumors and invasive carcinomas can be problematic and is further confounded by the inclusion of non-invasive mucinous carcinomas in the invasive carcinoma category in many North American centers but few European centers. Therefore, conclusions about histologic type in reports without centralized pathology review may be misleading.

Most epidemiologic studies of epithelial ovarian cancers group together the variety of different histologic types, but one cannot assume that epithelial ovarian cancers with different histologies necessarily share a common etiology. Three ovarian cancer studies that evaluated risk associations with parity and oral contraceptive use have demonstrated protective associations for serous and endometrioid tumors but not for mucinous tumors (50–52). In an Ontario-based case-control study, Risch demonstrated that parity and oral contraceptive use were protective for nonmucinous tumors but not for mucinous tumors and that saturated fat intake appeared to convey increased risk in patients with mucinous tumors compared with nonmucinous tumors (53). Use of noncontraceptive estrogens was associated with an increased risk of serous carcinomas ($p = 0.018$) and particularly endometrioid carcinomas ($p = 0.0041$). The hypothesis that the various histologic types of tumors may have different etiologies is also supported by studies of genetic abnormalities in tumors where mutations in *RAS* are much more common in borderline tumors and mucinous invasive tumors than in nonmucinous tumors (54).

Histology of Ovarian Cancers in High-Risk Families

Early studies of familial ovarian cancer demonstrated a trend toward a predominance of serous histology, with disproportionately few mucinous, endometrioid, or clear cell cancers. The Gilda Radner Familial Ovary Cancer Registry reported a high proportion of serous adenocarcinoma, and only 1.4% of the familial ovarian cancers were of the mucinous type compared with the 5% to 10% mucinous tumors predicted by SEER data (42). Recent studies (2,4,5) have confirmed that the majority of ovarian cancers in high-risk families are of serous histology.

Histology of Ovarian Cancer in Carriers of Mutations in BRCA1 and BRCA2

A compilation of reported cases of ovarian cancer arising in carriers of mutations in *BRCA1* showed that 138 of 155 (88.4%) are serous tumors, 5 of 155 (3%) are mucinous, 4 of 155 (2.6%) are undifferentiated, and 6 of 155 (3.8%) are endometrioid (23–25,34,47,48,55). Most of the series do not describe a centralized unbiased review by a gynecologic pathologist, so the classification of some of these cancers may be questioned. One study did report a blinded histologic review and found all 30 of the *BRCA1* cases and all 9 of the *BRCA2* cases to be invasive serous carcinomas (56). Risch and colleagues (27) found that women with both serous histology and a first-degree relative with ovarian cancer had a 25% frequency of *BRCA1* mutations. Mutations of either *BRCA1* or *BRCA2* were observed in 14% of all invasive serous carcinomas (27).

A more systematic pathology review is required to further qualify the histology of ovarian cancers arising in patients with germ-line mutations in *BRCA1* and *BRCA2*, but evidence to date indicates that serous carcinoma is the predominant histologic type. It is thus possible that germ-line mutations in *BRCA1* and *BRCA2* do not predispose to the development of tumors of mucinous, clear cell, or endometrioid histology.

Relatively few other histopathologic features have been documented in hereditary ovarian cancers. Bewtra and colleagues, in addition to assessing histologic type, documented grade, nuclear grade, nuclear pleomorphism, macronuclei, mitotic count, and number of abnormal mitoses (5). The only significant findings in addition to the aforementioned differences in

histologic type was the presence of more abnormal mitotic figures in patients with hereditary ovarian cancer compared with patients sporadic cancers. There was a trend toward higher-grade tumors (25% versus 3%), but the grading system in this paper was not specified, and there were only 3% grade 3 tumors in the control group, a figure that is very low compared with most studies of ovarian cancer. Johannsson and colleagues (55) reported a predominance of grade 3 tumors and an increased mitotic count in a report that included 13 patients with ovarian cancer with demonstrated mutations in *BRCA1*. The data must be considered preliminary owing to the small number of patients assessed, but it seems likely that ovarian cancers arising in association with germ-line mutations in *BRCA1* or *BRCA2* will be predominantly high grade, similar to what has already been documented for breast cancers in individuals with germ-line mutations in *BRCA1* (57,58).

Borderline Tumors

Borderline tumors have been consistently underrepresented in series of familial ovarian cancer cases. Schildkraut and Thompson (59) showed no increase in ovarian cancer in family members of patients with borderline tumors. Only 5 of 439 familial ovarian cancers in the Gilda Radner Familial Ovarian Cancer Registry were in the borderline category (42), 2 of 37 familial ovarian cancers in the Creighton Registry (5), and 1 of 31 familial ovarian cancers in an Ontario study (4). The estimated percentage of borderline tumors in unselected series of ovarian cancers is 10% to 15%, so these tumors are clearly underrepresented in individuals with abnormalities in *BRCA1*. In studies where the histologic type is defined, 5 borderline tumors, 3 serous (48) and 2 mucinous (25,48), have been described in association with *BRCA1* mutations, accounting for approximately 3% of the cases described. Patients present, on average, with borderline ovarian tumors a decade younger than those with invasive ovarian cancer. Because women referred to familial ovarian cancer clinics tend to be young, an increased incidence rather than a decreased incidence of borderline tumors would be anticipated. Thus, although borderline tumors have been reported to occur in individuals with germ-line abnormalities in *BRCA1*, they appear to be underrepresented.

It is of interest to note that ductal carcinoma in situ (DCIS) is seen less frequently in patients with hereditary breast cancer as compared with those with sporadic tumors (60). DCIS is believed to be a key step in tumor progression in breast cancer, suggesting that breast carcinomas that arise in individuals with abnormalities in *BRCA1* have a brief subclinical in situ phase or skip the in situ phase entirely. There is no well-defined model of tumor progression in ovarian cancer. Further, molecular genetics studies have demonstrated that serous invasive ovarian cancers do not have an obligatory borderline precursor (61). Borderline tumors, however, may be precursors to at least some invasive ovarian cancers (62). The paucity of borderline tumors in patients with abnormalities in *BRCA1* or *BRCA2* suggests either that borderline tumors are not a part of the spectrum of the syndrome or that, similar to DCIS, there may be a more rapid transition from borderline tumors to invasive ovarian cancer. Alternatively, borderline tumors may not be a precursor of invasive ovarian cancer in individuals with abnormalities in *BRCA1* or *BRCA2*.

Histology of Ovarian Cancer in Patients with the HNPCC Syndrome

Little is reported, yet, on the ovarian cancers that occur in HNPCC syndrome patients. Bewtra and colleagues (5) reported the histology of four HNPPC associated ovarian cancers: two clear cell carcinomas and one serous carcinoma (the type of the fourth was not specified), with all four of the tumors being low-grade or borderline tumors, an unusual finding in sporadic ovarian cancers. These numbers are much too small to draw conclusions, but it seems that serous carcinomas, the most common type of ovarian cancer, may not occur as frequently in the HNPCC–ovarian cancer syndrome as in sporadic tumors.

Importance of Histology in Assessment of Family History

Taken together, the data suggests that patients or families with nonserous histology or borderline tumors have a low risk of carrying a *BRCA1* or *BRCA2* germ-line mutation. Further, due to its relative rarity compared with breast cancer, ovarian cancer is a defining marker for the HBOC syndrome. In addition, historical recall of ovarian cancer, in contrast to breast cancer, has a high inaccuracy rate, frequently being confused with other intra-abdominal tumors or metastatic tumors. Hence accurate histology review of all cases of ovarian cancer in a family is critical for accurate risk assessment and genetic counseling.

Potential Precursor Lesions in Prophylactic Oophorectomy Specimens

Small, usually high-grade, carcinoma can present as an incidental finding in patients who have no clinical evidence of an ovarian lesion and undergo prophylactic oophorectomy. These tiny carcinomas may be only microscopic, a few millimeters in size, without a visible ovarian lesion. Most have been located in the superficial ovarian cortex, often with surface involvement. Bell and Scully (63) described 14 cases of early de novo ovarian carcinoma (mean age, 50 years), documenting that at least a subset of ovarian carcinomas arise in the absence of an apparent precursor lesion. Four women had first-degree relatives with ovarian and/or breast cancer; family history was unavailable on the remaining patients, and *BRCA* mutation status was unknown. In a histologic review of prophylactic oophorectomy specimens in 20 patients from 18 HBOC families (7 of whom had *BRCA1* mutations, either by mutation analysis or by linkage studies), Salazar and colleagues (64) found 2 early de novo ovarian carcinomas measuring 7 and 10 mm. Other histologic features also were common in these "cancer-prone" ovaries, including epithelial hyperplasia and atypia and stromal changes that Salazar and colleagues attributed to increased stromal activity. However, as the authors noted, this was not a blinded study, and further investigation is warranted to confirm these findings. Two subsequent studies have not confirmed the existence of distinct histologic phenotype of "high-risk" ovaries (64a, 64b). Nevertheless, these findings do introduce the important concept of a histologic phenotype of cancerprone ovaries in patients without a diagnosis of ovarian cancer. It also strongly suggests that all ovaries from patients undergoing prophylactic oophorectomy should be examined thoroughly histologically, and this requires that the increased risk of ovarian cancer in these women be communicated to the pathologist responsible for processing the specimen.

Molecular Diagnostics

A number of specific genetic changes have been demonstrated to occur and in some cases correlate with prognosis in sporadic ovarian cancers. The spectrum of additional genetic changes in tumors arising in individuals with abnormalities in *BRCA1* or *BRCA2* has not been studied extensively. Auranen and colleagues (65) reviewed 58 patients with familial ovarian cancer (defined in their study as at least two ovarian carcinoma cases per family). They reported increased percentages of cancers with *HER2/neu/erbB2* overexpression but no difference in *p53* overexpression or DNA aneuploidy as compared with sporadic tumors. Johannsson and colleagues (55) reported an increased frequency of overexpression of the *HER2/neu/erbB2* protooncogene and overexpression of the *p53* tumor-suppressor gene as assessed by immunohistochemistry in patients with abnormalities in *BRCA1* or *BRCA2*. Zweemer and colleagues (56) reported that 69% of *BRCA* mutation–associated ovarian cancers demonstrated p53 protein overexpression compared with a control group of 54%, a difference that was not statistically significant. Thus tumors that arise in patients with germ-line abnormalities in *BRCA1* or *BRCA2* may demonstrate a different frequency of associated genetic changes. This suggests that the outcome for these patients may be different from that for patients with sporadic tumors.

Survival

Survival differences have not yet been established definitively for breast or ovarian cancers in HBOC syndrome and specifically in carriers of mutations in *BRCA1* and *BRCA2*. In other syndromes, however, the outcome is different for individuals with inherited abnormalities in specific cancer-predisposition genes as compared

with sporadic cancers. For example, patients with colorectal cancers in HNPCC syndrome families have longer survival than those without HNPCC mutations (38,66–68). The observation of improved outcome in HNPCC syndrome patients is surprising given the adverse location of the tumors in this syndrome (right colon) and does not seem to be due to early detection or to differences in stage at presentation. Thus tumors arising in patients with an abnormality in a cancer-predisposition gene may demonstrate different pathophysiology than sporadic tumors. This could have important consequences for establishing prognosis as well as for selecting the most appropriate therapy for ovarian cancer patients.

Breast cancers that arise in carriers of abnormalities in *BRCA1* tend to demonstrate a higher grade and more frequent aneuploidy and occur in younger women. Although these features would suggest a poorer prognosis if found in sporadic tumors, this has not been demonstrated definitively to be the case in hereditary tumors. In fact, paradoxically, some studies have found survival in *BRCA1-associated* breast cancer patients to be better than for patients with sporadic breast cancers (41,69,70). One reason for this paradox may be the high incidence of medullary carcinoma among *BRCA1* cancers, a histologic type usually associated with a more prolonged survival (58,71). However, in a Swedish study, Johannsson and colleagues (72) reported a survival equal to or worse than their comparison group after correcting for age and calendar year of diagnosis. In a group of Ashkenazi Jewish women, Foulkes and colleagues (73) reported a 5-year disease-free survival of only 68.2% among *BRCA1* mutation carriers compared with 88.7% among noncarriers, suggesting that, at least in this homogeneous group of women, a germ-line *BRCA1* mutation is an adverse prognostic factor.

Early reports of survival in hereditary ovarian cancer are also conflicting. Rubin and colleagues (48) suggested that ovarian cancers in women with abnormalities in *BRCA1* have a favorable survival as compared with women with sporadic cancers. They identified 53 *BRCA1* ovarian carcinomas, and 43 showed serous histology, 37 were grade 3, and 38 were stage III. The median survival for the advanced-stage patients was 77 months, compared with 29 months for the controls. The 5-year survival of the *BRCA1* patients was 60%, and 10-year survival was 42%, rates much higher than for the general population. However, there was no documentation of the treatments received, and acquisition of the test and control cases differed. Furthermore, there was no pathology review for most of the tumors. Perhaps most important, a significant selection bias was introduced into the study because many of the patients survived long enough to be tested for mutations (74–78). However, there has been at least one other study reporting a survival advantage in patients with *BRCA1* mutations, and in this study, the *BRCA1* ovarian cancer cases were compared with age- and treatment-matched controls (47). The 5-year survival rate was 78.6% for the 25 *BRCA1-associated* ovarian cancer patients, the majority of whom were stage III or IV, compared with 30.3% in the control group. Median disease-free interval was 91.43 versus 40.92 months. Aida and colleagues (47) also suggested that response rates to chemotherapy were equal in the two groups but noted that there was a high incidence of complete response in *BRCA1* patients, as determined at second-look laparotomy, albeit in a very low number of patients ($n = 3$). The study patients in this report, however, are all Japanese and therefore represent a homogeneous population. Whether similar favorable outcomes will be demonstrated for different ethnic groups remains to be determined.

Other studies have failed to confirm a survival advantage for ovarian cancer in patients with abnormalities in *BRCA1*. Johannsson and colleagues (72) reported a survival equal to or worse than that of a stage- and age-matched control group, although there did appear to be an initial survival advantage for *BRCA1*-associated ovarian cancers. A study that attempted to eliminate selection bias by excluding probands reported a median survival of 2.6 years in *BRCA1*-associated ovarian cancers and a 10-year survival of 14.9%, rates similar to those of Rubin's control group and to those of other large studies of sporadic tumors (74). Larger, population-based prospective studies are urgently needed to determine whether there are differences in prognosis and potentially in response to specific therapies

in patients with abnormalities in *BRCA1* and *BRCA2* as compared with sporadic tumors.

Management of High-Risk Patients

Unfortunately, most of the ovarian cancers in high-risk patients present with the same vague symptoms or with a pelvic mass, as seen in the general population. There is as yet no evidence to suggest that patients known to be at increased risk for developing ovarian cancer are detected at an earlier stage than the general population. Indeed, as noted earlier, most of the tumors are detected at a late stage.

Early detection of ovarian cancer with serum CA-125 level determinations and/or transvaginal or transabdominal ultrasound has to date not shown these modalities to be effective in screening the general population. Fewer than 50% of stage I ovarian cancers are detected by CA-125 determinations, and there is a high false-positive rate. Transvaginal ultrasound may have a higher true-positive rate, but the false-positive rate and cost remain unacceptably high. However, these screening approaches may result in acceptable positive and negative predictive values when restricted to women with a genetic predisposition to ovarian cancer due to the higher prevalence of disease. An NIH consensus conference suggested that increased surveillance and screening are appropriate in women with a 7% risk of developing ovarian cancer; a risk frequently achieved in high-risk families and in individuals with abnormalities in *BRCA1* and *BRCA2*. Controlled trials are currently ongoing to attempt to determine whether screening will improve outcome in these high-risk individuals.

Because of the failure of current screening modalities to detect ovarian cancers at an early, curable stage and the lack of an effective chemopreventive, one option for high-risk patients is prophylactic oophorectomy. However, there is considerable debate about the value of prophylactic oophorectomy in high-risk patients because there are reports of these patients developing intraperitoneal carcinomatosis after the prophylactic surgery (79,80). Indeed, in a very small study, Streuwing and colleagues (81) suggested that prophylactic oophorectomy only decreased the incidence of intraperitoneal tumors by 50%. Some of these patients may have developed primary peritoneal carcinoma, a carcinoma that histologically resembles ovarian carcinoma but arises in an extra ovarian site. One possibility is that the risk of developing primary peritoneal carcinoma is greatly increased in patients with mutations in *BRCA1* or *BRCA2*. Given the observation of early tumors in ovaries removed during prophylactic oophorectomies described earlier, it is also possible that at least some of the patients had an early undetected ovarian cancer in the excised ovaries that had already spread to the peritoneal cavity. Of 324 women in the Gilda Radner Familial Ovarian Cancer Registry who underwent prophylactic oophorectomy, 1.8% developed peritoneal carcinoma 1 to 27 years after the prophylactic surgery (80). However, the *BRCA1* or *BRCA2* status of the patients undergoing prophylactic oophorectomy is unknown. Nevertheless, given the high lifetime risk for ovarian cancer in these high-risk families, it seems that a high proportion of these patients may have had their cancer prevented by this surgery. Because of the small risk that a clinically undetectable cancer already exists in the ovaries, pathologists must be alerted to this possibility and protocols adopted for the processing of these specimens. Models based on the controversial improved outcome of patients described in the analysis of Rubin and colleagues (48) and using the low level of protection afforded by prophylactic surgery proposed by Streuwing and colleagues (81) suggest that a prophylactic oophorectomy may provide only a minimal increase in survival. However, this study failed to consider an improvement in quality of life. Thus, at this time, definitive evidence regarding the efficacy of prophylactic oophorectomy is sorely lacking. The choice should be left to the patient, fully informed of the data described earlier, but making decisions based on her own family history, stress level, and personal circumstances.

References

1. Schildkraut J, Bastos E, Berchuk A. Relationship between lifetime ovulatory cycles and overexpression of mutant *p53* in epithelial ovarian cancer. J Natl Cancer Inst 1997;89(13):932–938.
2. Greggi S, Genuardi M, Benedetti-Panici P, et al. Analysis of 138 consecutive ovarian cancer patients: incidence and characteristics of familial cases. Gynecol Oncol 1990;39:300–304.
3. Houlston R, Collins A, Slack J, et al. Genetic epidemiology of ovarian cancer: segregation analysis. Ann Hum Genet 1991;55:291–299.
4. Narod S, Madlensky L, Bradley L, et al. Hereditary and familial ovarian cancer in southern Ontario. Cancer 1994;74:2341–2346.
5. Bewtra C, Watson P, Conway T, et al. Hereditary ovarian cancer: a clinicopathological study. Intl J Gynecol Pathol 1992;11:180–187.
6. Easton D, Bishop D, Ford D, et al. Genetic linkage analysis in familial breast and ovarian cancer: results from 214 families. The Breast Cancer Linkage Consortium. Am J Hum Genet 1993;52:678–701.
7. Narod S, Ford D, Devilee P, et al. An evaluation of genetic heterogeneity in 145 breast-ovarian cancer families. Am J Hum Genet 1995;56:254–264.
8. Wooster R, Neuhausen S, Manigion J, et al. Localization of a breast cancer susceptibility gene, *BRCA2*, to chromosome 13q12–13. Science 1994;265:2088–2090.
9. Narod S, Ford D, Devilee P, et al. Genetic heterogeneity of breast-ovarian cancer revisited. Am J Hum Genet 1995;57:957–958.
10. Steichen-Gersdorf E, Gallion H, Ford D, et al. Familial site-specific ovarian cancer is linked to *BRCA1* on 17q12–21. Am J Hum Genet 1994;55:870–875.
11. Liede A, Tonin PN, Sun CC, et al. Is hereditary site-specific ovarian cancer a distinct genetic condition. Am J Med Genet 1998;75(1):55–58.
12. Easton D, Ford D, Bishop D. Breast and ovarian cancer incidence in *BRCA1*-mutation carriers. Am J Hum Genet 1995;56:265–271.
13. Ford D, Easton D, Peto J. Estimates of the gene frequency of *BRCA1* and its contribution to breast and ovarian cancer incidence. Am J Hum Genet 1995;57:1457–1462.
14. Struewing J, Hartge P, Wacholder S, et al. The risk of cancer associated with specific mutations of *BRCA1* and *BRCA1* among Ashkenazi Jews. New Engl J Med 1997;336(20):1401–1408.
15. Gayther S, Mangion J, Russell P, et al. Variation of risks of breast and ovarian cancer associated with different germ-line mutations of the *BRCA2* gene. Nature Genet 1997;15:103–105.
16. Ford D, Easton D, Stratton M, et al. Genetic heterogeneity and penetrance analysis of the *BRCA1* and *BRCA2* genes in breast cancer families. Am J Hum Genet 1998;62:676–689.
17. Gayther S, Warren W, Mazoyer S, et al. Germline mutations of the *BRCA1* gene in breast and

ovarian cancer families provide evidence for a genotype-phenotype correlation. Nature Genet 1995;11:428–433.

18. Holt JT, Thompson ME, Szabo C, et al. Growth retardation and tumor inhibition by *BRCA1*. Nature Genet 1996;12:298–302.

19. Phelan CM, Rebbeck T, Weber B, et al. Ovarian cancer risk in *BRCA1* carriers is modified by the *HRAS1* variable number of tandem repeat (VNTR) locus. Nature Genet 1996;12:309–311.

20. Narod SA, Goldgar D, Cannon-Albright L, et al. Risk modifiers in carriers of *BRCA1* mutations. Int J Cancer 1995;64:394–398.

21. Narod SA, Risch H, Moslehi R, et al. Oral contraceptives and the risk of hereditary ovarian cancer. New Engl J Med 1998 (in press).

22. Ursin G, Henderson BE, Hail RW, et al. Does oral contraceptive use increase the risk of breast cancer in women with *BRCA1/BRCA2* mutations more than in other women. Cancer Res 1997;57:3678–3681.

23. Matsushima M, Kobayashi K, Emi M, et al. Mutations analysis of the *BRCA1* gene in 76 Japanese ovarian cancer patients: four germ-line mutations, but no evidence of somatic mutation. Hum Mol Genet 1995;5(10):1953–1956.

24. Takahashi H, Behbakht K, McGovern P, et al. Mutation analysis of the *BRCA1* gene in ovarian cancers. Cancer Res 1995;55:2998–3002.

25. Stratton J, Gayther S, Russell P, et al. Contribution of *BRCA1* mutations to ovarian cancer. New Engl J Med 1997;336(16):1125–1130.

26. Rubin S, Blackwood M, Bandera C, et al. *BRCA1, BRCA2*, and hereditary nonpolyposis colorectal cancer gene mutations in an unselected ovarian cancer population: relationship of family history and implications for genetic testing. Am J Obstet Gynecol 1998;178:670–677.

27. Risch H, Vesprini D, McLaughlin J, et al. High proportion of germ-line *BRCA1* and *BRCA2* mutations in a population series of ovarian-cancer cases. (submitted).

28. Simard J, Tonin P, Durocher F, et al. Common origins of *BRCA1* mutations in Canadian breast and ovarian cancer families. Nature Genet 1994;8:392–398.

29. Johannsson O, Ostermeyer E, Hakansson S, et al. Founding *BRCA1* mutations in hereditary breast and ovarian cancer in southern Sweden. Am J Hum Genet 1996;58:441–450.

30. Struewing J, Abeliovich D, Peretz T, et al. The carrier frequency of the *BRCA1* 185delAG mutation is approximately 1% in Ashkenazi Jewish individuals. Nature Genet 1995;11:198–200.

31. Fitzgerald M, MacDonald D, Krainer M, et al. Germ-line *BRCA1* mutations in Jewish and non-Jewish women with early-onset breast cancer. New Engl J Med 1996;334:143–149.

32. Roa B, Boyd A, Volcik K, Richards C. Ashkenazi Jewish population frequencies for common mutations in *BRCA1* and *BRCA2*. Nature Genet 1996;14:185–187.

33. Oddoux C, Struewing J, Clayton C, et al. The carrier frequency of the *BRCA2* 6174delT mutation among Ashkenazi Jewish individuals is approximately 1%. Nature Genet 1996;14:188–190.

34. Zweemer R, Verheijen R, Gille J, et al. Clinical and genetic evaluation of thirty ovarian cancer families. Am J Obstet Gynecol 1998;178(1):85–90.

35. Gudmundsson J, Johannesdottir G, Bergthorsson JT, et al. Different tumor types from *BRCA2* mutation carriers show wild-type chromosome deletions on 13q12-13. Cancer Res 1995;55:4830–4832.

35a. Tonin PM, Mes-Masson AM, Narod SA, et al. Founder *BRCA1* and *BRCA2* mutations in French Canadian ovarian cancer cases unselected for family history. Clin Genet 1999;55 (5):318–324.

36. Nuehausen S, Gilewski T, Norton L, et al. Recurrent *BRCA2* 6174delT mutations in Ashkenazi Jewish women affected by breast cancer. Nature Genet 1996;13:126–128.

37. Muto M, Cramer D, Tangir J, et al. Frequency of the *BRCA1* 185delAG mutation among Jewish women with ovarian cancer and matched population controls. Cancer Res 1996;56:1250–1252.

38. Lynch H, Smyrk T, Watson P, et al. Genetics, natural history, tumor spectrum, and pathology of hereditary nonpolyposis colorectal cancer. Gastroenterology 1993;104:1535–1549.

39. Watson P, Lynch H. Extracolonic cancer in herediatary nonpolyposis colorectal cancer. Cancer 1993;71:677–685.

40. Arzimanoglou II, Lallas T, Osborne M, et al. Microsatellite instability differences between familial and sporadic ovarian cancer. Carcinogenesis 1996;17(9):1799–1804.

41. Marcus J, Watson P, Page D, et al. Hereditary breast cancer: pathology, prognostic, and *BRCA1* and *BRCA2* gene linkage. Cancer 1996;77(4):697–709.

42. Piver M, Baker T, Jishi M, et al. Familial ovarian cancer: a report of 658 families from the Gilda Radner Familial Ovarian Cancer Registry, 1981–1991. Cancer 1993;71(suppl 2):582–588.

43. Piver M, Goldberg J, Jishi M, et al. Characteristics of familial ovarian cancer: a report of the first 1000 families in the Gilda Radner Familial Ovarian Cancer Registry. Eur J Obstet Gynaecol 1996;17:169–176.

44. Amos CI, Shaw GL, Tucker MA, Hartge P. Age at onset for familial epithelial ovarian cancer. JAMA 1992;268(14):1896–1899.

45. Houlston R, Bourne T, Collins W, et al. Risk of ovarian cancer and genetic relationship to other cancers in families. Hum Hered 1993; 43:111–115.

46. Goldberg JM, Piver SM, Jishi MF, Blumenson L. Age at onset of ovarian cancer in women with a strong family history of ovarian cancer. Gynecol Oncol 1997;66:3–9.

47. Aida H, Takakuwa K, Nagata H, et al. Clinical features of ovarian cancer in Japanese women with germ-line mutations of *BRCA1*. Clin Cancer Res 1998;4:235–240.

48. Rubin S, Benjamin I, Behbakht K, et al. Clinical and pathological features of ovarian cancer in women with germ-line mutations of *BRCA1*. New Engl J Med 1996;335(19):1413–1416.

49. Jiang X, Morland S, Hitchcock A, et al. Allelotyping of endometriosis with adjacent ovarian carcinoma reveals evidence of a common lineage. Cancer Res 1998;58:1707–1712.

50. Cramer D, Hutchison G, Welch W, et al. Determinants of ovarian cancer risk: I. Reproductive experiences and family history. J Natl Cancer Inst 1983;71:711–716.

51. Kvale G, Heuch I, Nilssen S, et al. Reproductive factors and risk of ovarian cancer: a prospective study. Int J Cancer 1988;42:246–251.

52. Cramer D, Hutchison D, Welch W, et al. Factors affecting the association of oral contraceptives and ovarian cancer. New Engl J Med 1982;307:1047–1051.

53. Risch HA, Marrett LD, Jain M, Howe GR. Differences in risk factors for epithelial ovarian cancer by histologic type: results of a case-study. Am J Epidemiol 1996;144(4):363–372.

54. Mok S, Bell D, Knapp R, et al. Mutation of *K-ras* protooncogene in human ovarian epithelial tumors of borderline malignancy. Cancer Res 1993;53:1489–1492.

55. Johannsson O, Idvall I, Anderson C, et al. Tumor biological features of *BRCA1*-induced breast and ovarian cancer. Eur J Cancer 1997;33(3):362–371.

56. Zweemer R, Shaw P, Verheijen R, et al. *p53* overexpression is a frequent event in ovarian cancers associated with *BRCA1* and *BRCA2* germ-line mutations. J Clin Pathol 1999;52(5):372–375.

57. Marcus JN, Watson P, Page DL, et al. *BRCA2* hereditary breast cancer pathophenotype. Breast Cancer Res Treat 1997;44(3):275–277.

58. Marcus JN, Page DL, Watson P, et al. *BRCA1* and *BRCA2* hereditary breast carcinoma phenotypes. J Am Cancer Soc 1997;80(3):543–556.

59. Schildkraut J, Thompson W. Familial ovarian cancer: a population-based case-control study. Am J Epidemiol 1988;128:456–466.

60. Sun CC, Lenoir G, Lynch H, Narod SA. In-situ breast cancer and *BRCA1*.Lancet 1996;348:408.

61. Berchuk A, Elbendary A, Havrilesky L, et al. Pathogenesis of ovarian cancers. J Soc Gynecol Invest 1994;1(3):181–190.

62. Puls LE, Powell DE, DePriest PD, et al. Transition from benign to malignant epithelium in mucinous and serous ovarian cystadenocarcinoma. Gynecol Oncol 1992;47:53–57.

63. Bell DA, Scully RE. Early de novo ovarian carcinoma: a study of fourteen cases. Cancer 1994;73(7):1859–1864.

64. Salazar H, Godwin A, Daly M, et al. Microscopic benign and invasive malignant neoplasms and a cancer prone phenotype in prophylactic oophorectomy. J Natl Cancer Inst 1996;88(24):1810–1820.

64a. Stratton JF, Buckley CH, Lowe D, Ponder BA. Comparison of prophylactic oophorectomy specimens from carriers and noncarriers of a *BRCA1* or *BRCA2* gene mutation. United Kingdom Coordinating Committee on Cancer Research (UKCCCR) Familial Ovarian Cancer Study Group. J Natl Cancer Inst 1999;91(7):626–628.

64b. Werness BA, Afify AM, Eltabbakh GH, et al. p53, c-erbB, and Ki-67 expression in ovaries removed prophylactically from women with a family history of ovarian cancer. Int J Gynecol Pathol 1999;18(4):338–343.

65. Auranen A, Grenman S, Klemi P-J. Immunohistochemically detected *p53* and *HER-2/neu* expression and nuclear DNA content in familial epithelial ovarian cancer. Cancer 1997; 79(11):2147–2153.

66. Lynch H, Albano W, Recabaren J, et al. Prolonged survival as a component of hereditary breast and nonpolyposis colon cancer. Med Hypotheses 1981;7:1201–1209.

67. Albano WA, Recabaren JA, Lynch HT, et al. Natural history of hereditary cancer of the breast and colon. Cancer 1982;50:360–363.

68. Watson P, Lin K, Rodriguez-Bigas M, et al. Colorectal carcinoma survival in hereditary nonpolyposis colorectal cancer family members. Cancer 1998;83(2):259–266.
69. Garcia-Patino E, Gomendia B, Provencio M, et al. Germ-line *BRCA1* mutations in women with sporadic breast cancer: clinical correlations. J Clin Oncol 1998;16(1):115–120.
70. Porter D, Cohen B, Wallace M, et al. Breast cancer incidence, penetrance and survival in probable carriers of *BRCA1* gene mutation in families linked to *BRCA1* on chromosome 17q12-21. Br J Surg 1994;81:1512–1515.
71. Pathology of familial breast cancer: differences between breast cancers in carriers of *BRCA1* or *BRCA2* mutations and sporadic cases. Breast Cancer Linkage Consortium. Lancet 1997;349(9064):1505–1510.
72. Johannsson OT, Ranstam J, Borg A, Olsson H. Survival of *BRCA1* breast and ovarian cancer patients: a population-based study from southern Sweden. Clin Oncol 1998;16(2):397–404.
73. Foulkes W, Wong N, Brunet J, et al. Germ-line *BRCA1* mutations is an adverse prognostic factor in Ashkenazi Jewish women in breast cancer. Clin Cancer Res 1997;3:2465–2469.
74. Brunet J, Narod S, Tonin P, Foulkes W. *BRCA1* mutations and survival in women with ovarian cancer. New Engl J Med 1997;336(17):1256. Letter.
75. Johannsson O, Ranstam J, Borg A, Olsson H. *BRCA1* mutations and survival in women with ovarian cancer. New Engl J Med 1997; 336:1255–1256. Letter.
76. Modan B. *BRCA1* mutations and survival in women with ovarian cancer. New Engl J Med 1997;336:1255. Letter.
77. Whitmore S. Letter. New Engl J Med 1997; 336:1254–1255.
78. Cannistra S. *BRCA1* mutations and survival in women with ovarian cancer. New Engl J Med 1997;336:1254. Letter.
79. Tobacman J, Tucker M, Kase R, et al. Intraabdominal carcinomatosis after prophylactic oophorectomy in ovarian cancer prone families. Lancet 1982;2:795–797.
80. Piver SM, Jishi MF, Tsukada Y, Nava G. Primary peritoneal carcinoma after prophylactic oophorectomy in women with a family history of ovarian cancer: a report of the Gilda Radner familial ovarian cancer registry. Cancer 1993;71(9):2751–2755.
81. Struewing J, Watson P, Easton D, et al. Prophylactic oophorectomy in inherited breast/ovary cancer families. J Natl Cancer Inst 1995;17: 33–35.

6

Genetic Screening for Ovarian Cancer Risk Assessment

Anita S. Y. Sit and Robert P. Edwards

As our understanding of the link of cancer-susceptibility genes and familial cancer syndrome has improved, the issue of genetic screening has become an integral part of our clinical practice. Providing information for effective screening for hereditary breast and ovarian cancer has become an important role of health care providers. However, the ability to offer appropriate counseling regarding the indications, benefits, and limitations of genetic testing to patients is of equal importance. It has been estimated that 5% to 7% of all breast and ovarian cancer is attributable to autosomal dominant germ-line mutations in the *BRCA1* and *BRCA2* genes (1). Women who inherit a *BRCA1* mutation have an 85% lifetime risk of developing breast cancer, and a 26% to 85% lifetime risk of developing ovarian cancer by age of 70 (1). With the advent of DNA-based testing for *BRCA1* and *BRCA2* mutations, there is the hope of improved outcome via early detection, risk-reduction measures, and well-timed interventions. However, this availability of *BRCA1* and *BRCA2* mutation genetic testing has raised several issues in the context of medical, social, psychological, and ethical implications. The question regarding offering genetic screening to high-risk individuals versus the general population is critical. The information obtained from the testing may lead to unnecessary and overzealous interventions, patient apprehension, and risk for discrimination in employment or insurance eligibility. Health care professionals should provide extensive counseling and a comprehensive approach to patients prior to commitment to testing.

Screening-Test Assessment

For a screening test to be effective, several screening criteria should be fulfilled. The condition of disease must have an asymptomatic period during which detection and treatment significantly reduce morbidity or mortality (2). Early screenings such as bimanual examinations, pelvic ultrasound, and CA-125 levels are aimed at early-stage detection of ovarian cancer in the asymptomatic period. Because of the lack of early symptoms in ovarian cancer, the goals of early screening and detection include probable improved prognosis and less radical treatment. On the other hand, the disadvantages of screening tests include the introduction of false reassurance to patients with false-negative testing and the subsequent decrease in health surveillance of individuals. Furthermore, for a screening test to be cost-effective, the cost of the test should be low, and it should be non-invasive and relatively easy to perform, hence allowing accessible application in a large population to identify high-risk individuals. In addition, the prevalence of disease in the pre-clinical state should be sufficient to justify the cost of screening. In a high-prevalence population such as the hereditary cancer syndromes families, the false-positive rates will decrease, hence improving the positive predictive value of testing. On the contrary, the screening test may not be cost-effective in the general population because of the low prevalence of the disease.

Familial Breast/Ovarian Cancer Syndromes: *BRCA1* and *BRCA2*

Among all the risk factors for the development of ovarian cancer in epidemiologic studies, family history of ovarian cancer is one of the strongest (3). It is currently estimated that 10% of all cases of ovarian cancer are attributable to familial ovarian cancer, whereas the remainder of cases occurs sporadically as a result of somatic mutations of oncogenes or tumor-suppressor genes (1). Familial ovarian cancer was noted to have an autosomal dominant pattern of inheritance (4). The age of onset of disease in these families was relatively early (4). This information further supports the genetic basis of germ-line mutation of ovarian cancer. Most familial ovarian cancer generally presents in the advanced stage of poorly differentiated serous subtypes (4). However, it was reported that familial ovarian cancer was associated with a better survival than the control group of sporadic occurrence (5,6).

Several population-based epidemiologic studies of familial clustering of ovarian cancer provide evidence that familial ovarian cancer is a dominant inheritance genetic disease with variable penetrance. Among the early work of Lynch and colleagues (7,8) in the 1970s, pedigree analysis demonstrated two distinct syndromes involving familial clustering of ovarian cancer: 1) the breast and ovarian cancer syndrome and 2) the hereditary non-polyposis colorectal cancer (HNPCC or Lynch II) syndrome, in which ovarian cancers occur with colorectal and endometrial cancers (9,10). Our understanding of familial ovarian cancer was furthered in the 1980s by the Gilda Radner Familial Ovarian Cancer Registry, in which several hundred families with ovarian cancer were accessioned (4). In the Cancer and Steroid Hormone (CASH) data base, the risk of ovarian cancer in the first-and second-degree relatives of women with ovarian cancer was found to be increased 3.6- and 2.9-fold, respectively, compared with women without a family history (11,12).

In 1990, genetic linkage analysis suggested that alterations in the long arm of chromosome 17 were associated with multiple cases of familial breast cancer (13). In 1994, Narod and colleagues (14) reported, based on linkage analysis studies, a gene on chromosome 17q21 (*BRCA1*) was closely linked to familial transmission of cancer in a given breast-ovarian cancer family. This *BRCA1* gene spans 100 kb on chromosome 17q21; however, the biologic function of the protein encoded by *BRCA1* is yet to be established. Mutations in *BRCA1* yield a prematurely truncated protein product. There is evidence to suggest that *BRCA1* acts as a tumor-suppressor gene despite the autosomal mode of inheritance of familial breast-ovarian cancer. Women who inherit a germ-line mutation of *BRCA1* invariably have lost the function of the normal copy of *BRCA1*. It was thought that the loss of both copies of the *BRCA1* gene initiates tumorigenesis when these women acquire the "second hit" of the mutation (15). As opposed to familial cancer syndromes, this acquired mutation of *BRCA1* does not appear to have a significant role in the development of sporadic ovarian cancers (16,17).

Approximately 75% to 90% of familial ovarian cancer occurrence is attributable to the inherited mutations of *BRCA1*, confirming that *BRCA1* is the gene associated with most breast-ovarian cancer susceptibility (18,19). The lifetime risks of developing breast and ovarian cancers in the carriers of *BRCA1* mutations were approximately 80% to 90% and 30% to 60%, respectively (1). The risk of developing ovarian cancer in affected families rises appreciably after age 30. In families with two or more individuals diagnosed with breast or ovarian cancer, the probability of finding a mutation of *BRCA1* is as high as 80% to 90% (20). However, it is important to interpret these estimated risks with an understanding that most of the studies were performed in selected families with exceedingly high penetrance of inheritance. Caution is recommended in extrapolating these calculations of estimated risk to low-risk individuals.

In 1995, *BRCA2* was identified as the second cancer-susceptibility gene when genetic linkage to chromosome 13q2 was observed in familial breast cancer patients in whom *BRCA1* mutations were not identified (21). The risk of developing ovarian cancer in individuals with *BRCA2* mutations appears to be increased to a lesser extent when compared with those carrying mutations in *BRCA1*. The cumulative risk of developing ovarian cancer is estimated to be approximately 10% by age 70 (22). Furthermore, an increased risk of male breast cancer was associated with *BRCA2* mutation (23).

Among all the different mutations of *BRCA1* and *BRCA2*, some recurrent mutations have reported to occur in a significantly higher frequency in particular ethnic groups. Two distinct deletion mutations, 185 delAG, a *BRCA1* mutation, and 617 delT, a *BRCA2* mutation, were found to occur at a frequency of approximately 1% and 1.4%, respectively in the Ashkenazi Jewish population (24,25). One study showed a 70% relative risk of breast or ovarian cancer in carriers of these deletion mutations in selected Jewish families (26). As many as 90% of the Ashkenazi Jewish families studied with two or more cases of ovarian cancer and two or more cases of early-onset breast cancer carry the *BRCA1* mutation (27). This finding contributes to the concept of *founder mutation*, in which a single mutation is unique to a high-risk ethnic population. Furthermore, it raises the question of universal genetic screening of the specific mutation of *BRCA1* or *BRCA2* by simple methods such as the polymerase chain reaction (PRC) in all Ashkenazi women with a family history. The limitation of specific mutation screening, however, is failure to recognize the existence of other sporadic mutations of *BRCA1* or *BRCA2* (28).

Currently Available Genetic Testing

Both *BRCA1* and *BRCA2* are relatively large genes. There are approximately 100 to 200 genetic mutations that can occur throughout *BRCA1* and *BRCA2* (29). DNA sequencing of the entire gene remains the "gold standard" for mutational testing to screen for all possible mutations. The disadvantage of complete gene sequencing is that it is very labor-intensive and costly. Furthermore, false-negative results are still not completely eliminated because splice-site mutations that lie outside the coding region potentially could be missed during DNA sequencing. Other genetic screening analyses that are less labor-intensive include single-stranded conformation analysis and the protein truncation test. Single-stranded conformation analysis screens mutations that

cause single strands of DNA to migrate abnormally during electrophoresis (30). The limitation of such analysis is the false-positive result of identifying shifted bands that are polymorphisms of the DNA but not disease-causing mutations. The protein truncation test, on the other hand, identifies truncated *BRCA1* and *BRCA2* proteins as a result of the translated RNA mutations (31). Missense mutations that occur in 10% to 15% of all hereditary cases are unlikely to be detected by the protein truncation test (32). In summary, based on the currently available technology, a simple, cost-effective genetic screening test of high specificity and sensitivity for *BRCA1* and *BRCA2* mutations has yet to be established. Furthermore, until there are proven benefits of improved morbidity and mortality from genetic screening, application of such costly genetic screening to the general population remains premature.

Genetic Screening in High-Risk Populations

The frequency of *BRCA1* mutations in the general population is approximately 1 in 800. However, the probability of finding a mutation in *BRCA1* or *BRCA2* in families with two cases of breast cancer and two cases of ovarian cancer is as high as 80% to 90% (20). The lifetime risk of ovarian cancer in women with a positive family history increases from 1.8% to 9.4% (3). Providing genetic counseling and screening for *BRCA1* and *BCRA2* mutations to individuals of families suspected of having increased susceptibility for ovarian cancer has become a very important aspect of clinical practice for oncologists. By identifying the genetic predisposition to ovarian cancer of these high-risk individuals, altered screening and risk-reduction strategies hopefully may improve the outcome for hereditary ovarian cancer syndrome, although this has yet to be proven. Reported risk of *BRCA1* mutation in specific diagnostic scenarios is shown in Table 6-1.

A multidisciplinary approach is the key feature in counseling patients with a significant family history of breast/ovarian cancer. Owing to the multi-faceted nature of genetic testing, which involves cancer risk assessment, cancer prevention, and social and psychological issues,

Table 6-1. Probability of a woman with breast or ovarian cancer bearing *BRCA1* mutation

Age of cancer diagnosis (years)	Probability of a woman bearing *BRCA1* mutation
Single Affected	
Breast CA <30	0.12
Breast CA <40	0.06
Breast CA 40–49	0.03
Ovarian CA <50	0.07
Families	
≥3 cases of breast CA diagnosed <50	0.40
≥2 breast CA with ≥1 ovarian CA	0.82
≥2 breast CA with ≥2 ovarian CA	0.91

Adapted from A Collaborative Survey of 80 Mutations in the *BRCA1* Breast and Ovarian Cancer Susceptibility Gene: Implications for Presymptomatic Testing and Screening. JAMA 1995;273:535–541, and Easton DF, Bishop T, Ford D, Crockford GP, and the Breast Cancer Linkage Consortium. Genetic linkage analysis in familial breast and ovarian cancer; results from 214 families. Am J Hum Genet 1993;52:678–701.

a team approach involving a genetic counselor in a research academic setting is recommended (33). The goals to be achieved during genetic counseling and testing include 1) confirming a strong family history, 2) performing a pedigree analysis to identify the genetic inheritance of the disease, 3) educating individuals about an informed decision to undergo testing, 4) performing genetic screening; 5) assessing the cancer risk of carriers and noncarriers of mutations, 6) presenting the availability of cancer prevention and early cancer detection, and finally, 7) posttest counseling.

With the advent of direct mutation analysis of *BRCA1* and *BRCA2* genes, the cumulative risk of developing ovarian cancer for subjects with *BRCA1* mutations is approximately 63% at age 70 (1). In offering risk assessment to carriers of *BRCA1* mutations, it must be remembered that these risk estimates are drawn from highly selected, population-specific family groups. The risk is most likely to be overestimated when data were derived from studies of families with very high penetrance. A good example is the specific mutations of *BRCA1* and *BRCA2* that occur at high frequency in the Ashkenazi Jewish population (24,25). Risk assessment by mutation analysis would be more meaningful if testing

panels were available specifically for individual ethnic groups.

In performing direct mutation analysis, interpretation of a negative test result (i.e., no known gene mutations are found) could be problematic. First, in selecting individuals within a family for screening, it is of paramount importance to initiate testing in the affected individuals. Once a mutation is identified in a family, specific mutation screening could then be offered to other unaffected individuals for cancer risk estimates (34). The problem arises when the affected individuals are not available for screening. Then, a negative screening test in unaffected individuals does not eliminate the possibility of other undiscovered causative mutations (30). The estimated risk based on evaluation of the pedigree remains unchanged despite this negative test result. In a recently published study by Rubin and colleagues (30), the prevalence of *BRCA1* and *BRCA2* mutations was determined in a large, unselected population of ovarian cancer patients. Eight-four percent of patients with a family history of breast or ovarian cancer tested negative for the known mutations. This finding raises the important question of the existence of other undiscovered genes predisposing to ovarian cancer in a less selected population. In sum, a negative test, unless in the setting in which known specific mutations have been identified in affected individuals, could reflect the following interpretations: 1) a lack of sensitivity of the molecular technique, 2) the existence of sporadic ovarian cancers in familial clusters, or 3) other, unidentified cancer-susceptibility gene mutations. The false assurance of a negative test result in the preceding setting should be carefully avoided during genetic screening.

In the event in which no *BRCA1* or *BRCA2* mutations are found in a strong family history, linkage analysis provides an alternative method of elucidating other cancer-susceptibility genes in the family. In linkage analysis, microsatellite markers that are close to the susceptibility gene are tested in family members. For example, the Lynch II syndrome is attributed to a set of inherited mutations of DNA repair genes (i.e., *MSH2*, *MLH1*, *PMS1*, and *PMS2*) identified during genetic linkage analysis (35). However, performing genetic linkage requires several affected and unaffected individuals undergoing analysis, which could be difficult from a practical perspective.

In addition to assessing the risk of inheriting mutations in either *BRCA1* or *BRCA2* genes, assessing the actual risk of developing ovarian cancer is also an integral part of genetic screening. Given the high variability of penetrance of *BRCA1*, it is crucial to individualize the penetrance of each family based on the pedigree analysis. An important point to remember in counseling patients is that risk estimates of cancer development are based on studies of families whose penetrance is probably very different from that of the tested individual.

Despite the commercial availability of *BRCA1* and *BRCA2* mutation screening, the administration of genetic screening to these high-risk individuals should be limited to a research academic setting. Until improved outcome from the genetic screening is proven, mutational analysis testing should be performed under strict research protocols that have met full institution review board approval. A multidisciplinary team that is capable of giving advice on psychological and social issues and appropriate interventions should manage clinical decisions based on the testing result. Full informed consent of individuals should be obtained prior to testing. It is absolutely vital that the patient has a full understanding of the scope, implications, and limitations of the molecular genetic screening. Patient confidentiality also is an important issue in terms of protection from possible insurance and employment discrimination. Identifier codes may offer some level of security of confidentiality.

The implications of the genetic testing result are tremendous. The benefit of a negative screening test of a known identified mutation offers assurance of no increased risk of developing ovarian cancer. Hence, no additional screening or risk reduction strategy is recommended in these individuals. On the other hand, a positive screening test for a known mutation in an unaffected individual will have significant impact on the individual's subsequent health care screening, psychological well-being, and the risk of social discrimination. Individuals who are carriers of a mutation are subjected to the

controversies of early ovarian cancer detection, including transvaginal ultrasound and CA-125 measurement, prophylactic surgeries, and intensive surveillance for colon and endometrial cancer development. Unfortunately, there is a paucity of substantial data to prove the efficacy of such screening in decreasing mortality and morbidity. The immense anxiety and emotional stress of the mutation carrier often require support group and psychological counseling prior to and following testing. The concern about transferring the inherited mutation to the next generation raises a new ethical issue. Discrimination in insurance coverage and employment is a potential concern because the presence of a genetic mutation may be considered as a "preexisting condition." Therefore, the importance of patient confidentiality cannot be over emphasized. Another difficulty encountered by such individuals is obtaining insurance approval for coverage of the indicated intensive cancer screening and interventions, such as transvaginal ultrasound and prophylactic oophorectomy.

Genetic Screening of the General Population

Application of mutation analysis screening for *BRCA1* and *BRCA2* mutations to the general population is still premature. As mentioned previously, an effective screening test should be a low-cost test that screens for a disease of relatively high prevalence (36). There should be potential benefits of improved outcome due to amenable therapy in the preclinical stage. The prevalence of ovarian cancer is 30 to 50 cases per 100,000 population. The frequency of mutations of *BRCA1* in the general population is estimated to be approximately 1 in 800. The probability of finding a *BRCA1* or *BRCA2* mutation in a woman who is the only affected individual in her family is less than 5% (20). Only 5% to 10% of all breast and ovarian cancers are due to hereditary syndromes (1). Predictive risks of ovarian cancer by *BRCA1* and *BRCA2* mutations are based on high-risk families group genetics and hence are unlikely to reflect general population risk. Furthermore, the efficacy of cancer surveillance and interventions to reduce the risk of ovarian cancer is still unknown. Although early detection may result in the diagnosis of earlier-stage ovarian cancer, a subset of stage I ovarian cancer patients may still have significant mortality and recurrence. Effective adjuvant therapy and ideal treatment for these patients have not been established (37). Hence, given the low incidence of *BRCA1* and *BRCA2* mutations in the general population and the lack of proven benefits of early cancer screening measures, general population screening for *BRCA1* and *BRCA2* mutations is not recommended.

Provisional Recommendations for Ovarian Cancer Surveillance for Carriers of Mutations

Genetic screening for mutations in *BRCA1*, *BRCA2*, and HNPCC genes may enable us to identify a subset of high-risk individuals who are more susceptible to the development of ovarian cancer. The next step is to answer the question of whether earlier intensive cancer surveillance and risk-reduction programs can improve the overall outcome of these patients. Unfortunately, the efficacy of these strategies remains controversial. The individual should be counseled comprehensively about the risks and benefits of undergoing these surveillance measures and interventions prior to the commitment of genetic testing.

The surveillance testing and diagnosis of ovarian carcinoma have always been challenging. The lack of specific symptoms means that the vast majority of women with ovarian cancer present with advanced disease. Most patients with early-stage ovarian cancer have no symptoms. Despite the advent of the CA-125 tumor marker determinations and transvaginal sonography with color Doppler, highly specific and sensitive screening modality for ovarian cancer is still lacking. In 1994, the National Institutes of Health (NIH) Consensus Development Conference concluded that "there is no evidence available yet that the current screening modalities of CA-125 and transvaginal ultrasonography can be effectively used for widespread screening to reduce mortality from ovarian cancer nor that their use will result in

decreased rather than increased morbidity and mortality" (38). However, in the event that an individual is at risk for hereditary ovarian syndromes, it is less controversial to apply these screening tests for surveillance purpose.

It has been recommended by the NIH Consensus Conference on Ovarian Cancer that annual or semiannual transvaginal sonography should be offered to carriers of the *BRCA1* gene mutations beginning at the ages of 25 to 35 (39) (Table 6-2). It is important to time the sonography during the nonovulatory period to avoid false-positive results (39). The advantage of transvaginal ultrasound over transabdominal sonography is the better discrimination of benign versus malignant pathology. The positive predictive value of transvaginal ultrasound alone is problematic, ranging from 3.1% to 7.7% (40). The use of color-flow Doppler and morphologic indices improves the specificity (41). In a study of 14,317 asymptomatic women, 54 of the 56 malignant ovarian lesions discovered had a low resistance index (Figs. 6-1, 6-2, and 6-3). However, the use of combined modalities of CA-125 determination and transvaginal ultrasound increases both the specificity and positive predictive value of screening for ovarian cancer. In a screening trial of 22,000 women aged 45 years or older using ultrasound and serum CA-125 determination, the specificity was increased from 97% to 98%, whereas the positive predictive value was increased from 7.7% to 26.8% (42). Owing to the early onset of hereditary ovarian cancer syndromes, such screening strategies are recommended as early as age 25 for mutation carriers. The justification of such intensive screening for carriers of *BRCA2* or HPNCC gene mutations is more controversial due to the lower risk of development of ovarian cancer. Second, the efficacy of such screening has not been assessed in reducing mortality, which is obviously a very important outcome of surveillance. Hopefully, randomized, prospective trials may soon answer these questions.

The tumor marker CA-125 has long been used as a marker in monitoring ovarian carcinoma. While most symptomatic ovarian cancer patients have elevated levels of this tumor-associated antigen, only 50% or fewer of patients with early-stage ovarian cancer have an elevated

20. Shattuck-Eidens D, McClure M, Simard J, et al. A collaborative survey of 80 mutations in the *BRCA1* breast and ovarian cancer susceptibility gene: implications of presymptomatic testing and screening. JAMA 1995;273:535–541.
21. Wooster R, Neuhausen S, Mangion J, et al. Localization of a breast cancer susceptibility gene, *BRCA2*, to chromosome 13q12-13. Science 1994;265:2088–2090.
22. Ford D, Easton D. The genetics of breast and ovarian cancer. Br J Cancer 1995;72:805–812.
23. Thorlacius S, Tryggvadottir L, Olafsdottir G, et al. Linkage to *BRCA2* region in hereditary male cancer. Lancet 1995;235:544–545.
24. Struewing J, Abeliovich D, Peretz T, et al. The carrier frequency of the *BRCA1* 185delAG mutation is approximately 1 percent in Ashkenazi Jewish individuals. Nature Genet 1995;11:198–200.
25. Oddoux C, Struewing J, Clayton C, et al. The carrier frequency of the *BRCA2* 617delT mutation among Ashkenazi Jewish individuals is approximately 1%. Nature Genet 1996;14:188–190.
26. Levy-Lahad E, Catane R, Eisenberg S, et al. Founder *BRCA1* and *BRCA2* mutations in Ashkenazi Jews in Israel: frequency and differential penetrance in ovarian cancer and in breast-ovarian cancer families. Am J Hum Genet 1997;60:1059–1067.
27. Tonin P, Weber B, Offit K, et al. Frequency of recurrent *BRCA1* and *BRCA2* mutations in Ashkenazi Jewish breast cancer families. Nature Med 1996;2:1179–1183.
28. Serova O, Mazoyer S, Puget N, et al. Mutations in *BRCA1* and *BRCA2* in breast cancer families: are there more breast cancer susceptibility genes? Am J Hum Genet 1997;60:486–495.
29. Couch F, Weber B. Mutations and polymorphisms in the familial early-onset breast cancer (*BRCA1*) gene. Hum Mutat 1996;8:8–18.
30. Rubin S, Blackwood A, Bandera C, et al. *BRCA1*, *BRCA2*, and hereditary nonpolyposis colorectal cancer gene mutations in an unselected ovarian cancer population: relationship to family history and implications for genetic testing. Am J Obstet Gynecol 1998;178:670–677.
31. Hogervorst F, Cornelis R, Bout M, et al. Rapid detection of *BRCA1* mutations by the protein truncation test. Nature Genet 1995;10:208–212.
32. Miki Y, Swensen J, Shattuck-Eidens D, et al. A strong candidate for the breast ovarian cancer susceptibility gene *BRCA1*. Science 1994;266:66–71.
33. Berchuck A, Cirisano F, Lancaster J, et al. Role of *BRCA1* mutation screening in the management of familial ovarian cancer. Am J Obstet Gynecol 1996;175:738–746.
34. Raffel L. Genetic counseling and genetic testing for cancer risk assessment. In: Pitkin R, Scott J, eds. Clinical obstetrics and gynecology. vol. 41. Philadelphia: Lippincott-Raven, 1998:141–156.
35. Kolodner R, Hall N, Lipford J, et al. Structure of the human *MSH2* locus and analysis to two Muir-Torre kindreds for *MSH2* mutations. Genome 1994;24:516–526.
36. American College of Obstetrics and Gynecology Committee Opinion: Routine Cancer Screening; Number 185, September 1997.
37. NIH Consensus Conference. Ovarian cancer: screening, treatment, and follow-up. JAMA 1995;273:491–497.
38. National Institutes of Health Consensus Development Conference. Statement, ovarian cancer screening, treatment, and follow-up. Gynecol Oncol 1994;55:S4–S14.
39. Burke W, Daly M, Garber J, et al. Recommendations for follow-up care of individuals with an inherited predisposition to cancer: II. *BRCA1* and *BRCA2*. JAMA 1997;277:997–1003.
40. Karlan B, Platt L. The current status of ultrasound and color Doppler imaging in screening for ovarian cancer. Gynecol Oncol 1994;55:S28–S33.
41. Daly M. The epidemiology of ovarian cancer. Hematol Oncol Clin North Am 1992;6:729–738.
42. Jacobs I, Davies A, Bridges J, et al. Prevalence screening for ovarian cancer in postmenopausal women by CA-125 measurement and ultrasonography. Br Med J 1993;306:1030–1034.
43. Jacobs I, Bridges J, Reynolds C, et al. Multimodal approaches to screening for ovarian cancer. Lancet 1988;1:269–271.
44. Jacobs I, Bast R. The CA-125 tumor-associated antigen: a review of the literature. Hum Reprod 1984;4:1–12.
45. Prentice R, Sheppard L. Dietary fat and cancer. Cancer Causes Control 1990;1:81–97.
46. Trock B, Lanza E, Greenwald P. Dietary fiber, vegetables, and colon cancer: critical review and meta-analyses of the epidemiologic evidence. J Natl Cancer Inst 1990;82:650–661.
47. Shushan A, Palteil O, Iscovich J, et al. Human menopausal gonadotropin and the risk of epithelial ovarian cancer. Fertil Steril 1996;65:13–18.
48. Bristow R, Karlan B. Ovulation induction, infertility and ovarian cancer risk. Fertil Steril 1996;66:499–507.

49. The Cancer and Steroid Hormone Study of the Centers for Disease Control and the National Institute of Child Health and Human Development. The reduction in risk of ovarian cancer associated with oral contraceptive use. New Engl J Med 1987;316:650–655.

50. Whittemore A, Harris R, Itnyre J, et al. Characteristics relating to ovarian cancer risk: collaborative analysis of 12 U.S. case-control studies: II. Invasive epithelial ovarian cancers in white women. Am J Epidemiol 1992;136:1184–1203.

51. Franceschi S, Parazzini F, Negri E, et al. Pooled analysis of 3 European case-control studies of epithelial ovarian cancer. III. Oral contraceptive use. Int J Cancer 1991;49:61–65.

52. Narod S, Risch H, Moslehi R, et al. Oral contraceptives and the risk of hereditary ovarian cancer. New Eng J Med 1998;339:424–428.

53. Combination oral contraceptive use and the risk of endometrial cancer. The Cancer and Steroid Hormone Study of the Centers for Disease Control and the National Institute of Child Health and Human Development. JAMA 1987;257:796–800.

54. Breast cancer and hormonal contraceptives. Lancet 1996;347:1713–1727.

55. Hankinson S, Huner D, Colditz G, et al. Tubal ligation, hysterectomy and risk of ovarian cancer. JAMA 1993;270:2813–2816.

56. Irwin K, Weiss N, Lee N, et al. Tubal sterilization, hysterectomy and the subsequent occurrence of epithelial ovarian cancer. Am J Epidemiol 1991;134:362–369, 681–684.

57. Schrag D, Kuntz KM, Garber J, Weeks J, et al. Decision analysis: effects of prophylactic mastectomy and oophorectomy among women with *BRCA1* or *BRCA2* mutations. New Engl J Med. 1997;336:1465–1471.

58. Piver M, Barlow J, Sawyer D. Familial ovarian cancer increasing in frequency? Obstet Gynecol 1982;60:397–400.

59. Graham J, Graham R, Schueller E. Preclinical detection of ovarian cancer. Cancer 1964;1: 1414.

60. Averette H, Nguyen H. The role of prophylactic oophorectomy in cancer screening. Gynecol Oncol 1994;55:S38–S41.

61. Sightler S, Boike G, Estage P, et al. Ovarian cancer in women with prior hysterectomy: a 14-year experience at the University of Miami. Obstet Gynecol 1991;78:681–684.

62. Schwartz P. The role of prophylactic oophorectomy in the avoidance of ovarian cancer. Int J Gynaecol Obstet 1992;39:175–184.

63. Jacobs I, Oram D. Prevention of ovarian cancer: a survey of the practice of prophylactic oophorectomy by fellows and members of the Royal College of Obstetricians and Gynecologist. Br J Obstet Gynaecol 1989;96:510–515.

64. Tobachman J, Tucker M, Kase R, et al. Intra-abdominal carcinomatosis after prophylactic oophorectomy in ovarian cancer prone families. Lancet 1982;2:795–797.

65. Piver M, Jishi M, Tsukada Y, Navs G. Primary peritoneal carcinoma after prophylactic oophorectomy in women with a family history of ovarian cancer: a report of the Gilda Radner Familial Ovarian Cancer Registry. Cancer 1993;71:2751–2755.

66. Nguyen H, Averette H, Janicek M. Ovarian carcinoma. A review of the significance of familial risk factors and the role of prophylactic oophorectomy in cancer prevention. Cancer 1994;74:545–555.

67. Steinberg K, Thacker S, Smith S, et al. A meta-analysis of the effect of estrogen replacement therapy on the risk of breast cancer. JAMA 1991;265:1985–1990.

68. Grady D, Rubin S, Petitti D, et al. Hormone therapy to prevent disease and prolong life in postmenopausal women. Ann Intern Med 1992;117:1016–1037.

69. Speroff T, Dawson, Speroff L, et al. A risk benefit analysis of elective bilateral oophorectomy: effect of changes in compliance with estrogen therapy on outcome. Am J Obstet Gynecol 1991:164:165–174.

70. Meijer W, van Linder A. Prophylactic oophorectomy. Eur J Obstet Gynecol Reprod Biol 1992;47:59–65.

71. Kerlikowske K, Brown J, Grady D. Should women with familial ovarian cancer undergo prophylactic oophorectomy? 1992;80:700–707. Obstet Gynecol 1992;80:700–707.

7

Contemporary Breast Imaging in the High-Risk Patient

Kathleen M. Harris

Screening mammography of asymptomatic high-risk young women and diagnostic evaluation of symptomatic women with special mammographic views and breast ultrasound are described in this chapter. The various imaging modalities used in everyday radiologic practice can help to differentiate the patients who have benign breast disease from those with breast cancer. The diagnostic information provided by the radiologic workup can decrease the number of surgical procedures for benign conditions, prevent delays in diagnosis of malignancy, and enable preoperative treatment planning and staging.

Mammography

Mammography is the single best method for the detection of clinically occult breast cancer (1). Mammographically, cancer can present as a soft tissue mass (Fig. 7-1a) an architectural distortion (Fig. 7-1b), microcalcifications (Fig. 7-1c), a focal asymmetric density, or a new or developing density. Microcalcifications can be the only sign of early-stage breast cancer (ductal carcinoma in situ; see Fig. 7-1c) (2,3) and are associated with 30% of invasive cancers. The ability of mammography to detect unsuspected malignant microcalcifications in asymptomatic women is one reason mammography is the single best method for detecting carcinoma. Increased compliance with screening guidelines has contributed to an increase in the detection of early-stage cancer and to a decrease in mortality of asymptomatic women whose cancers were detected at screening mammography. Screening of asymptomatic women from age 40 and older has been shown to decrease the mortality from breast cancer by approximately 30% (4).

For younger women who are at high risk for developing breast cancer (those with one or more first-degree relatives with breast cancer or those identified with one of the breast cancer genes *BRCA1* and *BRCA2*), screening mammography could begin earlier than age 40. The benefit of early detection of cancer would have to be weighed against any potential risk of radiation exposure (5–8). Screening mammography is often recommended to begin 10 years earlier than the age at which the woman's first-degree relative developed breast cancer. For example, a woman whose sister or mother developed breast cancer at age 42 could begin screening mammography at age 32 rather than waiting until she turns 40. Annual clinical breast examination in this high-risk group is also recommended. Another risk is exposure to radiation at a young age, which has been shown in Nagasaki and Hiroshima atomic bomb survivors (9). There is a higher incidence of breast cancer in young women who received mantle-type radiation therapy to the chest for Hodgkin's disease. The cancers of the breast may appear 10 or more years after the radiation therapy. Therefore, a young woman treated for Hodgkin's disease in her teens or 20s is at risk for developing breast cancer in her 30s. Also, women at risk for breast cancer include those who received multiple chest fluoroscopies and those

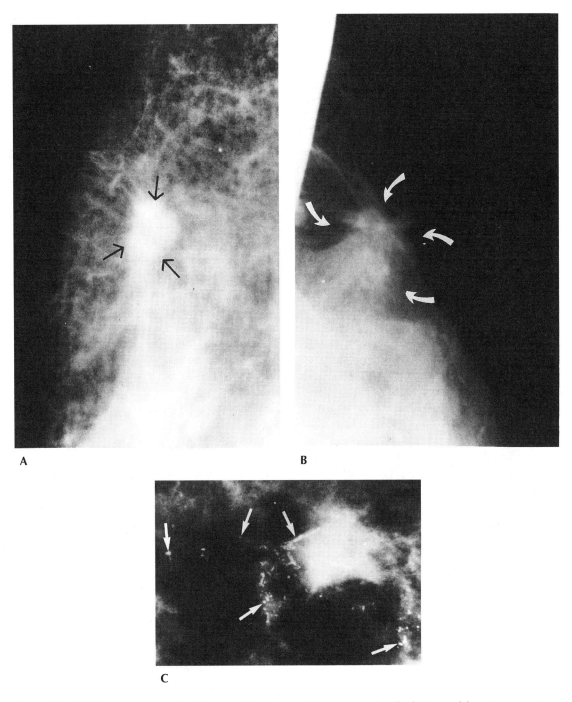

Figure 7-1. (**A**) This asymptomatic 36-year-old woman with a strong family history of breast cancer in a premenopausal sister and mother was referred for a baseline mammogram. The high-density mass with spiculated margins is highly suggestive of malignancy (*arrows*). Preoperative needle localization and surgical removal revealed an 0.8-cm infiltrating ductal carcinoma. (**B**) This 34-year-old woman with a subtle area of palpable thickening of the upper outer quadrant of the left breast was referred for diagnostic mammography. This irregular mass with spiculated margins and architectural distortion (*arrows*) is best seen on this special cone-down compression spot film. This mass was more difficult to see on the craniocaudal and mediolateral oblique views because of the adjacent dense glandular tissue. Mammography-guided needle localization and

treated with breast irradiation for postpartum mastitis at a young age (10).

Diagnostic mammograms, for symptomatic patients, can be performed at any age. Because the breast tissue is thought to be more sensitive to radiation in women under age 35 (11,12), only limited mammographic views are obtained in this young age group. For women below age 30, first ultrasound is performed to characterize a palpable mass because of the lack of ionizing radiation. A limited-focus mammogram of the area of concern may be needed to rule out microcalcifications that cannot be detected sonographically. If there is a strong suspicion of malignancy, however, mammograms may be performed at any age in order to make a diagnosis. Microcalcifications as a sign of malignancy can be detected even in the dense glandular tissue of young women or those who are lactating or pregnant. Approximately 2% to 5% of breast cancers occur in pregnant women (13). Mammographic density can be decreased in lactating women who nurse their infant just prior to the mammogram.

In young women, a higher proportion of cancer detected mammographically is ductal carcinoma in situ (DCIS) (14,15). DCIS is readily detectable, even in dense glandular breasts, because it often presents as microcalcifications mammographically (see Fig. 7-1c). DCIS can progress in time (5–15 years) to invasive carcinoma. Invasive cancers without associated microcalcifications are more difficult to detect in dense breast tissue because of the similar radiodensity of the carcinoma to the adjacent dense glandular tissue in younger women. Clinical breast examination and ultrasound for any palpable abnormalities can facilitate detection.

Although younger women in general have denser glandular tissue that lowers the sensitivity of mammography, not all young women have dense breasts. Some young women may have mostly fatty breasts that may be due to genetic differences, obesity, or multiple births at an early age. Conversely, not all older women have fatty breasts. Nulliparous women may maintain dense glandular tissue throughout life. Hormone replacement therapy can increase the density of the glandular tissue. There is no abrupt change in breast density at age 50 or at menopause but rather a gradual decrease in density with increasing age (16,17). Although the sensitivity for detecting soft tissue masses is greatest in fatty breasts, with good-quality mammograms, microcalcifications, developing densities, and masses can still be detected even in dense breasts. Jeffries and Adler found that half the women who had breast cancer under age 35 had fatty or mixed fatty-glandular breasts and that 86% of the cancers were seen mammographically (18). Unfortunately, tumors in younger, premenopausal women grow more rapidly than those in older, postmenopausal women (19,20). Therefore, it is recommended that screening be performed yearly rather than every other year for women aged 40 to 49 in order to detect tumors when they are smaller and to improve survival in this group (20). Also, annual clinical breast examination is important to detect a developing mass or thickening that could be a sign of malignancy.

Mammography is very sensitive in detecting an abnormality; sensitivity ranges from 85% to 90% (21). Because of the overlapping appearances of benign and malignant lesions, however, mammography is not very specific. Therefore, only 20% to 30% of suspicious lesions that are detected mammographically (clinically occult) and sent for surgical excision are actually malignant (21).

Figure 7-1. (*continued*) surgical removal revealed an infiltrating ductal carcinoma. (**C**) This asymptomatic 35-year-old woman had a baseline mammogram because of a history of a mother with breast cancer at age 46. Indeterminate microcalcifications were present in the right breast on the screening mammogram. The patient returned for magnification views of the microcalcifications that are highly suspicious for malignancy. The microcalcifications (*arrows*) are seen easily because of their greater radiodensity compared with the soft tissue density of the surrounding glandular and adipose tissue. The calcifications are pleomorphic in shape and are linear in distribution within the ducts extending toward the nipple. The calcifications were needle localized preoperatively and represented ductal carcinoma in situ, comedo type. Because of the extensive calcifications over a large area of the breast, the patient had a mastectomy and immediate reconstruction.

Further workup with other imaging modalities such as breast ultrasound and image-guided tissue sampling with ultrasound or stereotactic guided biopsy have reduced the false-positive rate, which is cost-effective. No test is 100% accurate, and unfortunately, mammography can miss 10% to 15% of cancers that can be obscured by dense glandular tissue (22,23). Therefore, clinical breast examination is important in conjunction with mammography to improve the cancer detection rate (1,24). Furthermore, the sensitivity of mammography in younger women may be lower because younger women have larger amounts of dense glandular tissue that can obscure a mass (25). Fortunately, microcalcifications (which may be the earliest sign of malignancy) can be detected because of their higher density even in the densest glandular tissue (2,3).

There are important differences between screening and diagnostic mammography. Screening mammography is performed for asymptomatic women, and diagnostic mammography is performed for women with signs or symptoms of breast disease. *Screening mammography* consists of two standard views of each breast: the mediolateral oblique view (MLO) and the craniocaudal (CC) view. In a screening examination, the technologist performs the two-view mammograms of each breast, develops the films, and checks for film quality. In order to improve efficiency and lower cost, the screening patient typically is sent home without the radiologist checking the films. At a later time, the films are loaded on a multiviewer and "batch read" by the radiologist, who reviews the clinical data sheet (pertinent history) and the mammograms and compares the current films with any previous studies. Because the incidence of breast cancer is low (i.e., between 3 and 7 cancers per 1000 women screened), most asymptomatic women will have a normal screening mammogram. Because the two-view screening mammogram cannot fully characterize an abnormality, the patient may be recalled for further workup if the mammogram is indeterminate. The recall rate is generally 10% or less when screening mammograms are interpreted by radiologists experienced in breast imaging (26). For those women who are recalled, whether for additional mammographic views, breast ultrasound, or image-guided biopsies, the majority will have

a benign condition, since fibrocystic changes such as cysts, fibroadenomas, or benign calcifications are more common than malignancy.

With *diagnostic mammography*, the radiologist is present to check the films, correlate the patient's symptoms and clinical findings with the mammographic findings, and perform additional tests such as ultrasound or percutaneous image-guided biopsies. Fortunately, palpable abnormalities are most often benign cysts, fibroadenomas, fat lobules, or "lumpy" glandular tissue. Further workup, however, is required to establish whether a palpable mass is likely to be benign or possibly may be malignant. Ultrasound is the best ancillary test to determine if the palpable mass is a cyst or a solid mass. Each diagnostic case requires an individualized imaging evaluation directly supervised by the radiologist. Indeterminate microcalcifications can be further evaluated with magnification views to determine the shape and distribution of the calcific particles to ascertain the likelihood of their being associated with benign or malignant disease. Mammographically detected asymmetric densities, architectural distortion, and masses can be characterized further with special views such as compression spot films, tangential views, roll views, and various other views (see Fig. 7-1b). Diagnostic mammography is indicated for symptomatic women who may present with a mass or thickening of the breast, acute onset of pain, change in the color or texture of the skin or nipple, change in the size or shape of the breast, or spontaneous unilateral nipple discharge. Diagnostic mammography is also indicated for patients who have been treated for breast cancer with segmental resection and radiation therapy and for those who have received preoperative "neoadjuvant" chemotherapy in order to shrink a malignant tumor. Women who have had implants placed for augmentation or reconstruction require extra views to better visualize the breast tissue (four views of each breast that include implant-displacement views) and may require breast ultrasound if silicone implant rupture is suspected or to evaluate a palpable breast mass. Patients with an abnormal screening mammogram (mass or microcalcifications) may be recalled for further diagnostic workup. Patients with metastases from an unknown primary tumor and those with large breasts that are difficult to examine require a thorough diagnostic study.

Communication between the radiologist and the referring physician and between the radiologist and the patient can improve patient care (27,28). Most radiologists are now using the standardized Breast Imaging Reporting and Data System (BI-RADS) (29,30) to standardize terminology and to help the referring physician understand the significance of the finding and the recommended action. Following is a summary of the BI-RADS reporting system for the final assessment category (levels 0, 1, 2, 3, 4, and 5) and recommendations:

- Level 1: Normal
  Recommendation: Routine mammographic follow-up according to the screening guidelines
- Level 2: Benign finding
  Recommendation: Routine mammographic follow-up as well as clinical follow-up.
- Level 3: Probably benign finding
  Recommendation: Short-interval follow-up (usually 6 months + 6 months + yearly for 3 years)
- Level 4: Suspicious abnormality
  Recommendation: Tissue sampling with percutaneous needle or core biopsy or surgical biopsy
- Level 5: Highly suggestive
  Recommendation: Appropriate action for suspected malignancy should be taken, such as surgical excision and definitive treatment
- Level 0: Incomplete
  Recommendation: Additional imaging evaluation needed

A level 1 finding with normal mammographic results prompts routine follow-up according to the screening guidelines for the patient's age. Level 2 lesions (Fig. 7-2) are benign, such as fibroadenomas, cysts, benign asymmetric densities, or benign calcifications, and are followed with routine mammograms (or ultrasound depending on the woman's age) usually in 1 year, as well as clinical follow-up. Level 3 lesions (Fig. 7-3) are "probably benign." It has been shown that malignancy is very rare in "probably benign" lesions—on the order of 0.5% to 2% of cases (31). Because of the low yield of malignancy in level 3 lesions, it is considered

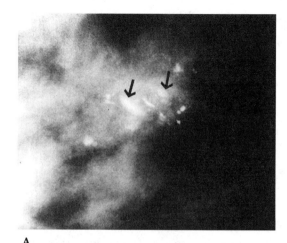

A

B

Figure 7-2. This asymptomatic woman has benign calcifications representing "milk of calcium." Magnification craniocaudal and 90-degree lateral views of the calcifications show a change in the configuration of the calcifications in the orthogonal views. (**A**) In the 90-degree lateral view, the calcifications are linear and semilunar in appearance, representing sedimentary layering of the calcific particles in the dependent portions of multiple small cysts as seen in the true lateral view with the x-ray beam parallel to the calcifications (*arrows*). (**B**) In the craniocaudal view, the calcifications (*arrow*) are more rounded with the x-ray beam perpendicular to the calcifications. These findings are characteristic of benign calcifications and do not require a short-interval follow-up or a biopsy. This patient can have a routine screening mammogram and was given a final assessment category of level 2.

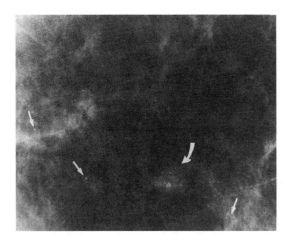

Figure 7-3. This cluster of microcalcifications (*curved arrow*) is within a small mass and probably represents calcifications within an involuting fibroadenoma. There are several benign scattered calcifications that are not in a cluster (*straight arrows*). If prior films are available showing stability over 3 or more years, this would be given a final assessment category of level 2 for a benign finding. Since no prior films were available in this patient, a short-interval follow-up was indicated to prove stability for this "probably benign" finding that has a less than 2% chance of malignancy. This was given a final assessment category of level 3 and was shown to be stable for more than 3 years follow-up and thus was proven to be benign by its stability.

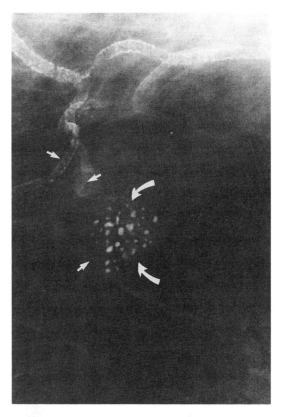

Figure 7-4. This cluster of microcalcifications in an asymptomatic woman is suspicious for malignancy (*curved arrows*). On this magnification view, the calcifications are pleomorphic, vary in size and shape, and are in a cluster. This was given a final assessment category of level 4, which indicates the need for a biopsy. Because of the fact the calcifications are close to a calcified artery (*short straight arrows*), it was decided not to perform a stereotactic biopsy in order to avoid the adjacent artery. Preoperative needle localization and surgical biopsy revealed ductal carcinoma in situ, comedo type.

safe to follow these women with short-interval follow-up at 6, 12, 24, and 36 months for closer observation. Any increase in size of a nodule, increase in the number of microcalcifications, or other suspicious changes would upgrade the final assessment category to level 4 and would require further evaluation with percutaneous image-guided or palpation-guided tissue sampling or surgical excision. Conversely, if stability is established over 3 or more years or the lesion decreases in size or disappears, the lesion can be downgraded to a level 2 ("benign") or level 1 ("normal"), and the patient can return to routine mammographic follow-up.

When breast cancer is suspected (level 4 or level 5), either by an abnormal clinical breast examination or by finding a suspicious mammographic or sonographic lesion, further workup is required to establish a definitive diagnosis and as an aid in staging and treatment planning. For level 4 (Fig. 7-4) or level 5 (Fig. 7-5)

lesions, a tissue diagnosis is indicated, such as image-guided or palpation-guided needle or core biopsy or surgical excision. Approximately 30% to 40% of level 4 abnormalities are malignant. Many of these undergo ultrasound-guided or stereotactic guided needle or core biopsies to establish the diagnosis. Percutaneous tissue sampling could avert surgical excision for benign lesions while identifying those with suspicious or malignant cytology (fine-needle aspiration) or histology (core biopsy) for surgical excision. Approximately 80% to 90% of level 5 lesions are

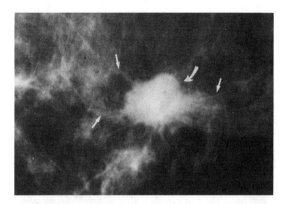

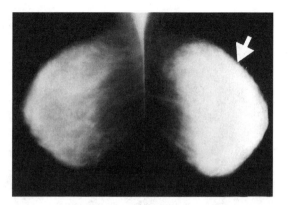

Figure 7-5. This high-density mass (*curved arrow*) with spiculated borders (*short arrows*) has the classic mammographic appearance of malignancy and was given a final assessment category of level 5. This was not palpable and was discovered at screening mammography. The patient had a mammography-guided preoperative needle localization followed by surgical removal of the entire mass and a rim of normal tissue. This represented a 1-cm infiltrating ductal carcinoma. The axillary lymph nodes were negative for metastatic tumor.

Figure 7-6. This 28-year-old woman who was 6 months postpartum discovered a swelling of her left breast. The patient's physician attributed the breast changes to mastitis and prescribed antibiotics. There was no improvement on antibiotic therapy, and 2 months later the patient was referred for a diagnostic imaging workup. The mammogram reveals overall asymmetric denser glandular tissue in the left breast (*large arrow*) compared with the right breast, which is shown in these side-by-side mediolateral oblique views. Ultrasound of the left breast did not reveal a mass, but there was skin thickening. On clinical breast examination, the left breast was mildly tender and was larger than the right breast. The skin of the left breast was reddened, warm, and had prominent skin pores. There was no dominant palpable mass, but the entire left breast felt thicker and heavier than the opposite breast. Based on the clinical findings, the patient was referred immediately to a surgeon. Palpation-guided needle biopsy revealed malignancy, confirming the clinical impression of inflammatory carcinoma. The patient was treated with "neoadjuvant" chemotherapy followed by left mastectomy and irradiation of the left chest wall. Despite the young age of the patient, clinical signs and symptoms must be investigated vigorously in order to make the diagnosis at the earliest time. Delays in diagnosis can adversely affect the patient's prognosis and could result in litigation.

malignant and require definitive surgical treatment, tumor staging, and appropriate oncologic management. A single malignant lesion may be treated with segmental resection and radiation therapy, depending on whether the surgeon can remove the entire carcinoma with a rim of normal tissue and still maintain good cosmesis. If there are multiple lesions (multifocal or multicentric carcinoma), or if the malignancy is too extensive to achieve a cosmetic result (depending on the size of the lesion relative to the size of the breast), the surgeon may elect to perform a mastectomy (see Fig. 7-1c). Since a two-view screening mammogram cannot evaluate all cases, those who are recalled for additional workup are given a final assessment category of level 0 temporarily until the areas of concern can be further evaluated in the near future. The great majority of the level 0 cases are proven to be benign findings such as cysts or benign calcifications or merely superimposition of normal glandular structures.

Concerning *malpractice litigation*, missed breast cancer is the most expensive medical condition (32). Breast cancer can occur at any age, although the incidence increases sharply from age 40 onward. Most cases that come to litigation

involve young women with a palpable mass or other breast abnormality for whom the physician incorrectly assumed the clinical findings to be benign because of the young age (33–36) (Fig. 7-6). Young patients with a palpable mass or thickening should have a diagnostic workup including mammography, ultrasound, and/or needle biopsy to establish a tissue diagnosis (Table 7-1). Fortunately, most masses in young women will be benign fibroadenomas or cysts, but women in their 20s and 30s can develop breast cancer. Whatever the patient's age, the physician

Table 7-1. Imaging strategies, age, and risk factors

Age	Risk Factors	Imaging Strategies

20–29	Low — clinical observation*
	High — annual clinical breast examination (CBE)
		None if negative clinical breast examination (CBE)
		Negative CBE
		  Begin screening mammogram (one view each breast)
		  10 years prior to age of first-degree relative with breast cancer
		Abnormal CBE
		  First: Ultrasound area of concern
		  Second: Limited mammogram area of concern
		  Third: Image-guided biopsy of abnormal area
		    Ultrasound-guided for mass
		    Stereotactic-guided for calcifications
		    If biopsy shows malignancy, consider bilateral breast MRI to look for multiple cancers
		Future considerations
		  For high-risk, especially with mutated *BRCA1, BRCA2* genes, consider annual bilateral breast ultrasound and consider annual MRI and/or sestamibi. The efficacy for MRI and sestamibi has not been proven in women with negative CBE, negative mammogram, and negative breast ultrasound.

30–39	Low — clinical observation*
	High — annual clinical breast examination (CBE)
		None if negative clinical breast examination (CBE)
		Negative CBE
		  Begin screening mammogram (2 views each breast)
		  10 years prior to age of first-degree relative with breast cancer
		Abnormal CBE
		  First: Diagnostic mammography (first) with special views
		  Second: Ultrasound area of concern
		  Third: Image-guided biopsy of abnormal area
		    Ultrasound-guided for mass
		    Stereotactic-guided for calcifications
		    If biopsy shows malignancy, consider bilateral breast MRI to look for multiple cancers
		Future considerations
		  For high risk, especially with mutated *BRCA1, BRCA2* genes, consider annual bilateral breast ultrasound and consider annual MRI and/or sestamibi. The efficacy for MRI and sestamibi has not been proven in women with negative CBE, negative mammogram, and negative breast ultrasound.

* Low-risk women with abnormal CBE: Refer for diagnostic evaluation the same as for high-risk women.

must treat the patient's complaints seriously and pursue all methods to make a diagnosis to rule out malignancy. The most effective approach is a combination of clinical breast examination by the physician, periodic screening for all women aged 40 and older (and younger for high-risk women), teaching women to perform monthly breast self-examination, and referring any women with symptoms for diagnostic imaging to include mammography, ultrasound, and tissue sampling as indicated. Despite a complete imaging evaluation, an unexplained dominant focal area of clinical concern could still be cancer, and referral to a surgeon for excisional biopsy is prudent.

Proper positioning and compression are important to obtain proper exposure of the breast at the lowest radiation dose (37,38). The dose depends on the thickness of the compressed breast and the type of glandular tissue (i.e., mostly dense glandular tissue versus mostly fatty tissue) (39). Proper compression should be firm in order to spread out the glandular tissue to enable detection of any underlying abnormality. Compression also decreases the radiation dose by shortening the time of exposure using phototiming techniques. The average glandular dose to an average breast (compressed to 4.2 cm) should not exceed 0.3 rad per view (3 mGy) for film-screen imaging using a grid and 0.1 rad (1 mGy) per view for nongrid film-screen images (38).

All women in the United States are assured optimal image quality at low radiation doses because of the American College of Radiology Mammography Accreditation Program and the Mammography Quality Standards Act (MQSA) of the Federal Food and Drug Administration (FDA) (40–42). All mammography facilities must be certified initially and then recertified annually by the FDA to be able to perform mammograms. To comply with the strict standards, the radiologic technologist conducts ongoing daily quality assurance tests to check the film processor and the mammography equipment (41). Phantom images consisting of tiny particles, fibers, and masses are exposed monthly to check the entire system. Quality-control tests performed by the technologist include testing the film processor daily and periodically checking the screens, film cassettes, and compression device, among others. The medical physicist is responsible for annual testing of the performance of the mammography equipment to ensure the lowest radiation dose while maintaining optimal image quality. The physicist checks the kVp accuracy and reproducibility, the focal spot and collimation performance, and the phototimer accuracy and assesses the beam quality and radiation dose (41). Actual patient mammograms are peer reviewed for each mammographic machine through the American College of Radiology Mammography Accreditation Program (41). Facilities that fail because of poor image quality must resubmit acceptable images before they can continue to perform mammograms. Annually, each mammography unit as well as the entire quality-assurance program of the facility is checked by a qualified medical physicist as part of maintaining FDA certification (42). It is

also required that the radiologist keep a medical audit of all patients who are suspected of having cancer (level 4 and level 5), including the final surgical results, which ensures patient follow-up (43). Each radiologist can calculate the number of cancers found (true positives) compared with the number of benign biopsies (false positives). Calculation of other statistics such as the positive predictive value, sensitivity, and specificity can be educational and potentially can result in improved patient care. Radiologists, technologists, and medical physicists are required to obtain initial training and to have ongoing experience and documented continued medical education in order to obtain and maintain certification under the MQSA regulations (42).

Breast Ultrasound

Breast ultrasound is the most useful adjunct to mammography. Ultrasound is used to evaluate palpable masses and to further characterize mammographically detected clinically occult masses. Ultrasound can differentiate whether a mass is a simple cyst (Fig. 7-7) or a solid lesion (Fig. 7-8)(11,12). In fact, ultrasound can diagnose a cyst with 96% to 100% accuracy (44). Some complex cysts, however, can mimic a solid mass sonographically, and ultrasound cannot differentiate benign solid from malignant masses in all cases (45). Therefore, another use for ultrasound is as a guide for fine-needle aspiration biopsy or larger-needle core biopsy in order to obtain a cytologic or histologic diagnosis.

Newer breast ultrasound equipment has high-resolution 7- to 10-MHz linear-array transducers and variable focal zones to better characterize the shape, borders, and acoustic properties of breast masses. Improved definition with newer ultrasound equipment allows better understanding of benign and malignant mass characteristics (46). With real-time breast ultrasound, the entire breast, including the skin, subcutaneous tissue, glandular tissue, chest wall, and axilla, can be scanned.

Breast ultrasound has the following uses:

- *To differentiate a simple cyst from a solid mass.* Fluid-filled cysts are anechoic, whereas solid masses contain internal echoes. Simple cysts have smooth walls, sharp anterior and posterior margins, no internal echoes, and usually (but not always) posterior acoustic enhancement (see Fig. 7-7). Proper gain settings are important in differentiating cysts from solid lesions.

- *To evaluate the underlying cause of an abnormal clinical breast examination.* Palpable masses or thickening, skin dimpling, or skin thickening can be evaluated with ultrasound (see Figs. 7-7 and 7-8). A palpable mass may be obscured mammographically by dense glandular tissue. Sonographically, malignant masses are most often hypoechoic (i.e., blacker, containing a few echoes) compared with the adipose tissue,

may have spiculated or lobulated borders, and may exhibit posterior acoustic shadowing (see Fig. 7-8). Fibroadenomas can be hypoechoic or isoechoic (i.e., having the same echogenicity as the adipose tissue), often with acoustic enhancement. Mammographically visible masses may be sonographically isoechoic and therefore not visible by ultrasound, especially when surrounded by adipose tissue. Therefore, an isoechoic lesion is assumed to be solid. Patients with "lumpy breasts" can be evaluated by ultrasound, and the "lumpy" areas could represent multiple cysts, multiple fibroadenomas, prominent fat lobules or prominent areas of dense glandular tissue. Ultrasound, however, cannot detect 100% of masses. Therefore, a

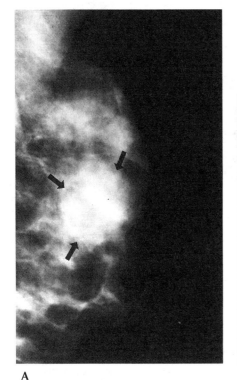

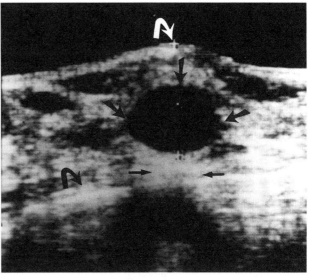

A **B**

Figure 7-7. This 30-year-old woman was sent for diagnostic imaging evaluation because of a firm moveable mass in her left breast in the upper outer quadrant. The patient's mother had breast cancer at age 50. (**A**) Diagnostic mammography reveals a mass with indeterminate features (*arrows*) that is partially obscured by adjacent dense glandular tissue. (**B**) Left breast ultrasound reveals an anechoic smooth-walled mass with increased through transmission (enhancement of sound deep to the mass, *thin black arrows*) characteristic of a simple cyst (*thick black arrows*). This cyst is deep near the pectoral muscle (*curved black arrow*) and elevates the skin overlying the cyst (*curved white arrow*). The patient can either be reassured that this is a cyst and followed, or ultrasound-guided or palpation-guided aspiration of the cyst can be performed the same day. Many women prefer to have a dominant palpable cyst aspirated for the benefit of having the symptomatic cyst disappear.

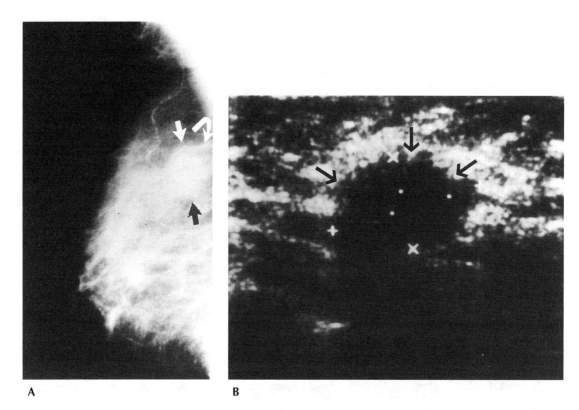

A   B

Figure 7-8. This 34-year-old woman was sent for diagnostic imaging because of a firm moveable mass in the right breast in the upper outer quadrant. (**A**) Diagnostic mammography reveals a mass with indeterminate mammographic features (*white and black straight arrows*). The mass is partially obscured by the adjacent dense glandular tissue and has a spiculated margin posteriorly (*curved arrow*). (**B**) Ultrasound reveals a hypoechoic mass with a microlobulated border (*arrows*) and acoustic shadowing deep to the mass. Cursers are noted (+ and ×) measuring this 1.5-cm mass, which is sonographically suspicious for malignancy. Ultrasound-guided core biopsy was performed to establish the diagnosis of malignancy preoperatively. Core samples revealed infiltrating ductal carcinoma. The patient underwent a one-stage procedure of segmental resection of the breast cancer and axillary node dissection. The cancer was completely excised, and the axillary nodes were negative for metastatic tumor. The patient opted for breast-conservation therapy including whole-breast irradiation. The patients in Figs. 7-7 and 7-8 had similar clinical presentations and similar mammographic findings. The ultrasound was helpful in differentiating a simple cyst in Fig. 7-7 from a solid suspicious mass in Fig. 7-8.

dominant palpable mass with a negative mammogram and a negative sonogram could still be a carcinoma, and surgical biopsy may be indicated. Clinical judgment must be used to prevent missing a cancer.

- *To evaluate patients with symptoms of breast infection.* In a patient with acute onset of a warm, tender, red breast, ultrasound can differentiate an infected breast cyst or an abscess from inflammatory carcinoma, which can mimic infection. Inflammatory carcinoma can present as a red, warm, tender breast with skin thickening (peau d'orange) (see Fig. 7-6).

- *To evaluate symptomatic patents with breast implants.* Ultrasound can differentiate a breast mass from a palpable portion of an implant or detect a ruptured silicone implant as the cause of a palpable mass.

- *To evaluate symptomatic young women with a palpable mass.* Since there is no ionizing radiation with ultrasound, breast masses in young women under age 30 can be evaluated primarily with ultrasound.

- *To evaluate symptomatic women whenever malignancy is suspected.* Ultrasound can evaluate the primary tumor and search for unsuspected multicentric or multifocal lesions or unsuspected axillary metastases, which can aid in staging and treatment planning. Ultrasound is especially useful in women with dense breast tissue that could mammographically obscure a palpable mass.

- *To assess a mass that cannot be completely evaluated with mammography.* Masses located peripherally may be outside the field of view of a mammogram and can be evaluated with ultrasound.
- *To guide interventional procedures.* During real-time ultrasound-guided fine-needle biopsy (FNAB) or core biopsy (CB), the needle can be visualized continuously within the mass, ensuring that the target lesion has been sampled.
- *To perform ultrasound-guided preoperative needle localization.* Whenever a suspicious lesion is seen by ultrasound and mammography or by ultrasound alone, ultrasound-guided needle localization (47) is preferred because of ease of performance and patient comfort. The patient is recumbent for both the ultrasound-guided needle localization and the surgical procedure, which provides a shorter distance from the skin entrance to the mass, and this is preferred by many surgeons.

Although ultrasound is complementary to clinical breast examination and mammography, it cannot be used for screening of asymptomatic women because it does not detect microcalcifications, which may be the only sign of an underlying malignancy. Furthermore, with older ultrasound equipment, false-positive (48) and false-negative results (49) were reported. With newer, higher-resolution ultrasound equipment, however, unsuspected cancers that were clinically and mammographically occult have been detected by ultrasound in 2.3% of cases (50,51). For a select group of women at high risk, especially those with one of the breast cancer genes (i.e., *BRCA1* or *BRCA2*), with dense breast tissue, with equivocal clinical breast examination, or young age, there may be a future role for screening with high-resolution bilateral breast ultrasound. A recent study of bilateral screening ultrasound found unsuspected occult carcinomas detected by ultrasound alone (not detected by clinical examination or mammography) in 0.3% of asymptomatic women with dense glandular tissue (52). The lack of ionizing radiation with ultrasound is an advantage over mammography, especially for young women under age 35.

Breast ultrasound is very operator-dependent and requires correlation of the mammographic abnormality and its location with the sonographic findings (12). Preferably, the radiologist who interprets the mammogram also performs the breast ultrasound in order to better correlate the mammographic and clinical findings with the ultrasound images and to guide any interventional procedures.

Breast Imaging Workup of Microcalcifications and Masses

The workup of microcalcifications is illustrated using a typical algorithm (Fig. 7-9). For indeterminate or suspicious microcalcifications, stereotactic core biopsy can establish a histologic diagnosis. An x-ray of the core samples ensures that some of the suspicious calcifications are included for histologic analysis.

The pathologist describes the histology of the tissue associated with the microcalcifications (see discussion in Chap. 8). If the calcifications are within benign tissue, the patient can be followed to ensure stability. If the calcifications are associated with malignant or atypical histology,

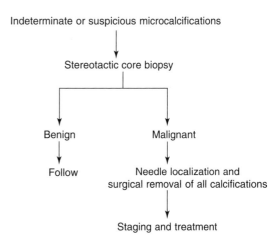

Figure 7-9. Algorithm for workup of indeterminate calcifications.

mammography-guided needle localization and surgical removal of the entire area of micro-calcifications are indicated. Definitive treatment will depend on the histologic analysis of the segmental resection. If the area is DCIS and the margins of resection are free of tumor, the patient could receive breast-conservation therapy. In some cases of DCIS, if the surgeon cannot obtain clear margins because of the large area of disease, or if good cosmesis cannot be achieved because of the size of the breast relative to the extent of the disease, a mastectomy may be required. If on histologic analysis there is microscopic inva-sive carcinoma as well as DCIS, axillary node dissection would be indicated, and the treatment would be the same for invasive cancer, which depends on the size and stage of the tumor.

The workup of a mass, whether it is pal-pable or found mammographically, includes sonographic evaluation (Fig. 7-10). If ultrasound reveals a simple cyst, the patient can be reas-sured and followed, or a dominant symptomatic cyst can be aspirated. If ultrasound reveals an indeterminate mass, fine-needle biopsy under

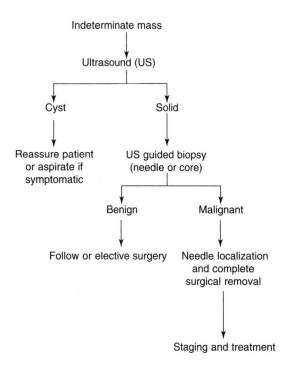

Figure 7-10. Algorithm for workup of a palpable mass, mammographic mass, or suspected mass.

ultrasound guidance can determine if this rep-resents a complex cyst (benign) or a solid mass. Ultrasound-guided core biopsy can diagnose a benign fibroadenoma with a high degree of accuracy, and this could be followed or be removed surgically, depending on the size and the patient's wishes. Malignant or atypical his-tology requires needle localization under ultra-sound guidance and complete surgical removal of the mass. The definitive treatment will depend on the stage of the tumor based on its size and the axillary node status.

Controversies Regarding Benefit and Optimal Intervals for Screening Young Women

Randomized, controlled clinical trials are the best method to determine whether a group of asymptomatic women undergoing periodic screening mammograms have fewer deaths from breast cancer compared with an unscreened control group. These trials require randomization of a large number of women into the "screening" or "control" groups and require follow-up of these women for many years to determine a statistically significant benefit. There have been many international controlled clinical trials that have shown a statistically significant benefit in the reduction of mortality from breast cancer for women age 50 and older (4).

Based on these data, in 1989, the Consensus Guidelines were accepted by the National Cancer Institute and the American Cancer Society and by 12 medical associations. These guidelines recommended a baseline mammogram by age 40, mammography every 1 to 2 years for women in their 40s, annual mammography for women aged 50 and older, and annual clinical breast examinations for all women aged 40 and older. Women aged 50 and older showed a statistically significant benefit after approximately 5 years of follow-up. Because of insufficient numbers of women in their 40s enrolled in the trials, and because younger women live more years after their breast cancer diagnosis, a longer follow-up period of approximately 10 years was needed to show a benefit from screening mammography.

This led to controversy over the "proof" of benefit for screening women aged 40 to 49 (53).

In 1993, the National Cancer Institute withdrew its recommendation for screening women in their 40s based on inconsistencies in the data (54,55). Subsequently, new data based on a meta-analysis that combined the numbers of younger women in eight randomized trials and looked at longer follow-up showed a significant benefit for younger women from screening mammography. Data also emerged that showed faster growth of breast cancers in younger women in their 40s compared with those aged 50 and older (56). The lead time for breast cancer in younger women aged 40 to 49 was shown to be 2 years or less than the approximately 4 years for women aged 50 and older (57). Tabar showed a mean sojourn time of 1.7 years for women aged 40 to 49 compared with 3.3 years for women aged 50 to 59 years, 3.8 for women aged 60 to 69, and 2.6 years for those aged 70 to 74 years (20,58). These results suggest that the smaller mortality reduction in women aged 40 to 49 years may be due to faster growth of some breast cancers as well as a rapid increase in the incidence of breast cancer during the decade of 40 to 49 years. These observations suggest that the interval between screening in the 40- to 49-year-old age group should be shortened to every year to achieve a greater benefit in this group rather than every 2 years. It is possible that annual screening in the 40- to 49-year-old group would result in a 19% reduction in mortality from breast cancer (20). Based on these new data, the American Cancer Society announced in 1997 that women in their 40s should have screening mammograms every year. The National Cancer Institute also reversed itself and recommended screening every 1 to 2 years, depending on risk factors, for women beginning at age 40. Many physicians believe that the intervals between screenings in women 40 to 49 years of age should be every year in order to reflect the biologic differences of faster tumor growth and the rapid increase in the incidence of breast cancer in this decade of life. Among younger women diagnosed with breast cancer before age 50, there is a 40% loss of years of life due to breast cancer (59).

The benefits of screening mammography of aysmptomatic women are the reduction of mortality from early-stage cancer and the increased use of breast-conservation treatment (i.e., segmental resection and whole-breast irradiation) for smaller cancers. Another benefit is a reduction in health care costs by reducing the number of advanced cancers (60–64). The survival is the same for women above and below age 50 when similar size, histologic grade, and stage are compared (65,66). Mammography has been shown to find early-stage breast tumors in women in their 40s as well as women in their 50s (53). There are no statistical differences in screen-detected cancers between women aged 40 to 49 and women aged 50 to 64 when comparing size, lymph node status, or stage of breast cancer (67). Thus annual screening of women aged 40 and older (and for even younger women who are at high risk) is the most prudent advice in order to decrease mortality from breast cancer and improve the quality of life (20,53,56).

Summary

For young women with an abnormal clinical breast examination, a combination of ultrasound and limited mammography (depending on the patient's age) can help to differentiate benign conditions from those which are likely to be malignant. Interventional procedures (discussed in Chap. 8) can establish a definitive tissue diagnosis.

There may be a future role for screening high-risk women under age 40 with periodic mammography and ultrasound. The role of screening these high-risk women with magnetic resonance imaging (MRI) and radionuclide scanning [sestamibi and positron-emission tomography (PET)] has yet to be defined. Each case should be individualized (see Table 7-1) depending on the severity of the risk and the patient's age in order to achieve the benefit of decreased mortality with the early detection of carcinoma.

References
1. Baker LH. Breast Cancer Detection Demonstration Project: Five-year summary report. CA 1982;32:196–225.
2. Ikeda DM, Andersson I. Ductal carcinoma in situ: atypical mammographic appearances. Radiology 1989;172:661–666.

entry to and exit from the preclinical detectable phase. Stat Med 1995;14:1531–1543.

59. Shapiro S, Venet W, Strax P, Veneth L. Periodic screening for breast cancer: the Health Insurance Plan Project and its sequelae, 1963–1986. Baltimore: Johns Hopkins University Press, 1988.

60. Solin LJ, Legoretta A, Schultz DJ, et al. The importance of mammographic screening relative to the treatment of women with carcinoma of the breast. Arch Intern Med 1994;154:745–752.

61. Feig SA. Cost-effectiveness of annual versus biennial mammographic screening of women age 40–49 years. Radiology 1996;198(suppl):206. Abstract RSNA.

62. Lindfors KK, Rosenquist J. The cost-effectiveness of mammographic screening strategies. JAMA 1995;274:881–884.

63. Tengs TO, Adams ME, Pliskin JS, et al. Five-hundred life-saving interventions and their cost-effectiveness. Risk Analysis 1995;15:369–384.

64. Kattlove H, Liberati A, Keeler E, Brook RH. Benefits and costs of screening and treatment for early breast cancer: Development of a basic benefit package. JAMA 1995;273:142–148.

65. Smart CR. Highlights of the evidence of benefit for women aged 40–49 years from the 14-year follow-up of the Breast Cancer Detection Demonstration Project. Cancer 1994;74:296–300.

66. Tabar L. New Swedish breast cancer detection results for women aged 40–49. Cancer 1993;72:1437–1448.

67. Curpen BN, Sickles EA, Sollitto RA, et al. The comparative value of mammographic screening for women 40–49 years old versus women 50–64 years old. AJR 1995;164:1099–1103.

8

Imaging-Guided Percutaneous Biopsies

Jules Sumkin and Kathleen M. Harris

For indeterminate masses or microcalcifications, percuctaneous image-guided biopsies with ultrasound or stereotactic guidance can establish a definitive diagnosis. This prevents delays in diagnosis and improves patient management. For malignant lesions, a one-stage surgical procedure can be performed (segmental resection and axillary node dissection), and for benign lesions, either elective surgery or close follow-up can be performed.

Ultrasound-Guided Biopsy

Breast ultrasound can identify simple cysts (1), but it cannot distinguish complex cysts from solid masses, nor can it always differentiate benign from malignant masses (2). Complex cysts can contain cellular material, proteinaceous material, cholesterol crystals, hemorrhage, or infection and can mimic a solid mass sonographically. Benign solid masses have sharp margins, few or no lobulations, and are oval in configuration with the longest axis parallel to the chest wall (3,4) and with acoustic enhancement. Malignant masses have irregular margins with spiculated or microlobulated borders, can be oriented perpendicular to the chest wall, and may have posterior acoustic shadowing (5,6). Not all masses, however, display these classic sonographic appearances. Carcinoma can have smooth borders with acoustic enhancement and mimic a fibroadenoma. Likewise, benign lesions such as fibroadenomas or complex cysts can appear irregular with acoustic shadowing and mimic a carcinoma. Therefore, for sonographically indeterminate lesions, ultrasound-guided percutaneous

biopsy is an important part of the diagnostic workup. Percutaneous tissue sampling of indeterminate breast lesions can differentiate benign from malignant lesions (7–9) (Fig. 8-1). Tissue sampling thus allows patients to be triaged into those who need definitive treatment for carcinoma or those who can be managed with elective surgery or close follow-up for benign conditions. Percutaneous tissue sampling eliminates delays in diagnosis for carcinoma and has been shown to be cost-effective.

If a suspicious lesion is proven to be malignant by needle biopsy, the surgeon can plan a one-stage procedure to completely remove the cancer and a rim of normal tissue (segmental resection, or "lumpectomy") and perform the axillary lymph node dissection for staging at the same time (one operation instead of two). Without a preoperative diagnosis with prior needle or core biopsy, two procedures would need to be performed, that is, one as an outpatient to remove the lesion and second to remove the axillary nodes for staging and to excise any possible residual tumor in the breast. Obtaining a definitive diagnosis of carcinoma by fine-needle aspiration biopsy (FNAB) or core biopsy (CB) allows the surgeon and the medical oncologist to discuss the treatment options with the patient. This is especially important in patients with large tumors that may require mastectomy rather than breast-conservation therapy or that may require neoadjuvant chemotherapy to shrink the tumor prior to any surgical intervention. Indications for ultrasound-guided tissue sampling instead of short-interval follow-up for "probably benign" lesions would include confirmation that a lesion is benign, elimination of patient anxiety, and

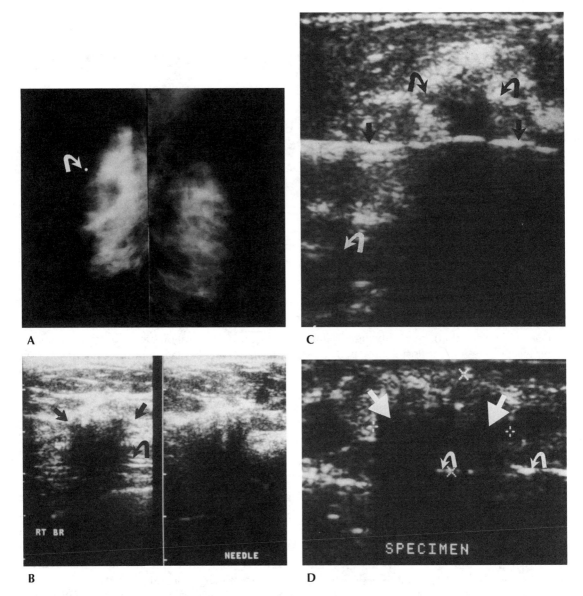

Figure 8-1. This 31-year-old nulliparous woman was referred for diagnostic imaging because of a palpable right breast mass. The patient's sister had breast cancer at age 34. (**A**) Mammographically, the glandular tissue is extremely dense bilaterally in the side-by-side mediolateral oblique views. Dense glandular tissue is common in young women. A metal marker (curved arrow) has been placed on the skin over the palpable mass in the upper outer quadrant. The dense glandular tissue obscures the lesion. There are no microcalcifications. (**B**) Ultrasound of the palpable mass revealed a simple cyst (now shown). Serendipitously, by ultrasound an unsuspected mass was present in the upper inner quadrant. The mass is hypoechoic, irregularly marginated (straight arrows), and is deep near the pectoral muscle (curved arrow). Note the acoustic shadowing posterior to the mass. Because of the high suspicion of malignancy, ultrasound-guided fine-needle aspiration was performed followed by ultrasound-guided core biopsy. (**C**) The needle shown as a straight echogenic line (straight arrows) has traversed the mass (curved black arrows), proving that the mass has been sampled. The needle is parallel to the chest wall in order to prevent entering the underlying lung. The pectoral muscle is shown (curved white arrow). The histology of the cores revealed infiltrating ductal carcinoma. (**D**) The patient had a one-stage segmental resection and axillary node dissection. A preoperative ultrasound-guided needle localization was performed because the cancer could not be seen mammographically and was not palpable. Ultrasound of the resected specimen shows the echogenic localization wire (curved arrows) within the mass (large straight arrows).

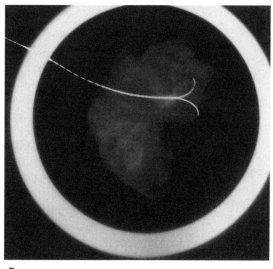

E

Figure 8-1. (*continued*) (**E**) A specimen radiograph of the resected mass reveals the double-hook localization wire to be within the spiculated mass. Pathology revealed a 1.5-cm infiltrating ductal carcinoma. All the axillary nodes were free of metastases. The patient was treated with breast conservation including whole-breast irradiation. This case illustrates an unsuspected cancer found by ultrasound in a high-risk woman who presented with a benign palpable cyst. Interventional ultrasound-guided core biopsy established the preoperative diagnosis.

avoiding delays in diagnosis for unsuspected malignant lesions.

Tissue sampling can be performed by palpation guidance (10), ultrasound guidance (8,9), or stereotactic guidance (11). Palpable lesions can be biopsied percutaneously by the surgeon, but palpable lesions that are deep near the chest wall or in a large breast are often referred by the surgeon to the radiologist for ultrasound-guided biopsy, which enables visualization of the needle in the mass, thus ensuring that the correct area has been sampled.

The choices for ultrasound-guided tissue sampling include fine-needle aspiration biopsy (FNAB), which yields a cytologic diagnosis, or core biopsy (CB) using a biopsy gun, which yields a histologic diagnosis. The decision as to which method to use (FNAB or CB) will depend on 1) the type of lesion and its location, 2) the experience and preferences of the radiologist, and 3) the expertise of the pathologist in interpreting cytology or histology. Most pathologists prefer core biopsies because they allow a histologic diagnosis, which is easier to interpret than breast cytology.

The advantage of ultrasound-guided biopsies is that any sonographically visible lesion can be biopsied, whether it is deep near the pectoral muscle, near a breast implant, or in the axilla. The disadvantage of ultrasound is the inability to visualize microcalcifications or isoechoic masses (i.e., masses with similar echogenicity to adipose tissue). Therefore, lesions that are mammographically visible and sonographically invisible can be sampled with mammography-guided stereotactic biopsies.

There are advantages and disadvantages to FNAB versus CB. Every mass does not need a core biopsy for diagnosis. FNAB is less invasive using 23- to 21-gauge "skinny" needles. There is no need for a skin incision with a fine needle, and local anesthesia is usually unnecessary unless the needle entrance is near the areola or the patient prefers local skin anesthesia. CB is more invasive, using a 14-gauge needle (sometimes with a 13-gauge coaxial guide), a small skin incision at the needle entry site, and local anesthesia. FNAB uses a shorter distance, has a simpler setup, is less time-consuming, and is easier to perform. Both FNAB and CB require an approach parallel to the chest wall to avoid entering the thorax. Visualizing the tip and shaft of the needle throughout the procedure can prevent inadvertently entering the lung. With the smaller needle used with FNAB, there are fewer complications, but hematoma, pneumothorax, and infection can occur. The complications with CB are the same as for FNAB except that tumor cells are more likely to be "seeded" into the breast during the forward thrust of a CB (12,13). This displaced tumor nidus potentially could grow if it remains within the breast, although this has not been documented. Additionally, milk fistula has been reported following CB of lesions in pregnant or lactating women (14).

In general, malignant lesions are very cellular and yield abundant cells with FNAB. Hypocellular malignancies such as infiltrating lobular carcinoma can have sparse cells and be difficult to diagnose with FNAB. Fibroadenomas that have become hyalinized are also hypocellular and may yield insufficient cells for diagnosis with FNAB. CB therefore may provide a specific diagnosis in these instances.

Cytopathology from FNAB can determine if a lesion is benign or malignant but cannot differentiate ductal carcinoma in situ (DCIS) from invasive carcinoma. Core histology is necessary to differentiate DCIS from invasive carcinoma and allows analysis of tumor receptors (estrogen and progesterone) and other tumor markers. It is not always possible to differentiate a papilloma from a papillary carcinoma by percutaneous tissue sampling (FNAB or CB), and surgical excision may be required for definitive diagnosis of papillary lesions. With spiculated masses, needle localization and surgical removal of the entire lesion are preferable to percutaneous biopsy. Core samples may not yield enough tissue for the pathologist to differentiate a benign radial scar from a well-differentiated tubular carcinoma because the entire lesion must be analyzed histologically to make the correct diagnosis.

Ultrasound guidance with free-hand technique (FNAB or CB) allows multiple lesions to be sampled, especially if multifocal or multicentric carcinoma is suspected.

Lesions for which FNAB is preferable include

● Any fluid-filled lesion (i.e., symptomatic simple cyst or complex cyst).
● Any abscess or infected cyst (to drain the lesion and obtain material for microbiology).
● Necrotic lesions.
● An intracystic mass. FNAB is also used to perform a pneumocystogram. Air is injected into the cyst after removal of the fluid, and the mammogram is repeated to outline an intracystic mass.
● Any lesions in pregnant or lactating woman (development of a milk fistula has been reported with CB).
● Enlarged axillary nodes (to diagnose metastases, lymphoma, or benign reactive nodes).
● Locally advanced breast cancer or inflammatory carcinoma where neoadjuvant chemotherapy is indicated and the diagnosis of malignancy is needed prior to chemotherapy.

Lesions for which CB is preferable include.

● Any lesion for which it is necessary to establish a specific benign diagnosis such as fibroadenoma in order to avoid surgery or short-interval follow-up.
● Any lesion for which it is necessary to establish a specific malignant diagnosis such as infiltrating ductal carcinoma or ductal carcinoma in situ.
● Any malignant lesion from which it is necessary to obtain ER and PR receptors.
● Any lesion for which it is necessary to establish a diagnosis after an insufficient cytology following FNAB.

It is not necessary to send all cyst fluid for cytologic analysis. We discard cyst fluid that has the typical appearance of a benign cyst (straw colored). Whenever a cyst does not disappear completely, or if an intracystic mass is suspected, or if the fluid is bloody or thick, the aspirate is sent for cytologic analysis.

Limitations of ultrasound-guided biopsies can be insufficient samples (too few cells to make a diagnosis), difficulty in visualizing the needle during the biopsy, and movable lesions.

Ultrasound-guided FNAB or CB can reliably sample indeterminate lesions, identifying benign or malignant lesions with a high sensitivity and specificity (8,15,16). Teamwork is required among the radiologist, cytopathologist, histopathologist, and surgeon to correlate any discrepancy. Good clinical judgment of each individual patient is imperative. The radiologist who performs the biopsy correlates the prebiopsy radiologic prediction (prediction of a probably benign lesion or suspected malignant lesion) with the pathology report (cytology following FNAB or histology following CB). When there is *concordance* between the prebiopsy radiologic prediction and cytologic or histologic diagnosis, benign lesions can be followed or electively surgically removed and malignant lesions can be referred for definitive surgical and/or oncologic treatment. When the prebiopsy radiologic prediction and cytologic or histologic diagnosis are *discordant*, surgical biopsy is recommended. False-negative results can occur with sampling errors or insufficient cells for diagnosis. Atypical ductal hyperplasia requires surgical excision for further identification of a possible adjacent malignancy (16,17).

Stereotaxic Breast Biopsy

As a direct result of increasing compliance with screening mammography guidelines and increased sensitivity of mammography, increasing numbers of suspicious, nonpalpable lesions are being discovered. In the past, many of these lesions were evaluated by needle localization and surgical excisional biopsy. Unfortunately, there is a significant cost and morbidity for a surgery that historically has been performed for benign lesions approximately 80% of the time (18).

In 1988, stereotaxic biopsy was introduced as a nonsurgical method of sampling mammographically visible, nonpalpable breast lesions. Although not totally accepted at first, stereotaxic biopsy is now considered to be a highly accurate, less invasive, and less expensive alternative to surgical biopsy (11,19–26).

Equipment and Procedure

The devices necessary to perform this type of biopsy consist of a computer, a needle holder, a biopsy device, and a method of obtaining stereotaxic mammograms (two projections separated by 30 degrees from one another) (Fig. 8-2). These mammograms are obtained either by a device added onto a standard mammography machine in which the biopsy is performed in the seated position or obtained with the patient lying prone on a dedicated table with the breast

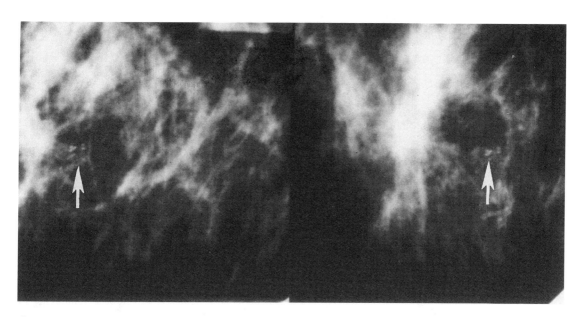

Figure 8-2. Stereotaxic views each taken 15 degrees off center. Note how the calcifications move in opposite directions relative to the center of the image (arrows).

suspended beneath the patient (Fig. 8-3). The computer allows rapid calculation of the three-dimensional location of a lesion within the breast based on movement of the lesion during the stereotaxic mammographic views. These coordinates are then used to position a needle, with the assistance of a needle holder, in the desired lesion (see Fig. 8-3).

FNAB has been used for years with both palpation guidance for palpable lesions and ultrasound guidance for nonpalpable lesions. With the introduction of stereotaxic technology, initially FNAB was employed, but it was quickly replaced by large-needle CB. CB is considered by most workers to be preferable because there is a smaller number of insufficient specimens and a lower false-negative rate (27–29). In addition, cytologic evaluation requires an experienced cytopathologist. Most pathologists feel more comfortable interpreting the histologic

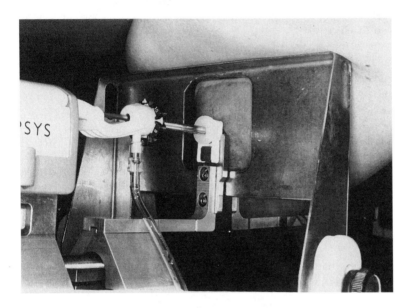

Figure 8-3. Dedicated stereotaxic table. The breast is suspended beneath the table through a hole in the table. The needle can be placed from any breast surface. The needle holder is visible beneath the patient.

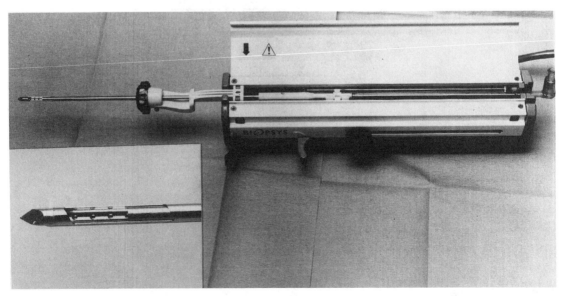

Figure 8-4. An 11-gauge mammotome needle. Inset reveals detail of sampling chamber. Note fenestration for tissue suction.

specimens from a CB. The first large CBs were performed with 18- and 14-gauge Tru-Cut needles. The smaller 18-gauge needles were abandoned in favor of the larger 14-gauge needles. More recently, newer devices are being used such as the mammotome device (Biopsys). This is a vacuum-assisted directional device with a hollow cutting cannula that allows for the removal of multiple 11-gauge core specimens with only one entry and removal of the needle into and from the breast (Fig. 8-4). A specimen harvested with an 11-gauge mammotome device (or mammotomy, as some call it) in general is two times the weight per each core specimen compared with a standard 14-gauge core needle. (30–32).

Another device recently introduced to compete with the mammotome is the ABBI (U.S. Surgical). This is an instrument capable of removing large cylinders of tissue up to 2 cm in diameter. It consists of a 20-mm plastic cannula containing a rotating blade that is powered by an electric motor that cuts in an oscillating fashion. Initial reports suggest that this technique may be an alternative to traditional needle localization and excisional biopsy. However, currently the device is approved by the FDA only as a diagnostic biopsy device (33).

Stereotaxic biopsy is performed as an outpatient procedure with local anesthesia. The only patient preparation is that no aspirin should be taken for a week prior to the procedure, and no nonsteroidal anti-inflammatory drugs should be taken for 2 days prior to the biopsy. Images are performed to document that the needle is within the lesion. In addition, specimen radiographs are taken when the biopsy is performed for calcification to ensure that calcium has indeed been obtained and is visible in the specimen (Fig. 8-5).

Indications

Initially, the major indication for stereotaxic biopsy was considered to be lesions with an intermediate probability of being malignant. These lesions would be considered to be BIRADS (Breast Imaging Reporting and Data System of the American College of Radiology) category 4, such as a round mass with a partially indistinct border or indeterminate microcalcifications. Lesions considered to be "probably benign" (BIRADS category 3) are safely followed with

6-month follow-up imaging (24,34). However, there are patients with "probably benign" lesions who find waiting 6 months intolerable. For these patients, stereotaxic biopsy is a viable option.

Increasingly, investigators have been advocating stereotaxic biopsy for evaluating "probably malignant" masses (BIRADS category 5). A preoperative diagnosis of breast cancer offers the advantage of a surgeon being able to discuss treatment options with the patient prior to surgery. It also allows a two-stage surgical procedure to be converted to a single-stage procedure. In other words, it would be possible to remove the tumor with clear margins and dissect the axillary lymph nodes in one operation (17,25,35) (Fig. 8-6). Liberman and colleagues (35) have shown that stereotaxic biopsy of nonpalpable spiculated masses decreased the number of surgical procedures in 77% of cases. Jackman and colleagues (25) demonstrated that the histologic concordance of CB and surgical excision is good enough that decision making can be made for a definitive treatment. The histologic concordance between DCIS versus invasive cancer and the determination of extensive intraductal components are excellent. In addition, the distinction between lobular carcinoma and intraductal carcinoma is very good (25).

Accuracy

The concordance between stereotaxic CB and surgery ranges between 87% and 97% (11, 19–23). Sensitivity is generally reported to be approximately 98%, with a specificity of 100% (false-positive results are distinctly unusual) (16,17,20–23,36). Most workers would concede that large-needle CB and needle localization with surgical excision are equally accurate (11, 16,20–22,37).

Problems

Atypical ductal hyperplasia (ADH) is problematic with large-needle CB. Indeed, lesions that reveal this histology at CB have an approximately 50% chance of proving to be carcinoma after surgical excision. (19,25,30,38–40). Even with newer acquisition devices such as the mammotome, there is a 44% risk of ADH being upgraded to carcinoma at final pathology if surgery is

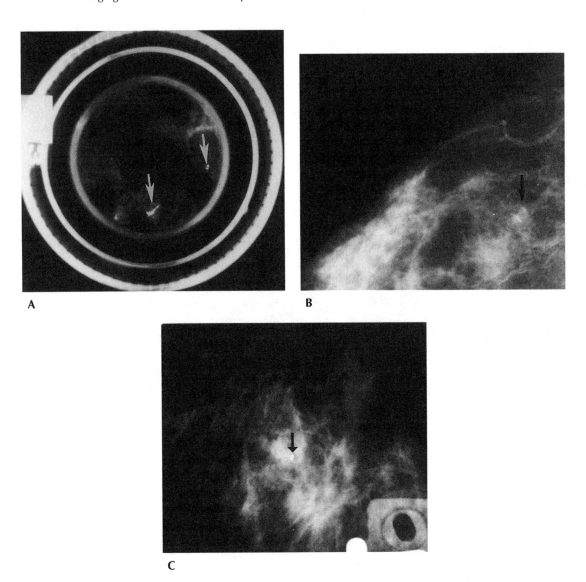

Figure 8-5. (**A**) Specimen of calcifications from a hylanized fibroadenoma (white arrows). (**B**) Note calcifications seen on MLO view of mammogram (black arrows). Specimen was obtained with 11-gauge mammotome needle. (**C**) Since all of the calcifications were removed a metallic marker was placed at the time of the biopsy (arrow).

performed. It appears that part of this problem may be sampling error, but another part of the problem rests with subjective difficulties the pathologist has in distinguishing between ADH and low-grade noncomedo DCIS. It appears prudent, therefore, to recommend surgical excision when the diagnosis of ADH is made by large-needle CB.

Although seeding of the needle track is considered possible, it is estimated to occur with similar infrequency as in other parts of the body (from 0.003% to 0.009%) (27,41). The significance of this complication is further minimized by the fact that when cancer is diagnosed by CB, the needle track can be removed during surgical excision. Although hematomas occur approximately 40% of the time, they are superficial and are rarely symptomatic (42).

Cost-Effectiveness

Cost-effectiveness has been evaluated carefully by numerous investigators. In an evaluation of

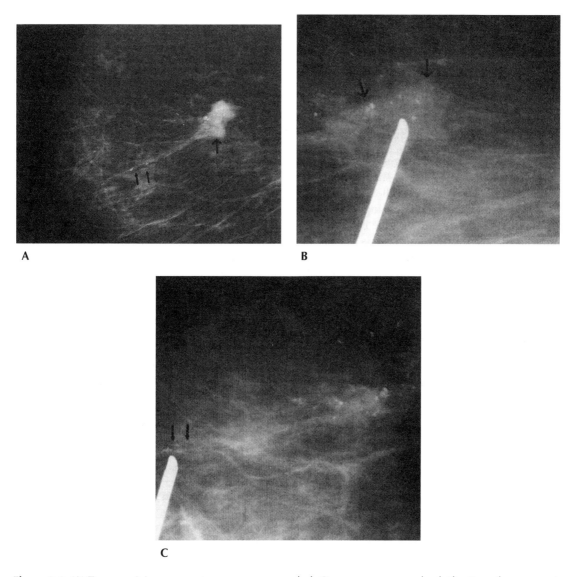

Figure 8-6. (**A**) Two suspicious separate areas were sampled. One was a mass and calcifications (large arrow), the other was calcifications (small arrows). (**B** and **C**) Biopsy of both areas was performed. Both demonstrated invasive infiltration ductal carcinoma and DCIS. Mastectomy was performed.

405 lesions in 356 women, Lee and colleagues (43) noted that open surgical biopsy could be averted in 81% of these patients. Overall cost savings for stereotaxic CB over open surgical biopsy were $741 per patient, slightly more in patients with masses and less for those with calcifications. Others have found similar cost savings, such as the study by Liberman and colleagues (24), in which the mean adjusted direct savings in cost per stereotaxic CB was $893 using Medicare compensation. Extrapolating these results at the national level would result in annual savings of approximately $200 million.

Outcomes

Despite proven cost-effectiveness, an improved outcome in patient care is the desirable goal. In a study by Rubin and colleagues (38), the introduction of stereotaxic biopsy into the breast care program more than doubled the yield of cancer at surgical biopsy from 21% prior to

9

New Horizons in Breast Imaging

Jules Sumkin and Lara A. Hardesty

Nuclear Medicine in Breast Imaging

Mammography in combination with sonography is currently the best method for the early detection of breast cancer, but it has limitations, especially in dense breasts, post-operative breasts, and implant-containing breasts. Complementary new techniques with which to image breast cancer include nuclear medicine techniques such as positron-emission tomography (PET) and scintimammography.

PET

Positron-emission tomography (PET) is an imaging modality approved by the Food and Drug Administration (FDA). PET uses positron-emitting radionuclides that decay by emitting two photons that travel in opposite directions. PET scanning works by detecting these two photons, called *coincidence detection* (1). The radionuclides used in PET scanning are short-lived and must be manufactured by a cyclotron.

PET in Tumor Imaging

PET has the ability to image primary, axillary, and systemic breast carcinoma. PET tumor imaging uses specific metabolic tracers labeled with positron emitters and relies on the physiologic changes in tumors relative to normal tissue.

Tumors have increased consumption of glucose. Fluorine-18 (a positron emitter) is incorporated into fluorodeoxyglucose (FDG), a structural analogue of glucose. FDG is transported into the tumor cell like glucose, and once phosphorylated, it cannot recross the cell membrane (1).

FDG is the most commonly used radiopharmaceutical for PET breast cancer imaging, but other metabolic tracers are used, including DNA precursors such as thymidine (2), protein precursors such as amino acids (3), and estradiol, a ligand for the estrogen receptor that is expressed on the surface of many breast carcinomas (4).

Protocol

For PET imaging of the breast with FDG, the patient must have fasted for 4 hours to lower insulin and blood glucose levels. Blood glucose could compete with the radioactive FDG for uptake into tumor cells, thus lowering the sensitivity of the study (5).

Although variations exist, the protocol at our institution is a common one. First, 20 mCi of FDG are injected into an antecubital vein. The patient rests quietly for 2 hours to allow the tracer to distribute throughout the body. Then the patient lies supine on the PET scanner, which looks similar to a computed tomographic (CT) scanner, with her arms held above her head. A 15-minute *transmission scan* is performed to correct for body thickness (6). Then a 30-minute dynamic three-dimensional (3-D) *emission scan* is performed with the scanner's detectors sensing the emissions from the ^{18}F in the FDG molecules. Finally, a 60-minute two-dimensional (2-D) *whole-body scan* is performed to assess whether systemic metastatic disease is present.

There is no known adverse reaction to PET scanning using FDG. The whole-body effective radiation dose is 2 rem. This represents approximately one-third of the dose to which radiation workers may be exposed annually (5 rem) under current federal guidelines.

Study Interpretation

The data from the scans are reconstructed onto a computer monitor, and the images can be viewed as cross-sectional images in the transverse, coronal, or sagittal planes (Figs. 9-1, 9-2). Interpretation of the images is a form of "hot spot" interpretation. Areas of increased tracer activity indicate increased glucose use and suggest the presence of tumor at that location.

Uses

PET's most common use in breast imaging currently is as an adjunct to mammography and sonography in situations where mammography is notoriously unreliable. These situations include

1. *Breasts that contain dense glandular breast tissue* (7). This use for PET will likely increase as testing for the breast cancer genes increases and women at high risk need to have breast imaging performed at a younger age when their breasts are more dense.

2. *Breasts that contain implants for augmentation* (8). Despite the widespread use of implant-displacement (Eklund) mammographic views, the sensitivity of mammography in implant-containing breasts is lower than in other breasts. The photons used in PET scanning easily penetrate the silicone implants, unlike x-ray photons, so cancers are not obscured by the implants.

3. *Postoperative breasts*, whether from benign surgical biopsy or from segmental resection for carcinoma. Because PET images detect alterations in physiology, not alterations in anatomy, PET can determine whether an area of increased mammographic density represents postoperative scar or residual or recurrent tumor. Tumor has abnormally increased uptake of FDG, whereas scar does not.

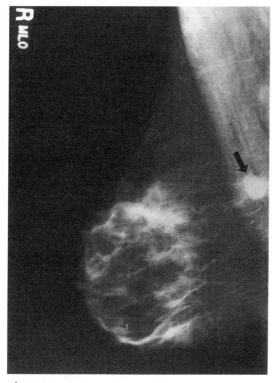
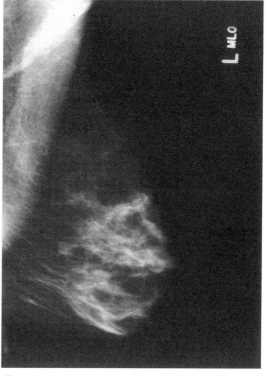

A   B

Figure 9-1. Mammography shows irregular new density at 1 o'clock in the right breast (**A**), near the pectoral muscle (arrow). Needle biopsy proved this to be infiltrating ductal carcinoma. (**B**) Normal left breast.

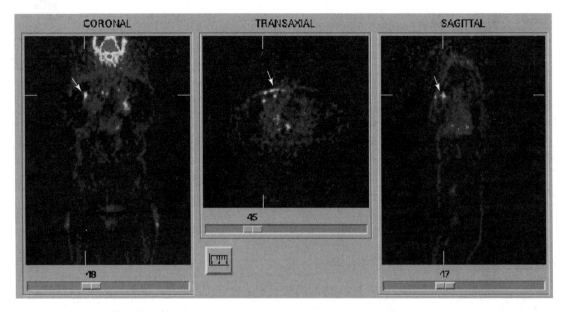

Figure 9-2. PET scan shows the breast carcinoma as an area of focally increased activity at 1 o'clock near the right pectoral muscle (arrows). The normal level of activity in the right axilla suggests that there are no axillary metastases. At axillary dissection, 19/19 nodes were negative for tumor.

PET can help determine which mammographic abnormalities should be biopsied and which can undergo short-interval (6-month) follow-up (9,10). Only 33% of mammographic lesions referred to biopsy are malignant (11–13). Benign breast lesions take up significantly less FDG than do malignant breast lesions (6). One published report shows PET to have a greater than 90% accuracy for this indication (10).

FDG PET can evaluate the response of locally advanced breast cancers to chemotherapy. Tumor response to treatment is currently assessed by sequential measurement of tumor or lymph node size on mammography, sonography, and physical examination. This method can be misleading with regard to the amount of remaining viable tumor because measurements often lag behind the actual decrease in viable tumor volume. FDG uptake occurs only in viable tumor cells, not in necrotic portions of a tumor. As early as 8 days after the initiation of chemotherapy, a significant decrease in tumor uptake of FDG compared with baseline pretreatment levels is seen in breast cancers that will eventually show a clinical response to that chemotherapeutic agent. This decrease in FDG uptake precedes decreases in tumor size that are

detectable by physical examination, mammography, or sonography (14,15). In contrast, the tumors that show no decrease in FDG uptake will show no clinical response even after completion of the course of chemotherapy (14,16,17). Once published study reports similar findings for the response of axillary node metastases to treatment (15). The use of PET to monitor response to treatment will allow early discontinuation or alteration of ineffective treatments in tumors that are not responsive (1).

Potential Uses

PET's ability to assess the status of the axillary lymph nodes in a noninvasive manner is being studied (10,18–21). This use of PET shows promise as a way to decrease the number of negative axillary node dissections in the future. Published results vary, showing sensitivities of 70% to 100% and specificities of 66% to 100% for the detection of axillary lymph node metastases. PET cannot detect micrometastases that can be found histologically by axillary dissection (20,22). One task force abstract (23) estimated that if axillary lymph node dissections were avoided based on negative PET scans, up to $160 million per year could be saved in the United States,

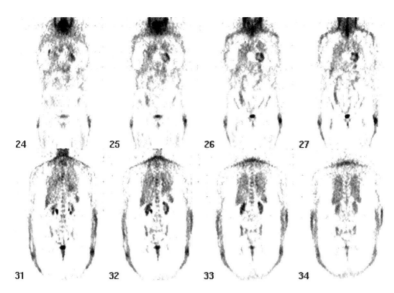

Figure 9-3. Total body PET scan of the patient in Figure 9-1 shows no evidence of distant metastatic disease from the known breast carcinoma.

with only 3% of axillae falsely classified as negative on PET scan and with the overall lower morbidity due to the avoided axillary dissections "far outweighing" the false-negative results (23). Larger-scale studies are needed to determine whether PET will enable us to decrease the number of axillary dissections without an adverse affect on patient survival.

Because the entire body can be scanned, PET shows potential as a single imaging study for the staging of breast carcinoma (Fig. 9-3). FDG PET can detect the primary, axillary or internal mammary lymphadenopathy, and distant metastases (e.g., bone, liver, lung, etc.) (7,9,22,24,25). PET's ability to detect regional spread of tumor to the internal mammary lymph nodes is important because the presence of tumor within the internal mammary lymph nodes has an impact on prognosis and treatment, yet these nodes are not assessed by axillary lymph node dissection. One report concluded that "FDG PET is able to identify local recurrence, lymph node involvement, and distant metastases with high sensitivity, and acceptable specificity" and reported sensitivity and specificity for distant metastases as 100% and 98% in bone, 83% and 97% in lung, and 100% and 97% in liver (25). Two other studies showed 100% sensitivity and 100% specificity for PET detection of distant metastases from breast cancer (7,9). Eventually, whole-body PET may

replace the current series of chest x-ray, abdominal CT, and total-body bone scan. This staging application of PET will need to undergo additional prospective clinical trials to determine its clinical usefulness.

Accuracy

Reported sensitivities and specificities reported for PET scanning in detecting primary breast carcinoma range from 80% to 100% and 86% to 100% respectively (Table 9-1). This wide variation is seen because most of the earlier studies did not include small, nonpalpable lesions. The resolution of most modern PET scanners is approximately 1 cm (1). This makes detection of lesions smaller than 1 cm very difficult. While some smaller tumors are detected (10,22), most tumors smaller than 1 cm are not. For primary breast tumors 1 cm or larger, the sensitivity of PET is nearly 100% (7,10), but for smaller tumors, the sensitivity is unknown (6) because such smaller tumors have not been studied extensively with PET (1). The ability of PET to detect axillary metastases and systemic metastases smaller than 1 cm is similarly limited and not adequately studied. Currently, the sensitivity and specificity of PET in the detection of axillary lymph node metastases range from 70% to 100% and 66% to 100%, respectively (Table 9-2).

Table 9-1. FDG PET scanning of primary breast lesions

Author	Year	No. of Patients	No. of Breast Lesions	Size (cm) of Breast Lesions	Sensitivity, %	Specificity, %	Ref.
Wahl	1991	10	10	3.2–12.0	100	—	7
Adler	1993	28	35	0.9–6.3	96	100	10
Nieweg	1993	20	20	$\geqslant$1.0	91		27
Wahl	1994	2[a]	2[a]	<1.5	100	100	8
Bassa	1996	16	17	0.6–5.0	100	100	15
Scheidhauer	1996	30	30	Stages T_1–T_4	91	86	9
Bender	1997	75	16[b]	Not given	80	96	25
Range					80–100	86–100	

[a] Both patients had silicone breast implants.
[b] All breast masses were recurrences of treated breast cancer.

Table 9-2. FDG PET scanning of axillary lymph nodes

Author	Year	No. of Axillae Scanned	Sensitivity, %	Specificity, %	Ref.
Tse	1992	—	70	100	22
Adler	1993	20	90	100	10
Bassa	1996	17	77	100	15
Avril	1996	37	79 overall	96 overall	20
Avril	1996	37	94 primary >2 cm	100 primary >2 cm	20
Avril	1996	37	33 primary <2 cm	100 primary <2 cm	20
Scheidhauer	1996	18	100	89	9
Adler	1997	52	95	66	21
Bender	1997	75	97	91	25
Range			70–100*	66–100	

*Excluding the 33% if primary <2 cm.

Limitations

PET scanning is expensive. Current PET scanners cost between $1 million and $2 million (1). Although not entirely necessary, an on-site cyclotron is ideal to produce the short-lived positron-emitting radiopharmaceuticals because time prohibits their production at a central cyclotron that is shared by several PET scanners (20). Cyclotrons have inherently high capital and operating costs.

A method is needed with which to localize PET-detected lesions for needle biopsy or open surgical biopsy. One method has been tested successfully on phantom breast lesions (28). This uses raw data from PET scans obtained at two different angles to calculate the x, y, and z axis coordinates of the lesions in a manner similar to mammographic stereotaxic biopsy. Further experimentation with design and clinical trials are needed urgently.

Future Developments

PET's limited ability to detect lesions smaller than 1 cm in size will likely improve in the near future with the development of dedicated breast PET scanners (29) and with improvements in the resolution of the most recently developed PET scanners (6). The newest PET scanners have 5-mm resolution in all three planes (26).

agreed that MRI of the breast had little to offer over conventional imaging techniques such as mammography. Conventional MRI relies on the water content of tumors to make them conspicuous. Since there is not a significant difference in water content between benign and malignant tumors, they exhibited similar behavior. In the middle 1980s, gadopentetate dimeglumine was introduced in Europe as a contrast agent. Several groups began experimenting with contrast-enhanced MRI (CE MRI). They discovered that CE MRI was a very sensitive technique for detecting cancer. Malignant tumors enhanced consistently and rapidly within the first minutes after injection of contrast material, whereas benign entities either did not enhance or enhanced more slowly (59–61). The earliest studies focused mainly on the enhancement characteristics of lesions. As experience grew and imaging protocols became more refined, morphologic evaluation assumed a more important role in attempts to improve the specificity of an already extremely sensitive technique (62–66).

Current Imaging Protocols and Equipment Considerations

Most breast MRI to date has been performed using standard 1.5-T magnets and specially designed surface coils placed around the breast for increased resolution. Recently, a lower-priced dedicated breast MRI unit operating at 0.5 T has been introduced. It is hoped that by making the equipment more affordable and placing it in the breast-imaging environment, utilization will become more practical (Fig. 9-6).

Multiple imaging protocols have been employed. In general, they take less than 10 minutes (53,57,67). Most institutions start with standard T_1- and T_2-weighted scout films without contrast enhancement. After administration of contrast material, multiple strategies are used. Initially, 2-D gradient-echo sequences were employed (59–61). Two-dimensional sequences excite protons within a single slice of tissue. These sequences allow evaluation of multiple slices over time with good demonstration of contrast kinetics. More recently, however, 3-D

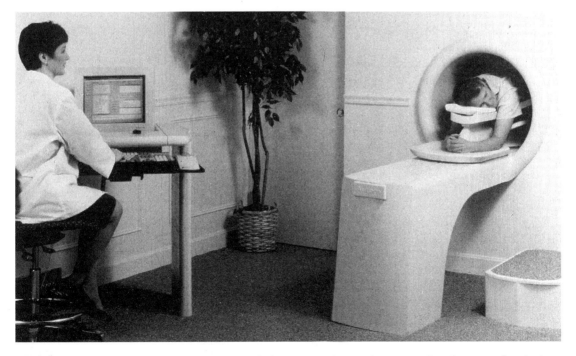

Figure 9-6. A 0.5-T dedicated breast magnet. With this magnet design, the patient's head is not within the bore of the magnet, which eliminates claustrophobia as a problem. Also, both breasts are imaged simultaneously, which is currently not possible on traditional machines with 1.5-T magnets.

gradient-echo sequences have been used. These sequences excite protons within a large volume of tissue, making it possible to obtain many slices simultaneously. With 3-D techniques, it is possible to re-format images in various planes, allowing spatial relationships to be determined. There is also improved spatial resolution, which results in better depiction of breast and tumor morphology. Investigators also discovered that removing fat from the image improves the conspicuity of tumors. Essentially there are two methods to remove fat from images: *fat-saturation pulses* and *subtraction*. Fat-saturation sequences take advantage of the different precession frequencies of fat and water protons, allowing differentiation of these types of tissues. With subtraction techniques, each voxel of the precontrast image is mathmatically subtracted from the postcontrast image. This leaves bright areas of increased signal intensity, which represent contrast-enhanced lesions. Slice thickness in the range of 2 to 3 mm is considered standard. This allows for the demonstration of very small tumors.

MRI Characteristics of Breast Cancer

The basis of tumor conspicuity by MRI is contrast enhancement. The histopathologic basis for tumor enhancement is thought to be related to tumor angiogenesis. Studies have demonstrated that once tumors attain a size of more than several millimeters, the growth of small blood vessels becomes necessary for continued tumor growth. These tiny blood vessels have been demonstrated in the stroma of breast cancers (68–70).

Most invasive breast cancers enhance focally, early, rapidly, and intensely. There does appear to be overlap, however, between benign and malignant disease. For instance, proliferative fibrocystic disease and sclerosing adenosis may enhance in a manner similar to cancer, whereas nonproliferative fibrocystic disease and fat necrosis do not (67) (Fig. 9-7). Morphologic features most specific for cancer include a mass with an irregular border and rim enhancement (Fig. 9-8). These features are 88% predictive of malignancy. Conversely, masses with smooth borders have a 97% negative predictive value (62) (see Fig. 9-7). Other features are also helpful; for instance,

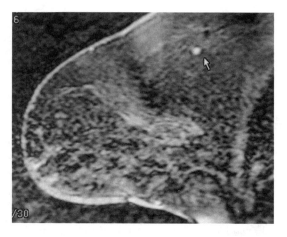

Figure 9-7. Gadolinium-enhanced breast MRI obtained with a 1.5-T magnet shows an enhancing benign intramammary lymph node in the upper outer quadrant of the breast. Despite early enhancement, smooth margins suggest benignity.

nonenhancing septations are very specific for fibroadenoma.

Characterization of cancer has been problematic. Similar to invasive cancer, ductal carcinoma in situ (DCIS) tends to enhance early in most cases. Reported sensitivities for the identification of DCIS have ranged from 40% to 100% (67,68,71–73). Enhancement patterns can be linear (ductal), regional, or peripheral (68). In 10% to 15% of patients, DCIS may not enhance at all (53,74,75). Variable detection of DCIS undoubtedly results from the small size of some DCIS lesions and to the variable histopathologic characteristics of the lesion.

Accuracy

Currently, the sensitivity of breast MRI is reported to range from 94% to 100%. Specificities from 37% to 97% have been reported (50,53,57,63,77–79). Experience has demonstrated that MRI is capable of detecting nonpalpable tumors, particularly in the dense breast, not detected by any other means. The introduction of interpretation models that take tumor morphology into consideration, along with rate and intensity of enhancement, has increased specificity to approximately 78%. Specificity may be limited by the fact that some cancers may enhance moderately, slowly, or diffusely. Some histologic types of cancer may be less likely to

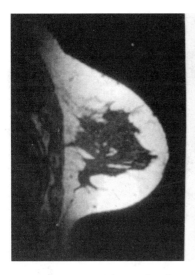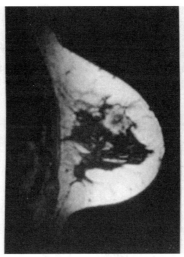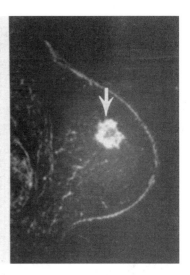

Figure 9-8. Images obtained with a 0.5-T dedicated breast magnet. The carcinoma is not seen on the unenhanced image. It is seen with gadolinium enhancement as a rapidly enhancing, irregularly marginated mass, best seen on the subtraction images (unenhanced image pixels are substracted from enhanced image pixels; arrows).

enhance, such as lobular, tubular, mucinous, and ductal carcinoma (65,74). Variable accuracy of MRI is likely due to differing imaging equipment (types of magnets and surface coils) and multiple imaging protocols. The experience of observers and the type of interpretation algorithm employed undoubtedly also affect accuracy. Hormonal factors may influence the accuracy of breast MRI as well. It has been noted that there may be diffuse and focal transient enhancement before and during menses. It has been suggested, therefore, that scans be performed between day 6 and 17 of the menstrual cycle. In addition, hormone-replacement therapy may cause false-positive scans. Scans may need to be repeated 2 to 3 months following the cessation of therapy (53).

Current Indications

MRI, like other modalities, such as ultrasound, sestamibi scintimammography, and PET scanning, should be considered an ancillary test to be used in selected patients in addition to a standard mammographic evaluation.

MRI may be of considerable help in surgical planning for patients with diagnosed breast cancer. Unsuspected multifocal disease is found in 44% to 60% of patients with clinically occult,

nonpalpable breast cancers detected at mammography (67,80–83). Because of its high sensitivity, MRI should prove to be of great value in helping plan for breast conservation therapy. For example, Harms and colleagues (67) detected additional cancers in 37% of patients with MRI that were not suspected by mammography (Fig. 9-9). In addition, because of its ability to more accurately depict tumor size, particularly in the dense breast, MRI is helpful to the surgeon in planning the lumpectomy size and should decrease the number of patients with positive margins (59) (Fig. 9-10).

MRI is a valuable tool in the evaluation of carcinoma of unknown primary in patients who present with isolated axillary nodal metastasis. This presentation is known to occur in 0.3% to 0.8% of patients who present with operable breast cancer (84,85). Morris and colleagues (84) found the primary tumor with MRI in 75% of patients who presented in this manner.

Other indications for MRI include the evaluation of tumor size in patients with locally advanced breast cancer before and after treatment with induction chemotherapy. It has been shown that MRI is more accurate than mammography, particularly in the dense breast, for the estimation of tumor size and hence tumor response to chemotherapy (53,67,86–91). MRI is also helpful as an adjunct to mammography in

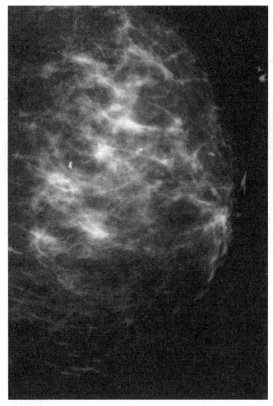

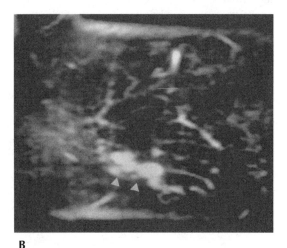

B

Figure 9-9. (**A**) MLO view from a mammogram and (**B**) corresponding view from an MRI showing an irregularly enhancing cancer (arrowheads) not visible on the mammogram.

the evaluation of suspicious lesions seen on only one mammographic view. MRI is helpful with clinical dilemmas such as unilateral spontaneous

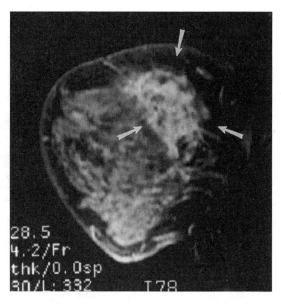

Figure 9-10. The saggital MRI projection demonstrates a large, enhancing, irregularly marginated area (arrows) that was biopsy-proven invasive lobular carcinoma. The mammogram (not shown) greatly underestimated the size of the palpable mass.

nipple discharge with a negative mammogram and palpable abnormalities in patients with negative conventional imaging (Fig. 9-11). Another clinical indication is in distinguishing post operative scarring from tumor recurrence (53,92).

The use of breast MRI in the evaluation of the high-risk patient has not yet been tested. Particularly in women with dense breasts, because of its high sensitivity, MRI holds considerable promise. Trials are ongoing world wide. Models have been designed to test the cost-effectiveness of breast MRI. Plevitris and colleagues (93) demonstrated that breast MRI, with reasonable assumptions, was cost-effective for screening young, high-risk populations at 3- or 4-year intervals. This certainly seems to justify large multi-institutional trials in this country, which will be necessary if screening is to become a standard of care. The challenge will be distinguishing MRI's false-positive results from benign disease such as proliferative fibrocystic disease and the ability to resolve them with biopsy capability.

Contra Indications

Currently, MRI is not indicated as a screening tool or in instances where conventional imaging

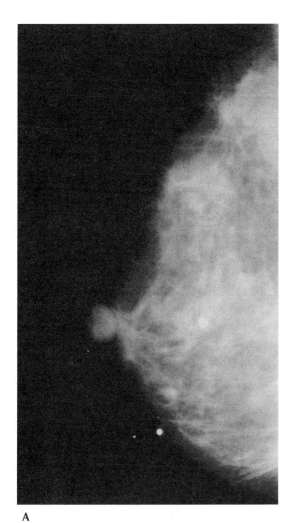

A

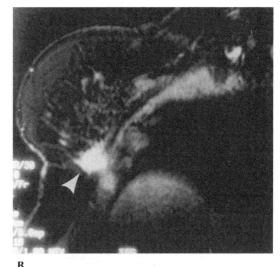

B

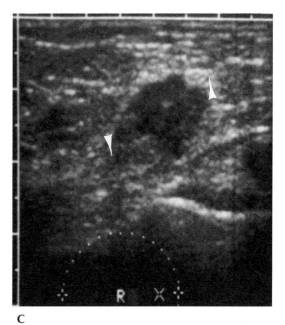

C

Figure 9-11. (**A**) MRI performed on a patient with a negative mammogram and palpable mass. (**B**) A "bb" on the skin marks palpable area. MRI images show an enhancing, irregularly marginated mass (arrows) that (**C**) could be demonstrated by ultrasound after the MRI.

tests such as mammography or ultrasound are sufficient. MRI is not indicated for the detection of malignancy in patients known to have benign diseases such as proliferative fibrocystic disease or benign inflammatory conditions such as mastitis, which are known to enhance. For example, MRI is not recommended to evaluate indeterminate microcalcifications because of the known difficulty in distinguishing DCIS from benign proliferative fibrocystic disease. This is particularly true in light of the extremely high specificity of stereotaxic core biopsy in this situation (53).

MRI-Directed Interventions

Because of the known false-positive results associated with breast MRI, it is important to be able to biopsy or needle localize for surgical excision any suspicious enhancing lesions. Although prototype MRI-directed core biopsy devices have been described in the literature, their efficacy has not been confirmed, nor are devices commercially available (94). There are technical hurdles to overcome. For instance, the contrast enhancement that makes a lesion visible lasts for approximately 6 minutes. Another problem relating to needle localization for excisional biopsy is that unlike conventional mammographic localization, there is no way to confirm that the lesion is within the biopsy material specimen.

Summary

MRI holds great promise as an additional problem-solving tool for diagnosing breast cancer. By virtue of its extremely high sensitivity, it will help us find nonpalpable cancers previously undetectable by conventional means. Because it is expensive and there is a significant incidence of false-positive results, it should be used in carefully chosen patients. The role that it will play in screening young patients with dense breast tissue who are at high risk for breast cancer remains to be elucidated.

References

1. Wahl RL. Nulcear medicine techniques in breast imaging. Semin Ultrasound CT MRI 1996; 17(5):494–505.
2. Larson SM, Grunbaum Z, Rasey JS. Positron imaging feasibility studies: selective tumor concentration of ^{3}H-thymidine, ^{3}H-uridine, and ^{14}C-2-deoxyglucose. Radiology 1980;134:771–773.
3. Leskinen-Kallio S, Nagren K, Lehikoinen P, et al. Uptake of ^{11}C-methionine in breast cancer studied by PET: an association with the size of S-phase fraction. Br J Cancer 1991;64:1121–1124.
4. Mintun MA, Welch MJ, Siegel BA, et al. Breast cancer: PET imaging of estrogen receptors. Radiology 1988;169:45–48.
5. Wahl RL, Henry CA, Ethier SP. Serum glucose: effects on tumor and normal tissue accumulation of 2-fluoro-2-deoxy-D-glucose in rodents with mammary carcinoma. Radiology 1992;183:643–647.
6. Adler DD, Wahl RL. New methods for imaging the breast: techniques, findings, and potential. AJR 1995;164:19–30.
7. Wahl RL, Cody R, Hutchins GD, et al. Primary and metastatic breast carcinoma: initial clinical evaluation with PET with the radiolabeled glucose analogue 2-[^{18}F]-fluoro-deoxy-2-D-glucose (FDG). Radiology 1991;179:765–770.
8. Wahl RL, Helvie MA, Chang AE, et al. Detection of breast cancer in women after agumentation mammoplasty using fluorine-18-fluorodeoxyglucose-PET. J Nucl Med 1994; 35:872–875.
9. Scheidhauer K, Scharl A, Pietrzyk U, et al. Qualitative [^{18}F]FDG positron emission tomography in primary breast cancer: clinical relevance and practicability. Eur J Nucl Med 1996;23:618–623.
10. Adler LP, Crowe JP, Al-Kaisi NK, et al. Evaluation of breast masses and axillary lymph nodes with with [^{18}F] 2-deoxy-2-fluoro-D-glucose PET. Radiology 1993;187:743–750.
11. Meyer JE, Eberlein TJ, Stomper PC, et al. Biopsy of occult breast lesions: analysis of 1261 abnormalities. JAMA 1990;263:2341–2343.
12. Kopans DB, Swann CA. Observations on mammographic screening and the false-positive mammograms. AJR 1988;150:785–786.
13. Tabar L, Gad A. Screening for breast cancer: the Swedish trial. Radiology 1981;138:221–222.
14. Wahl RL, Zasadny K, Helvie M, et al. Metabolic monitoring of breast cancer chemohormonotherapy using positron emission tomography: initial evaluation. J Clin Oncol 1993;11:2101–2111.
15. Bassa P, Kim EE, Inoue T, et al. Evaluation of preoperative chemotherapy using PET with fluorine-18-fluorodeoxyglucose in breast cancer. J Nucl Med 1996;37:931–938.
16. Jansson T, Westlin JE, Ahlstrom H, et al. Positron emission tomography studies in patients with locally advanced and/or metastatic breast cancer: a method for early therapy evaluation? J Clin Oncol 1995;13(6):1470–1477.
17. Bruce DM, Evans NTS, Heys SD, et al. Positron emission tomography: 2-deoxy-2[^{18}F]-fluoro-D-glucose uptake in locally advanced breast cancers. Eur J Surg Oncol 1995;21:280–283.
18. Wahl RL, Cody RL, August D. Initial evaluation of FDG PET for the staging of the axilla in newly diagnosed breast carcinoma patients. J Nucl Med 1991;32:981.
19. Crowe JP, Adler LP, Shenk RR, et al. Positron emission tomography and breast masses: comparison with clinical, ammographic, and pathological findings. Ann Surg Oncol 1994;1:132–140.
20. Avril N, Dose J, Janicke F, et al. Assessment of axillary lymph node involvement in breast cancer patients with positron emission tomography using radiolabeled 2-(fluorine-18)-fluoro-2-deoxy-D-glucose. J Natl Cancer Inst 1996; 88(17):1204–1209.
21. Adler LP, Fahulhaber PF, Schnur KC, et al. Axillary lymph node metastases: screening with [^{18}F]

2-deoxy-2-fluoro-D-glucose (FDG) PET. Radiology 1997;203:323–2327.

22. Tse NY, Hoh CK, Hawkins RA, et al. The application of positron emission tomographic imaging with fluorodeoxyglucose to the evaluation of breast disease. Ann Surg 1992;216:27–34.

23. ICP Breast Cancer Task Force. Positron emission tomography: clinical application and economic implications of PET in the assessment of axillary lymph node involvement in breast cancer. A retrsopective study. In: Proceedings of 1994 Institute for Clinical PET Meeting, ICP Breast Cancer Task Force. Fairfax, VA: Institute for Clinical PET, 1994. Abstract.

24. Hoh CK, Hawkins RA, Glaspy JA, et al. Cancer detection with whole-body PET using 2-[18F] fluoro-2-deoxy-D-glucose. J Comput Assist Tomogr 1993;17:582–589.

25. Bender H, Kirst J, Palmedo H, et al. Value of 18fluoro-deoxyglucose positron emission tomography in staging of recurrent breast carcinoma. Anticancer Res 1997;17Z:1687–1692.

26. Powe JE. Positron emission tomography (PET) scanning in breast cancer. Br J Radiol 1997; 70:668–670.

27. Nieweg OE, Kim EE, Wong WH, et al. Positron emission tomography with fluorine-18-deoxyglucose in the detection and staging of breast cancer. Cancer 1993;71:3920–3925.

28. Raylman RR, Ficaro EP, Wahl RL. Stereotactic coordinates from ECT sinograms for radionuclide-guided breast biopsy. J Nucl Med 1996;37:1562–1567.

29. Williams MB, Pisano ED, Schnall MD, et al. Future directions in imaging of breast disease. Radiology 1998;206:297–300.

30. O'Tuama LA, Packard AG, Treves SD, et al. SPECT imaging of pediatric brain tumor with hexakis methoxyisobutyl isonitrile 99mTc. J Nucl Med 1990;31:2040–2041.

31. Caner B, Kitapel M, Unlu M, et al. Technetium-99m MIBI uptake in benign and malignant bone lesions: a comparative study with technetium-99m MDP. J Nucl Med 1992;33:319–324.

32. Balon HR, Fink-Bennett DM, Stoffer SS. Technetium-99m uptake by recurrent Hurtle cell carcinoma of the thyroid. J Nucl Med 1992;33: 1393–1395.

33. O'Driscoll CM, Baker F, Casey M, et al. Localization of recurrent medullary thyroid carcinoma with technetium-99m-methoxyisobutylnitrile scintigraphy: a case report. J Nucl Med 1991; 32:2281–2283.

34. Kitapci MT, Tastekin G, Turgut M, et al. Preoperative localization of parathyroid carcinoma using Tc-99m MIBI. Clin Nucl Med 1993;18:217–219.

35. Taillifer R, Boucher Y, Potrin C, et al. Detection and localization of parathyroid adenomas in patients with hyperparathyroidism using a single radionuclide imaging procedure with technetium-99m sestamibi (double-phase study). J Nucl Med 1992;33:1801–1807.

36. Hassan IM, Sahweli A, Constantinides C, et al. Uptake and kinetics of Tc-99m hexakis 2-methoxyisobutyl isonitrile in benign and malignant lesions in the lungs. Clin Nucl Med 1989;14:333–340.

37. Khalkhali I, Mena I, Jouanne E, et al. Prone scintimammography in patients with suspicion of carcinoma of the breast. J Am Col Surg 1994;178:491–497.

38. Palmer EL, Scott JA, Strauss HW. Cardiovascular imaging. In: Bralow L, ed. Practical Nuclear Medicine. Philadelphia: WB Saunders, 1992: 71–120.

39. Khalkhali I, Cutrone JA, Mena IG, et al. Scintimammography: the complementary role of Tc-99m sestamibi prone breast imaging for the diagnosis of breast carcinoma. Radiology 1995;196:421–426.

40. Khalkhali I, Mena I, Diggles L. Review of imaging techniques for the diagnosis of breast cancer: a new role of prone scintimammography using technetium-99m sestamibi. Eur J Nucl Med 1994;21:357–362.

41. Hall FM. Technological advances in breast imaging: current and future strategies, controversies, and opportunities. Surg Oncol Clin North Am 1997;6:403–409.

42. Helbich TH, Becherer A, Trattnig S, et al. Differentiation of benign and malignant breast lesions: MR imaging versus Tc-99m sestamibi scintimammography. Radiology 1997;202:421–429.

43. Fenlon HM, Phelan NC, O'Sullivan PO, et al. Benign versus malignant breast disease: comparison of contrast-enhanced MR imaging and Tc-99m tetrosfosmin scintimammography. Radiology 1997;205:214–220.

44. Jackson VP, Hendrick RE, Kerg SA, et al. Imaging of the radiographically dense breast. Radiology 1993;1983:297–301.

45. Mena FJ, Mena I, Diggles L, et al. Design and assessment of a scintigraphy-guided biplane localization technique for breast tumours: a phantom study. Nucl Med Commun 1996; 17:717–723.

46. Scopinaro F, Ierardi M, Porfiri LM, et al. Tc-99m MIBI prone scintimammography in patients with high and intermediate risk mammography. Anticancer Res 1997;17:1635–1638.

47. Carril JM, Gomez-Barquin R, Quirce R, et al. Contribution of Tc-99m MIBI scintimammography to the diagnosis of non-palpable breast lesions in relation to mammographic probability of malignancy. Anticancer Res 1997; 17:1677–1682.

48. Kao CH, Wang SJ, Liu TJ. The use of technetium-99m methoxyisobutylisonitrile breast scintigraphy to evaluate palpable breast masses. Eur J Nucl Med 1994;21:432–436.

49. Lam WW, Yang WT, Chan YL, et al. Role of MIBI breast scintigraphy in evaluation of palpable breast lesions. Br J Radiol 1996;69:1152–1158.

50. Servais F, Blocklet DC, Seret AE, et al. Differentiation between benign and malignant breast lesions with MR imaging and scintimammography. Radiology 1997;205–283.

51. Delpassant ES, Jackson EF. Differentiation between benign and malignant breast lesions with MR imaging and scintimammogrpahy. Radiology 1997;205:283–284.

52. Khalkhali I. Differentiation between benign and malignant breast lesions with MR imaging and scintimammography. Radiology 1997; 205:284–285.

53. Heywang-Kobrunner SH, Viehweg P, Heinig A, Kuchler Ch. Contrast-enhanced MRI of the breast: accuracy, value, controversies, solutions. Eur J Radiol 1997; 24:94–108.

54. Van Dijck JAAM, Verbeek ALM, Hendriks IHCL, Holland R. The current detectability of breast cancer in a mammographic screening program. Cancer 1993; 72:1933.

55. Harvey JA, Fajardo LL, Inhis CA. Previous mammograms in patients with impalpable breast cacrinoma: retrospective versus blinded interpretation. AJR 1993;161:1167.

56. Bird RE, Wallace TW, Yankaskas BC. Analysis of cancers missed at screening mammography. Radiology 1992;184:613.

57. Coons TA. MRI's role in assessing and managing breast disease. Radio Tech 1996;67(4):311–336.

58. Mansfield P, Morris PG, Ordidge R. Carcinoma of the breast imaged by NMR. Br J Radiol 1979;52:242–243.

59. Harms SE. MRI in breast cancer diagnosis and treatment. Curr Probl Diagn Radiol 1996; 25:193–215.

60. Heywang SH, Wolf A, Pruss E, et al. MR imaging of the breast with Gd-DTPA: use and limitations. Radiology 1989;171:95–103.

61. Stack JP, Redmond OM, Codd MB, et al. Breast disease: tissue characterization with Gd-DTPA enhancement profiles. Radiology 1990;174: 491–494.

62. Nunes LW, Schnall MD, Siegelman ES, et al. Diagnostic performance characteristics of architectural features revealed by high spatial-resolution MR imaging of the breast. AJR 1997;169:409–415.

63. Nunes LW, Schnall MD, Orel SG, et al. Breast MR imaging: interpretation model. Radiology 1997;202:833–841.

64. Orel SG, Schnall MD, LiVolsi VA, et al. Suspicious breast lesions: MR imaging with radiologic-pathologic correlation. Radiology 1994; 190:485–493.

65. Orel SG, Hochman MG, Schnall MD, et al. High-resolution MR imaging of the breast: clinical context. RadioGraphics 1996;16(6):1385–1401.

66. Frankel SD, Sickles EA. Morphologic criteria for interpreting abnormalities seen at breast MR imaging. Radiology 1997;202:633–634.

67. Harms SE, Flamig DP, Hesley KL, et al. MR imaging of the breast with rotating delivery of excitation off resonance: clinical experience with pathologic correlation. Radiology 1993;187:493–501.

68. Orel SG, Mendonca MH, Reynolds C, et al. MR imaging of ductal carcinoma in situ. Breast Imaging 1997;202(2):413–420.

69. Folkman J. What is the evidence that tumors are angiogensis dependent? J Natl Cancer Inst 1990;82:4–6.

70. Weidner N, Semple JP, Welch WR, et al. Tumor angiogenesis and metastasis: correlation in invasive breast carcinoma. New Engl J Med 1991;324:1–8.

71. Gilles R, Zafrani B, Guinebretiere JM, et al. Ductal carcinoma in situ: MR imaging-histopathologic correlation. Radiology 1995;196(2):415–419.

72. Piccoli CW, Matteucci T, Outwater EK, et al. Breast cancer diagnosis with MR imaging: effect of clinical and mammographic findings on recommendations for biopsy. Radiology 1995;197(P):372.

73. Heywang SH. Contrast-enhanced magnetic resonance imaging of the breast. Invest Radiol 1994;29:94–104.

74. Gilles R, Guinebretiere J, Lucidarme O, et al. Non-palpable breast tumors: diagnosis with contrast-enhanced subtraction dynamic MR imaging. Radiology 1994;191:625–631.

75. Orel SG, Schnall MD, Powell CM, et al. Staging of suspected breast cancer: effect of MR

imaging and MR guided biopsy. Radiology 1995;196:115–122.

76. Hewang-Kobrunner SH, Viehweg P. Sensitivity of contrast-enhanced MR imaging of the breast. Breast Imaging 1994;2(4):527–536.

77. Hulka CA, Edmister WB, Smith BL, et al. Dynamic echo-planar imaging of the breast: experience in diagnosing breast carcinoma and correlation with tumor angiogenesis. Radiology 1997;205:837–842.

78. Kaiser WA, Zeitler E. MR imaging of the breast: fast imaging sequences with and without Gd-DTPA. Radiology 1989;170:681–686.

79. Hulka CA, Smith BL, Sgroi DC, et al. Benign and malignant breast lesions: differentiation with echo-planar MR imaging. Radiology 1995; 197:33–38.

80. Rosen PP, Fracchia AA, Urban JA, et al. "Residual" mammary carcinoma following simulated partial mastectomy. Cancer 1975;35:739–747.

81. Holland R, Veling SHJ, Mravunac M, et al. Histologic multifocality of Tis, T1–2 breast carcinomas: implication for clinical trials of breast-conserving surgery. Cancer 1985;56:979–990.

82. Lagios MD, Westdahy PR, Rose MR. The concept and implications of multicentricity in breast carcinoma. In: Sommers SG, Rosen PP, eds. Pathology Annual. New York: Appleton-Century-Crofts, 1981:83–102.

83. Schwartz GF, Patchesfsky AS, Feig SA, et al. Multicentricity of nonpalpable breast cancer. Cancer 1980;45:2913–2916.

84. Morris EA, Schwartz LH, Dershaw DD, et al. MR imaging of the breast in patients with occult primary breast carcinoma. Radiology 1997;205:437–440.

85. Fourquet A, De la Rochefordiere A, Campana F. Occult primary cancer with axillary metastases. In: Harris JR, Hellman S, Henderson CI, et al, eds. Breast Diseases. 3rd ed. Philadelphia: JB Lippincott, 199X:892–896.

86. Knopp MV, Junkermann HI, Heb T, et al. MR-Mammographie zum. Monitoring von neoadjuvanter Therapie beim Mammakarzinom. Radiologe 1995;35/4:81.

87. Degani H, Fields S, Catane R, et al. Evaluation of breast cancer therapy with contrast-enhanced MRI at high spatial resolution. J Magn Reson Imag 1994;4(P):116.

88. Gilles R, Guinebretiere J, Toussaint C, et al. Locally advanced breast cancer: contrast-enhanced subtraction MR imaging of response to preoperative chemotherapy. Radiology 1994; 191:633–638.

89. Przetak C, Audretsch W, Schnabel T, et al. Therapie-Monitoring des Mamma Carcinoms durch Kernspintomographie bei neoadjuvanter therpie. Radiologe 1995;35(4)(1):581.

90. Rieber A, Tomczak R, Rosenthal H, et al. Mamma-MRT nach chemotherapierten Mammakarzinomen. Radiologe 1995;35(4):82.

91. Kurtz B, Achten C, Audretsch W, et al. MR-mammographische Beurteilung des Tumoransprechverhaltens nach neoadjuvanter Radiochemotherapie lokal fortgeschrittener Mammakarzinome. Roe Fo 1996;164(6):469–474.

92. Heywang-Kobrunner SH, Beck R. Contrast-Enhanced MRI of the Breast. New York: Springer, 1996.

93. Plevritis SK, Garber AM, Macovski A, et al. Cost-effective analysis of MRI in screening for breast cancer. Med Decision Making 1996;16:456.

94. Kuhl CK, Elevelt A, Leutner CC, et al. Interventional breast MR imaging: clinical use of a stereotactic localization and biopsy device. Radiology 1997;204:667–675.

10

Development of a Risk Assessment Clinic

Constance A. Roche, Michele R. Lucas, and Kevin S. Hughes

Cancer Genetics: The Promise and the Challenge

The nineties may be remembered as the decade of genetics research and revolution, a movement driven by the media as well as by the scientific community. Media attention to the familial component of breast cancer has led to heightened public interest and demand for cancer risk information, generating expectations for identification and management of at-risk individuals as well as prevention.

Until recently, health care professionals had little interest in trying to identify the high-risk patient because inadequate methods existed for assessing risk and there was no clear course of action for those identified as high risk. Understanding hereditary risk has remained at such a rudimentary level that many have failed to answer their patients' questions or have offered them misplaced reassurance. For example, women with a strong paternal family history of breast cancer were likely to be told incorrectly that they were not at increased risk because they had no affected first-degree relatives or that risk was only passed on by the mother. At the same time, women with a few minor risk factors, such as nulliparity or early menarche, received reinforcement of their belief that they were at high risk. Even in dedicated cancer centers, awareness of the need for hereditary cancer services is quite recent. In 1994, a survey revealed that only 17 of 34 responding National Cancer Institute–supported cancer centers offered genetic services for familial cancer. Five of these were described as new or in the development phase, and only five reported seeing more than 100 patients per year (1).

The explosion of cancer genetics information has allowed for more accurate identification of high-risk individuals, for a better understanding of the natural history of hereditary breast and ovarian cancer, and for developing management strategies for individuals at risk. There is now a critical need for hereditary cancer services in view of this rapidly expanding body of knowledge and surge in the numbers of individuals seeking genetic information about cancer. Primary care providers and oncologists are increasingly aware of the value of obtaining and evaluating family cancer history, but with the demands on their time, they only may be able to perform limited cancer risk assessment and counseling. The medical community must now determine who is trained and available to meet this need. Who will monitor the provision of cancer risk information?

The new economic restraints on the provision of medical care dictate ever-improved efficiency. We must continue to provide the optimal service in the most cost-conserving manner. It is the responsibility of a health care system to provide appropriate screening for all patients, and therefore, identification of high-risk individuals is imperative. Identification and intensive screening of the highest-risk patients will most likely save lives. Preliminary data from Canada (2) and from New York's Columbia-Presbyterian Medical Center (3) provide evidence that surveillance of women at increased risk may be useful in detecting disease at an earlier stage.

Are today's health care providers able to identify individuals at increased risk for cancer? Are they prepared to discuss the risks and benefits of genetic testing? Do they have a sufficient level of understanding to advise their patients? Research in this area indicates that there is a knowledge deficit even among physicians who proceed with genetic-predisposition testing. In one study (4), among 77 patients who underwent genetic testing for familial adenomatous polyposis, testing was not indicated for 17%. For 21%, an unaffected patient was inappropriately tested before affected relatives were tested. In all, 82% did not receive pretest counseling, and 83% did not sign a consent form. Moreover, 31% of the results were misinterpreted by physicians.

While obstetricians and gynecologists would be expected to have a greater understanding of genetics because of their involvement in prenatal counseling and testing for genetic disorders, they appear to lack sufficient education in cancer genetics. A survey performed in 1996 (5) found that obstetricians and gynecologists often were ill-informed regarding hereditary breast cancer. Of the obstetricians and gynecologists surveyed, 22% were unaware that ovarian cancer was related to hereditary breast cancer, 22% did not realize that cancer-susceptibility genes could be transmitted by men or women, 25% did not realize that the syndrome was characterized by early age at onset, 40% did not realize that this syndrome was related to a dominant gene, 64% did not realize that multiple primary cancers in a patient were an indicator of the syndrome, and, 65% did not realize that male breast cancers are related to the syndrome. The findings of these two studies highlight the need for specific education and training in the area of cancer genetics.

Why a Risk Assessment Clinic?

Recent advances in cancer genetics have sparked interest in the development of clinics for cancer risk assessment to provide services for high-risk individuals. For women at increased risk for breast cancer, the clinic can provide evaluation, education, counseling, screening services, and genetic testing (when appropriate). Additionally, the risk assessment clinic serves as a focal point for cancer genetics education for an entire health care network and as a resource for the development of relevant guidelines and standards. It serves as a repository of information to help track the latest data in a rapidly evolving field and serves as a consultation resource for clinicians, centralizing the effort to identify high-risk individuals. This specialized clinic's multidisciplinary team centralizes a highly complex function, relieving the health care network by managing the high-risk patient in a more cost- and time-efficient manner.

The recent surge of interest in developing breast cancer risk assessment clinics has been generated largely by the desire to institute genetic testing programs. While this is an important objective, genetic testing should be considered as a tool in risk assessment rather than as an end in itself. The more important goal is to establish a program to identify women at increased risk, to educate and counsel them, and to facilitate appropriate management and screening measures. Another goal of risk assessment should be universal appropriate screening acknowledging that all women are at risk for breast cancer. There is a need to institute a standard method of screening for all, and individuals identified at highest risk will require modification of the standard guidelines to a more intense level.

The concept of breast cancer risk-assessment and high-risk clinics is not new. However, until recently, there have been few such programs. Notable pioneers in the field were ahead of their time in recognizing hereditary cancer syndromes and developing approaches to identify and provide surveillance and risk-reduction strategies for women at high risk. Clinicians in the field of cancer genetics are indebted to Dr. Henry Lynch, who developed the Institute for Familial Cancer Management and Control at Creighton University in Omaha, Nebraska, in the midsixties (6). Patricia Kelly, Ph.D., a medical geneticist, established a program for cancer risk analysis at the University of California at San Francisco in the early eighties (7) and later developed an extensive program at the Salick Cancer Centers. At the University of Wisconsin, Dr. Richard Love developed the Cancer Prevention Clinic in 1981, focusing on a spectrum of interventions for risk reduction (8). In New York, Memorial Sloan-Kettering Cancer

Center offers a Special Surveillance Breast Program that began in 1983 as a research protocol to determine if screening affected outcome in women at increased risk (Cynthia Knauer, R.N., personal communication, February 1995) (9).

Tomorrow's risk assessment clinic must expand on the foundations already established, responding to the promise and the challenge that accompany the new era of cancer genetics.

The Fundamentals

Medical professionals who consider development of a risk-assessment clinic can find justification in the preceding discussion and in their own experience. The process should begin with development of a mission statement and identification of objectives. What will be the scope of the clinic? Which patients are candidates for risk assessment? Which staff will provide the service? What knowledge base should staff members possess? What are the components of cancer risk counseling? Should services be consultative or comprehensive? Should genetic testing be offered? The following discussion presents some of the areas to be addressed.

Candidates for the Clinic

A cancer risk assessment clinic may be limited to a single cancer type or may endeavor to evaluate and manage all hereditary cancer syndromes. The focus will depend on the expertise and interest of the staff and the availability of expert consultation. Eligibility for the breast cancer risk assessment clinic may be limited to individuals whose families demonstrate a high likelihood of hereditary cancer or may be more inclusive, with services for any woman who perceives herself to be at increased risk. In some settings, a research focus or limited resources may necessitate limiting eligibility to those who fit high-risk criteria. Candidates also may include women with nongenetic risk factors such as a biopsy diagnosis of atypical hyperplasia or lobular carcinoma in situ.

A family pedigree may reveal cancers other than that for which the woman seeks counseling. The staff of the breast cancer risk-assessment clinic must be knowledgeable about risk factors

and screening and detection of ovarian cancer because it is now evident that women who carry *BRCA1* or *BRCA2* mutations also are at increased risk for ovarian cancer (10). Even in the disease-focused clinic, the staff should be able to recognize other hereditary cancer syndromes and should be aware of standard screening guidelines for other common cancers. For example, in a breast cancer risk assessment clinic, a woman's extended family history may reveal many relatives with colon cancer. The counselor must be prepared to evaluate the risk of a hereditary colon cancer syndrome and make appropriate recommendations for screening. Alternatively, the clinic should develop a network of experts to consult with or refer to regarding hereditary cancer syndromes involving other cancers.

While the primary goal of the clinic may be to identify the women at high risk for breast cancer, the clinic also should be prepared to provide services for women who have been diagnosed with breast or ovarian cancer. These women may wish to learn whether their cancer was caused by a genetic predisposition, or about risk for their relatives. They may be interested in genetic testing, or they may be seeking advice about risk for other cancers.

In summary, the risk assessment clinic should be prepared to evaluate and counsel women who have been diagnosed with breast and ovarian cancer as well as those who are at increased risk. These women also may be at increased risk for other cancers.

Staffing

The staff of a breast cancer risk-assessment clinic must have substantial expertise in cancer etiology, screening, diagnosis, and treatment, as well as in basic genetics and cancer genetics. They also must possess the skills to provide counseling related to cancer experience and fear of the disease. Considering the recent evolution and growth in the field of cancer genetics, it is unlikely that any one member of a specific professional discipline will have the necessary expertise by virtue of formal education or usual practice. Cancer risk counseling has been described as inherently multidisciplinary. The information is sophisticated and difficult to communicate in a meaningful fashion, requiring a team with skills in medicine, genetics, nursing, and mental health (11). Each discipline possesses different skill sets that are complementary in providing cancer risk counseling.

Hiring of new staff may be desirable or necessary, or staff may be recruited from existing personnel. Staffing might include physicians (e.g., medical, surgical, radiation, or gynecologic oncologist or medical geneticist), nurses, genetic counselors, mental health professionals (e.g., social worker, psychologist, or psychiatrist), and health educators. Each discipline likely will need supplementary education. Medical, surgical, and radiation oncologists are well versed in the screening, diagnosis, and treatment of cancer but are less skilled in genetics and counseling strategies. Geneticists and genetic counselors are expert in pedigree analysis and counseling about hereditary risks in the setting of preconception and prenatal counseling but are likely to need enhanced understanding about cancer, hereditary cancer syndromes, nongenetic risk factors, and counseling about adult-onset disease. Advanced-practice oncology nurses with experience in the care, education, and counseling of cancer patients and their families require additional education in genetics and counseling about hereditary risk. Mental health professionals with experience in counseling oncology patients and their families also need to have an understanding about genetics and hereditary risk. Whether using existing professionals or hiring new staff, it is essential to provide for initial and frequent staff education and training.

A number of institutions have offered short courses on cancer genetics, and professional organizations are responding to the need for professional education in this rapidly evolving field. The American Society of Clinical Oncology has taken the position that cancer risk counseling is part of the mission of clinical oncologists (12) and has organized educational programs as part of its commitment to develop courses to educate oncologists and other medical professionals who are called on to provide these services. The International Society of Nurses in Genetics and the special interest group of the Oncology Nursing Society are resources for nurses interested in this field, and both organizations regularly

offer educational programs. The Oncology Nursing Society also has released position papers on cancer genetic testing, risk assessment counseling (13), and the role of the oncology nurse in cancer genetic counseling (14). The American Nurses Association officially recognizes genetics as a nursing specialty. The National Society of Genetic Counselors has formed a special interest group to address the educational, research, clinical, and networking needs of genetic counselors specializing in cancer genetics (15).

A cancer risk-assessment clinic requires a multidisciplinary team with expertise in the areas of cancer, genetics, and counseling. The makeup of the team can follow several models (Table 10-1). Staffing model 1 uses a genetic counselor, an oncologist, and a mental health professional to provide these services. The genetic counselor obtains the family history, constructs the pedigree, and counsels about hereditary risk. The oncologist provides additional information about cancer and cancer risk, makes screening recommendations, and performs a physical examination. And the mental health professional assesses the woman's level of anxiety and coping skills and offers strategies for coping and stress reduction.

Staffing model 2 uses an oncology nurse to provide the range of education and counseling services, and a medical geneticist serves as a resource for genetic evaluation. This model does not provide for physical examination or clinical services.

In staffing model 3, the oncologist provides the risk assessment and counseling within the office setting. Some comprehensive centers include the services of nutritionists and physical therapists, who assist in healthy lifestyle modification.

Our experience, staffing model 4, with staffing provided by a nurse practitioner, social worker, and breast surgeon as medical consultant will be described in detail later.

Whatever the staffing configuration, the objective is to identify women at increased risk, recommend appropriate surveillance, provide information regarding cancer and cancer genetics, and properly counsel and comfort patients. In this evolving field, whatever the discipline of the cancer risk counselor, as Peters and Stopfer

Table 10-1. Cancer risk-assessment clinic examples of staffing models

Areas to be Addressed in Risk-Assessment Clinic	Staffing Model 1	Staffing Model 2[a]	Staffing Model 3	Staffing Model 4[a]
Cancer	M.D.[b]	R.N.[c]	M.D.[b]	Nurse practitioner[d]
Genetics	Genetic counselor	R.N.[c]	M.D.[b]	Nurse practitioner[d]
Counseling	Psychologist/ genetic counselor	R.N.[c]	M.D.[b]	Social worker
Examination	M.D.[b]	(Not provided)	M.D.[b]	Nurse practitioner[d]

[a]Non-M.D. professional models require consultation with M.D.'s (e.g., medical or surgical oncologist, medical geneticist).
[b]Oncologist.
[c]Oncology nurse.
[d]Oncology specialist.

(16, p. 164) point out: "It is the individual training, experience, and skill of the counselor that contribute to the art of cancer risk counseling."

Location

The breast cancer risk assessment clinic may be developed in one of a variety of settings: a dedicated familial cancer clinic, a clinical genetics clinic, a breast center, or the department of medical, surgical, or radiation oncology in a hospital. The choice of location may be determined by the goals and strategic plan of the institution or by the interests of clinicians in these specialties. Oncology departments or disease-specific clinics have the advantage of access to screening, preventive, and treatment services, whereas the genetics department will have greater experience with analyzing pedigrees and identifying uncommon hereditary syndromes.

Space allocation may be determined by external factors, but consideration should be given to proximity to associated screening services and accessibility for the multidisciplinary staff. Special attention should be paid to the surroundings, since women who arrive for risk-assessment counseling are likely to be anxious about the nature of the visit. For example, it may be distressing for a woman who is anxious about her risk to be in a waiting room with acutely ill patients or individuals undergoing chemotherapy. Even the use of a clinical examination room

may engender unpleasant memories of accompanying family members when they were undergoing treatment for cancer. Peters (17, p. 22) states that the room needs to be "quiet, private, safe, esthetically pleasing, comfortable for lengthy discussion, [and] large enough to accommodate several family members." The risk assessment session can take place in a consultation room or office, although an examination room is necessary if a clinical examination is to be performed. Space also should be allocated for administrative and clerical personnel, computer, printer, fax machine, phones, files, and a reference library.

Scheduling

Scheduling plans should take into account staff availability, the number of staff members who interact with the woman at the visit, space allocation, the expected length of visits, and the number of visits to complete the risk assessment. Thompson's (1) survey of cancer centers revealed a range of from one to three visits and an average total consultation time of 129 minutes. Josten and Love (8) at the University of Wisconsin describe one 3-hour visit. Time can be saved if the woman has received and completed a risk-assessment questionnaire prior to the visit and has been instructed to verify family history and obtain medical records of affected family members. Some centers schedule the appointment only after the woman has returned her questionnaire and obtained all available documentation of family medical history. Others schedule a second visit once cancer history documentation has been obtained.

Visits can be scheduled within the normal appointment schedule, or a block of time can be designated for the clinic. The latter may be preferable particularly when multiple staff members are involved. This also may facilitate the timing of a postclinic conference. It is probably best to start slowly with a few appointments per week, allowing the staff to hone their skills and strengthen their team approach.

Cancer Risk Counseling

Stefanek (18, p. 31) stated that the goal of counseling women at high risk for breast cancer is "to increase awareness of risk and emphasize the benefit of early detection, without creating levels of anxiety that might reduce compliance with screening exams." The process includes collecting the family history and other risk data, assessing the woman's beliefs and understanding about cancer, assessing her level of anxiety and coping skills, constructing a pedigree, assessing cancer risk, providing recommendations for surveillance and risk reduction, and counseling about managing risk and the attendant stress. The focus is on education tailored to the needs, concerns, and educational level of the individual, taking into account her experience with cancer and her coping style. The expertise of the counselor is critical. As Kelly (19, p. 291) points out, the woman must "make informed health care decisions based on sophisticated scientific and medical information."

It is important to begin by ascertaining the woman's own perception of risk and her reason for attending the clinic. She may want to understand the risk associated with her family history or the effects of other risk factors, or she may want to receive advice or reassurance. She may be attending only at the direction of her physician or family. The woman affected with breast cancer may want to know if her cancer is hereditary and if her sisters and daughters are at risk, or she may want to know if she is at risk for ovarian cancer. She may have been approached by family members to undergo genetic testing to clarify risk for the family. An understanding

of her agenda and needs will help the staff to individualize the focus and content of the visit.

Unless eligibility criteria are very selective, the majority of women evaluated will not be assessed as high risk. The woman who is at average or moderate risk and unlikely to be a member of a hereditary cancer family has particular needs. She may benefit from an overview of hereditary cancer syndromes and a description of the breast cancer–susceptibility genes. She may gain a more realistic perception of her risk if she can compare her own pedigree with that of a hereditary cancer family. However, as Entreken and Summerlot (20, p. 187) point out, "in a time when the media defines who is at risk, reassuring statistics may not be enough to allay her fears." Taking time to interview the patient in a sensitive and supportive manner, the staff may be able to ascertain the source of her anxiety and overestimation of risk and then help to determine how best to allay her fears. She may be comforted and reassured, and she may avoid embarking on an intensive screening program that is unwarranted with her level of risk.

Ideally, the woman arrives at her visit with accurate information about her family's cancer history. A questionnaire or phone call prior to the visit can explain to her the importance of contacting family members and obtaining medical records. The pedigree can be constructed in the woman's presence as she provides information about the cancers in the family and describes relationships. This interactive process allows the counselor to assess the woman's understanding about the cancer diagnosis and treatments, her level of anxiety, and elements of family dynamics.

While assessing cancer risk based on family history is likely to be the primary focus of the clinic, it is essential that the staff be knowledgeable about other potential risk factors. The cancer risk counselor should be able to interpret study findings for individuals and identify when risk factors can or should be modified. The woman who is anxious about her breast cancer risk is likely to be confused by conflicting reports of research findings and the magnitude of risk as interpreted on the morning news. It is important, for example, to help a woman understand the difference between the magnitude of the risk of lung cancer associated with cigarette smoking (relative risk 12) (21) compared with the weak association between breast cancer and estrogen replacement therapy (relative risk 1.4) (22).

Assessing Risk

Despite technological advances in cancer genetics, in practice, the cancer risk counselor has rather crude tools for assessing risk. Indeed, most women who develop breast cancer have no major risk factors, resulting historically in our poor track record at predicting risk. Some general guidelines will apply. If there is no family history and no risk factors, the woman is at population risk. If the pedigree suggests a classic Mendelian pattern of hereditary breast and ovarian cancer, then counseling can begin with a description of hereditary cancer and what is known about breast cancer–susceptibility genes, and the woman can be provided with a percentage risk based on her position in the family. If the woman has had lobular carcinoma in situ (23) or atypical hyperplasia (24), risk can be estimated by reference to published work on these diagnoses.

More often, however, there is not a definite pattern of cancer in the family, and other approaches are used to assess risk. Several empirical models are available to assess risk for the moderate-risk individual. In practice, these are commonly calculated to provide the counselor with a reference, or confirmation, of an intuitive assessment, but they may have limited use in predicting risk for the individual. The Gail model (25) considers age at menarche, age at first live birth, number of breast biopsies, number of affected first-degree relatives, and the current age of the individual. While frequently used, this model ignores paternal transmission and probably overestimates the effect of minor risk factors. It is not useful for assessing individual risk for women under age 40 (26) and should be used cautiously. The Claus model (27) calculates risk based on family history alone, taking into account the woman's current age, affected first- and second-degree relatives, and their ages at diagnosis. It cannot accommodate more than two relatives, and it does not consider other features of hereditary cancer such as bilaterality, ovarian cancer, or male breast cancer. It is probably most useful for calculating risk for families at moderate risk and often can provide reassuring

numbers. The more recently developed Berry model (BRCAPRO) (28) allows for a more refined risk calculation based on a larger pedigree, taking into account affected and unaffected relatives and considering bilaterality, ovarian cancer, and ethnicity.

Communicating Risk Information

There has been much discussion in the literature about the best approach for presenting risk information (8,29–33). Options include lifetime risk, relative risk, absolute risk, and comparison with baseline general population risk. While numerical data can facilitate rational discussion (34) and can provide boundaries (8), many individuals have a poor understanding of numbers (31) and find numerical information confusing (35). Richards and colleagues (32) found that while providing an estimation of risk was central for the counselor, the counselee's primary issue was what to do about risk. Ponder (33) cautions that we should not assume that the woman wants to know everything.

It is the responsibility of the professional team to convey risk information in a sensitive manner, taking into account the woman's preconceived estimation of her risk and her response to the risk information as it is provided. Is she interested in a numerical calculation, or would she prefer a general categorization of her risk? It is important to frame the information in the most positive way; for example, "a 30% risk means that you have a 70% chance of not developing breast cancer." The woman in a hereditary cancer family should be told that high risk does not mean that she will definitely develop cancer. The language employed to convey risk may affect interpretation. For example, Richards and colleagues (32, p. 229) recommend using neutral terms whenever possible, suggesting that it may be preferable to refer to "chance of occurrence" rather than "risk." Women also should be reminded that risk of breast cancer is not the same as risk of death from the disease and that most women with breast cancer survive.

Whatever the method of risk calculation used by the counselor, the result is most likely a categorization of high risk in the hereditary cancer family, moderate risk in the family whose cancer history does not exhibit all the criteria for

Mendelian inheritance, or close to average risk for the family whose cancer appears to be sporadic. This categorization may be useful for the woman being counseled, and it also will allow the clinic to maintain a data set that will reflect the risk level of the population.

Genetics: To Test or Not to Test?

The identification and cloning of the *BRCA1* (36) and *BRCA2* (37) genes led to dramatic improvement in our ability to estimate cancer risk for individuals with a family history of breast and ovarian cancer. Early research enhanced our ability to identify high-risk families, whereas later studies have helped to determine the prevalence of mutations in these genes and the risk of developing cancer in carriers of these mutations (penetrance). The understanding of hereditary cancer gained from these studies allows us to better counsel and manage high-risk individuals, whether or not they themselves elect genetic testing.

The risk-assessment clinic is likely to evaluate many more individuals who are at moderate risk than individuals who are members of hereditary breast and ovarian cancer families. Of those identified as high-risk, only a subset will wish to undergo testing, and, in most cases, testing must begin with a living family member who has breast or ovarian cancer. The risk-assessment clinic should either provide genetic testing or be able to make appropriate referrals for testing following cancer risk counseling and preliminary discussion about testing.

There is no medical parallel to genetic testing for cancer susceptibility. Couch and Hartmann (38, p. 956) caution that "clinical application of (*BRCA1*) testing is most appropriate when trained health care professionals use the available clinical and statistical tools to identify high-risk families in which testing may be clinically beneficial." Unlike other medical procedures, the decision to undergo testing is made by the individual, but the decision affects the entire family, even those who are not tested. The result is not diagnostic but probabilistic and may be entirely indeterminate. It is the responsibility of the cancer risk counselor to provide the individual and family with sufficient information

to make an informed choice and to be adequately prepared for the possible results.

If the clinic offers genetic testing, provision must be made for 1) adequate education of staff, 2) investment of sufficient time for pre- and posttest counseling, and 3) establishment of procedures for maintaining confidentiality and providing for informed consent.

Standardizing Recommendations

It is important for the risk-assessment clinic to develop a consistent method of categorizing risk and providing appropriate management recommendations. With the exception of those who have undergone genetic testing, categorization of risk will be based on pedigree analysis and other risk models. The resulting categorization should reflect the current scientific evidence and the theories about risk and management held by the clinic staff.

The current recommendations for intensive breast cancer screening for the highest-risk patients (those who carry mutations in *BRCA1* or *BRCA2*) are outlined by Burke and colleagues (39) and include physical examinations every 6 months beginning between the ages of 25 and 35, with mammography yearly beginning between the ages of 25 and 35, and monthly breast self-examinations beginning at age 20. Prophylactic mastectomy will substantially reduce the risk of breast cancer (40,41), but this strategy should be considered only for those with very high risk and would be acceptable only to a subset of that group. Chemoprevention may be an additional approach for the high-risk patient, but there are currently no standard guidelines. Results from the Breast Cancer Prevention Trial (42) indicate that tamoxifen reduces the incidence of breast cancer in a group of women determined to be at higher risk (see Chapter 12). The value of lifestyle modifications, such as restriction of dietary fat (43,44) and limited alcohol intake (45,46), is uncertain, but it is wise to counsel patients about the possibility that these may contribute to risk and advise according to the American Cancer Society guidelines (47), the findings of well-designed research studies, and studies of risk related to other diseases.

Since women who are carriers of a mutation in a breast cancer–susceptibility gene are also at high risk for ovarian cancer, the clinic also must have a strategy for categorizing ovarian cancer risk and providing management and screening recommendations. Oral contraceptives have been found to reduce the risk of ovarian cancer (48,49) and should be considered unless medically contraindicated. Prophylactic oophorectomy will reduce the risk substantially for women at highest risk for ovarian cancer, although the procedure is not 100% effective (50,51). Ovarian cancer screening with twice-yearly transvaginal ultrasonography, and, in postmenopausal women, CA-125 testing will be the most likely recommended course for those at moderate risk and those at highest risk who do not opt for surgical prophylaxis. However, the efficacy of this screening has not been proven. It is useful to counsel the high-risk woman who is past childbearing that oophorectomy should be considered if she undergoes abdominal surgery for other indications.

Guidelines for women who carry mutations in breast cancer–susceptibility genes (39) can be used for women who have not been tested but are at high risk by virtue of their position in a hereditary cancer family. Since there are no standardized guidelines for women at moderate risk, these should be developed with the guidance of the team's oncology expert. Recommendations may include breast examinations every 6 months and starting mammography before age 40 if a relative has been diagnosed at a young age.

Staff Activities in Addition to the Scheduled Visit Time

The staff should plan time to discuss patients seen in the clinic, ideally on the day of the patient's visit. Time also should be allocated for consultation with other experts about pedigree analysis or screening recommendations for other cancers. One member of the team should send a summary letter to the patient and her referring provider (if the patient wishes). Administrative time should be allocated to enter and analyze data, to formulate clinic guidelines, to review current literature, and to develop and participate in research protocols. Since part of the mission of the risk-assessment clinic is to educate the public and medical providers, the staff will need

time to plan and participate in these educational programs.

The Risk Assessment Clinic at Lahey Clinic

Lahey Clinic is a multispecialty medical group practice of 470 physicians located in 2 full-service sites and 33 community-practice settings in eastern Massachusetts. A dedicated Breast Center was developed when the second site was opened in October 1994. Planning for the breast cancer Risk Assessment Clinic began at that time, with the goal of enhancing the spectrum of services in the Breast Center. After months of developing a business plan and strategy and building our knowledge base, our first patient was seen in April 1995.

The clinic is staffed by a nurse practitioner (CAR) who also works in the Breast Center evaluating and managing the care of breast cancer patients and women with benign breast problems, and a social worker (MRL) who has extensive experience counseling cancer patients and their families. The medical director (KSH) is a breast surgeon with an interest in cancer genetics. Additional services are provided by an administrative assistant, a research assistant, and consulting gynecologic oncologists Anne Shapter, M.D., and Robert McLellan, M.D. Our preparation for entering the field of cancer genetics involved attending national meetings and special courses, joining national professional organizations, reading the published literature, making visits and phone calls to existing clinics, and collaborating with local and national experts in the field. We have found that professionals involved in this new field are enthusiastic and have been quite willing to share their experiences and resources.

As a resource of the Breast Center, we initially limited our service to breast cancer risk assessment. Our eligibility criteria were listed on brochures that were displayed in the Breast Center and distributed to medical practices. Candidates for the clinic included women with a family history of breast cancer, women who had a biopsy diagnosis of atypical hyperplasia or lobular carcinoma in situ, women with concerns about breast cancer risk, and women with questions regarding particular risk factors such as use of hormone replacement therapy. Despite this eligibility listing, our third patient presented with concerns about her mother's history of ovarian cancer at age 68 (and no family history of breast cancer). One week later we saw a man whose father had three primary cancers including breast cancer. Thus our experience becomes an admonition to be knowledgeable and have resources for the spectrum of cancers that may be encountered.

Within a year of opening the clinic, we expanded our services to women with a family history of ovarian cancer, women affected with breast or ovarian cancer, and individuals with a personal or family history of melanoma. Of interest to us was the fact that the woman whose mother had ovarian cancer at age 68 (and was advised against ovarian cancer screening) returned 18 months later when her 40-year-old sister was diagnosed with breast cancer. Her first clinic visit had made her aware of the increased risk associated with breast and ovarian cancer, and she is now under closer surveillance.

Referral sources include surgeons, primary care providers, gynecologists, and gynecologic oncologists. Many women refer themselves or initiate referral by asking their primary care providers about risk assessment. During the first year, over 60% of the referrals were from the breast practice of the medical director. This has changed over time so that now, as our network of physicians has become aware of the services of the clinic, other medical providers account for 70% of the referrals.

After almost 5 years of operation, the Risk Assessment Clinic has evaluated 623 patients. As would be expected, the majority (61%) were referred because of a family history of breast cancer, 13% had a family history of breast and ovarian cancer, and 4% had a family history of ovarian cancer. A history of atypical hyperplasia (AH) accounted for 17%, and lobular carcinoma in situ (LCIS) accounted for 5% of patients (Fig. 10-1). Of those with a family history of breast and or ovarian cancer, 26% had families that appeared to have hereditary predisposition, 53% were assessed to be at moderate risk, and

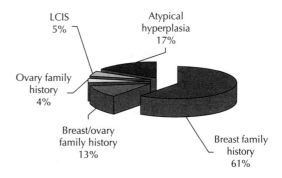

Figure 10-1. Risk assessment clinic patients. Of the 623 (excluding 9 patients seen for family history of melanoma) patients seen at the Lahey Clinic Risk Assessment Clinic from April 1995 through January 2000, 61% were seen for a family history of breast cancer, 13% were seen for a family history of breast and ovarian cancer, 3% were seen for a family history of ovarian cancer, 17% were seen for atypical hyperplasia (AH), and 6% were seen for lobular carcinoma in situ (LCIS).

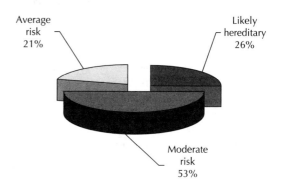

Figure 10-2. Family history of breast cancer. Of the patients presenting with family history of breast and/or ovarian cancer seen at the Lahey Clinic Risk Assessment Clinic form April 1995 through January 2000, 26% were members of families likely to be hereditary cancer families, 53% were assessed to be at moderate risk, and 21% were assessed to have average risk for breast cancer.

21% were assessed to be at close to average risk (Fig. 10-2).

The clinic staff is committed to educating health care providers and the public regarding the identification of the "high-risk woman." We schedule regular lectures for the medical community and for the general public. Patient summary letters to the referring and primary provider also serve as educational tools. We have developed and distributed brochures and flyers describing our services, and we have established our own Web page that is available as an educational resource to the public (*www.familycancer.org*).

Two weeks prior to a patient's first appointment, a letter explaining the format of the clinic and a questionnaire (Appendix A) are mailed to the patient. A few days before the appointment, the administrative assistant phones the patient reminding her of the appointment, encouraging her to complete the questionnaire and to obtain family history information, and answering any questions she may have. This is done in a very sensitive and empathetic manner, which is especially helpful for women who are anxious or who are unsure about what to expect from the visit. Initially, we found that many women canceled or failed to keep their appointments. Mailing the questionnaires and instituting the previsit phone call have almost eliminated the no-show rate, although we still have a high rate of cancellations within a few days of an appointment. Some women have demonstrated a pattern of canceling and rescheduling, leading us to believe that for many women, anxiety is so intense that it renders them unable to attend. Researchers in this field similarly have noted that psychological stress associated with perception of high risk may affect adherence to screening recommendations (52). Ultimately, the majority of women seen in a risk-assessment clinic may be a self-selected, proactive group.

We began with a schedule of four appointments on Wednesday morning, and a year later, we added two visits on Tuesday afternoon. On Wednesday afternoon, the team meets for discussion of each case and to reach agreement about risk assessment and screening recommendations. Any woman who has abnormal findings on her mammogram or breast examination is seen by the breast surgeon/medical director. Any woman who is considering prophylactic mastectomy is seen by the breast surgeon and a plastic surgeon. The gynecologic oncologist is consulted about each patient with a family history of ovarian cancer and will see any patient with abnormal ovarian screening and any woman who is considering prophylactic oophorectomy.

The nurse practitioner has the responsibility of obtaining the family history and analyzing the pedigree. We are currently experimenting with a format in which the administrative assistant sees the patient first and creates a computer-generated pedigree (Cyrillic 2, Cherwell Scientific Publishing, Ltd., Oxford, England). This saves time for the assessment and education portions of the visit, and it eliminates the step where previously the nurse practitioner gave the hand-drawn pedigree to the administrative assistant to then enter into the computer. The patient sees the pedigree developing and can be more aware of patterns when the description of hereditary cancer is presented. It is possible that with this format, the nurse practitioner will miss some indicators as to the woman's understanding about cancer and her level of anxiety and details about family dynamics. However, the administrative assistant is aware of these issues and communicates relevant information after the pedigree is drawn.

The Nurse Practitioner's Visit

The patient sees our nurse practitioner for a 1-hour appointment. She begins by assessing the reason for the visit and inquiring about what issues the patient would like to address during the visit. Many patients assume that they are at very high risk, and they want only to learn how to reduce or manage their risk. Others have specific concerns about various risk factors that might contribute to their risk or want to understand the implications of their family history. The family pedigree is reviewed, and relevant information is verified. The patient is asked how each affected member of the family was diagnosed, what treatment she received, current health status, or cause of death. The recounting of this information helps provide insight into the patient's theories about screening practices and cancer development, why she feels some survive and others do not, and her knowledge about treatment plans. It is important to have a sense of the woman's belief system prior to embarking on a scientific explanation of cancer development and genetics.

The visit generally continues with discussion of basic information about breast cancer, theories of cancer development, the value of screening and early detection, and a description of hereditary cancer and cancer-susceptibility genes. The extent of the discussion of cancer genetics varies depending on the level of risk, the degree of interest, and the woman's ability to understand this information. We feel that this discussion is beneficial even for women at moderate risk. The availability of genetic-susceptibility testing has been widely publicized in the media, and this discussion serves to explain to most women that they are not at very high risk and why testing would not be useful. Those who appear to be in a hereditary cancer family and are candidates for testing can begin to think about the implications of testing and the major issues involved, including the impact this may have on herself and her family members, how this may affect her management plan, and the possibility of incurring employment or insurance discrimination.

The discussion about hereditary risk is followed by review of the effects of other common risk factors associated with breast and ovarian cancer. The discussion focuses on those risk factors which are relevant to the individual woman. Emphasis is placed on the value of adhering to screening recommendations and the multitude of benefits associated with a healthy diet, regular exercise, moderate alcohol intake, and stress management.

A clinical breast examination is performed along with instruction in the technique of breast self-examination. The visit concludes with screening recommendations and an offer to higher-risk women to be followed for breast examinations and for those at high risk for ovarian cancer to have their screening coordinated by the clinic. About 70% of the higher-risk women continue their follow-up in the Breast Center, providing an ongoing opportunity to update information and continue counseling services. This is always done with the approval of the primary care provider. Even in this age of capitation and cost containment, most providers feel more reassured by having their high-risk patients followed in the Breast Center.

The Social Worker's Visit

The social worker sees each patient for a visit lasting 30 minutes on average. She begins by explaining that she and the nurse practitioner have reviewed the history and family pedigree, the estimated level of risk, and relevant recommendations. Next, she evaluates the patient's understanding of the information received and the impact this has made. The patient is encouraged to discuss her experience with cancer and her fears associated with the disease, often as it relates to losses to cancer suffered by the family and the significance of each to the patient. This enables the social worker to define the patient's areas of fear and her level of success at resolving her losses. For some, there is fear of death, while for others, there is fear of disfigurement or of having passed the risk on to their children. It is often helpful to remind the patient that improvements in early detection and treatments for breast cancer have led to less extensive surgery and greater chance for survival. An assessment of the patient's coping skills and support network relevant to these issues is a vital part of the visit. Treatment recommendations may be made, for example, referral to a psychotherapist or to a bereavement group, if the patient is highly anxious, appears to be clinically depressed, or has unresolved issues involving illness and death.

The second half of the session is aimed at empowering the patient. The benefit of healthy lifestyle choices is reinforced, and suggestions are made in areas needing improvement. Advice may include a review of smoking-cessation techniques, strategies for improved dietary habits, encouragement to develop an ongoing structured exercise regime, and strategies to lessen the fear of conducting a self breast examination. Some patients are taught basic relaxation techniques within the context of the visit. All patients are allowed sufficient time in a therapeutic milieu that encourages expression of concerns about cancer, loss, and death, as well as any other issues affecting psychological well-being.

Genetic Testing

A woman is considered a candidate for genetic testing if she is affected with breast or ovarian cancer and has a family history suggestive of hereditary breast or breast and ovarian cancer. An unaffected woman may be tested if she is of Ashkenazi heritage and has a family history suggesting a hereditary predisposition. Unaffected women who are not Ashkenazi are counseled to discuss testing with appropriate family members. Once a mutation has been identified in an affected relative, the unaffected woman can proceed with testing if she wishes.

If a woman elects to undergo genetic testing, we schedule an additional visit, and we encourage her to bring a companion along at that time. The purpose of this visit is to provide the woman with sufficient information to understand the potential benefits as well as the risks and limitations of testing. Critical elements of this session are the assessment of her psychological stability and her capacity to cope with receiving test results and discussing them with family members.

This second visit provides the woman with more detailed information about the testing process. The educational component addresses the topics outlined by Lerman and colleagues (53): 1) inheritance of breast/ovarian cancer susceptibility, 2) cancer risks associated with mutations, 3) tests for mutation status, 4) benefits of genetic testing, 5) limitations of genetic testing, 6) risks of genetic testing, 7) options for prevention and surveillance, and 8) assurance of confidentiality. The individual's interest in testing is likely generated by a strong desire to understand her risk and a plan to make management decisions based on the results of testing. It is critical for her to understand the limitations of testing, particularly the possibility of indeterminate results, the uncertainty of cancer risk prediction, and the lack of proven prevention strategies. We assist the woman in articulating her motives for testing and help her consider and prepare for the effects the results will have on her and other family members.

If the patient consents to testing, the blood sample is obtained, and a follow-up visit is arranged. This next visit is for results disclosure; however, the patient is made aware that she has the option to postpone or to decide against learning the results. Thus far each woman who has undergone testing through our clinic has chosen to receive her results, and we believe that this is so because of the preparatory work prior to the decision to have testing. Women who have chosen to be tested have done so because they wish to know the results and generally because they plan to make management decisions based on testing results. Despite this preparation, we

encourage the woman to explore her feelings about learning her results and to discuss her plans to relay this information to her family.

An additional visit is planned for approximately 2 months later, when the patient is given the opportunity to reflect on her experience after learning her results. The social worker assesses the woman's psychological response and determines if additional counseling sessions are indicated or if she needs referral for further psychotherapy.

Since genetic-susceptibility testing remains new and is relatively uncharted territory, we believe that it is important to provide this service in the context of a research protocol whenever possible.

Conclusion

Recent developments in molecular genetics have increased our understanding of hereditary breast and ovarian cancer dramatically. Applying this knowledge to clinical practice and adjusting management strategies based on this knowledge are challenges that must be met by our health systems today.

The establishment of a risk-assessment clinic is a reasonable first step to bring a health care system into the genetic age. Such a clinic functions not just to care for patients at the highest risk but also as a focal point of genetic education for patients and clinicians and as a central resource for the latest findings in genetic research.

The clinic must have personnel with the knowledge and experience to care for high-risk patients, the expertise to translate new information into management strategies for patients, and the ability to develop educational programs and materials for patients and clinicians. Since few individuals possess these qualifications, a reasonable approach is to identify professionals with relevant experience and interest and provide them with the time and resources to become expert. In their educational and organizational endeavors, they should use the experiences of others who have undertaken the same tasks. In this area, sharing of information and procedures is the norm, and contacting and working with existing centers are expected. In this, as in almost no other area of medicine, cooperation among clinics is essential. As more women present for genetic testing, clinicians will need to be prepared to facilitate the testing process for relatives who live at a distance. It behooves the risk assessment clinic to have contacts in other states who can undertake the counseling and testing and cooperate in the genetic services for the geographically separated family.

The development of a risk assessment clinic will allow a health care system to take advantage of new genetic information as it becomes available and incorporate it into daily medical practice. Since the area of breast cancer genetics is making significant advances and involves a common disease of concern to many, this is a reasonable place to start. It could then be relatively straightforward to expand the breast/ovarian risk-assessment clinic to evaluate for other cancers as more information becomes available.

References

1. Thompson JA, Wiesner GL, Sellers T, et al. Genetic services for familial cancer patients: a survey of national cancer institute cancer centers. J Natl Cancer Inst 1995;87:1446–1455.
2. Chart PL, Franssen E. Management of women at increased risk for breast cancer: preliminary results from a new program. Can Med Assoc J 1997;157:1235–1242.
3. Schnabel FR, Estabrook A. Surveillance for breast cancer: benefits of participation in a high risk program. Breast Cancer Res Treat 1997;46:64.
4. Giardiello FM, Brensinger JD, Petersen GM, et al. The use and interpretation of commercial *APC* gene testing for familial adenomatous polyposis. New Engl J Med 1997;336:823–827.
5. Rowley PT, Loader S. Attitudes of obstetrician-gynecologists toward DNA testing for a genetic susceptibility to breast cancer. Obstet Gynecol 1996;88:611–615.
6. Albano WA, Lynch HT, Recabaren JA, et al. Familial cancer in an oncology clinic. Cancer 1981;47:2113–2118.
7. Kelly PT. Refinements in breast cancer risk analysis. Arch Surg 1981;116:364–365.
8. Josten DM, Evans AM, Love RR. The cancer prevention clinic: a service program for cancer-prone families. J Psychosoc Oncol 1986;3:5–20.
9. Sclafani L. Management of the high-risk patient. Semin Surg Oncol 1991;7:261–266.
10. Struewing JP, Hartge P, Wacholder S, et al. The risk of cancer associated with specific mutations of *BRCA1* and *BRCA2* among Ashkenazi Jews. New Engl J Med 1997;336:1401–1408.
11. Kelly PT. Cancer risk information services: promise and pitfalls. Breast J 1996;2:233–237.
12. American Society of Clinical Oncology. Statement of the American Society of Clinical Oncology. J Clin Oncol 1996;14:1730–1736.
13. Oncology Nursing Society. Cancer genetic testing and risk assessment counseling: a position paper, 1997. Oncol Nurs Forum 1998;25:464.
14. Oncology Nursing Society. The role of the oncology nurse in cancer genetic counseling: a position paper, 1997. Oncol Nurs Forum 1998;25:463.
15. Peters JA, Biesecker BB. Genetic counseling and hereditary cancer. Cancer Suppl 1997; 80:576–586.
16. Peters JA, Stopfer JE. Role of genetic counselor in familial cancer. Oncology 1996;10(2):159–182.
17. Peters JA. Familial cancer risk: I. Impact on today's oncology practice. J Oncol Manage 1994;Sept-Oct:20–30.
18. Stefanek ME. Counseling women at high risk for breast cancer. Oncology 1990;4:27–38.
19. Kelly PT. Informational needs of individuals and families with hereditary cancers. Semin Oncol Nurs 1992;8:288–292.
20. Entrekin N, Summerlot L. Nurses' role in educating women on risks. In: Stoll BA, ed. Reducing Breast Cancer Risk in Women. The Netherlands: Kluwer Academic Publishers, 1995:185–192.
21. Newcomb PA, Carbone PP. The Health consequences of smoking: cancer. In: Fiore MC, ed. Cigarette Smoking: A Clinical Guide to Assessment and Treatment. Philadelphia: WB Saunders Co, Med Clin N Am 1992:305–331.
22. Colditz GA, Stampfor MJ, Willett WC, et al. Prospective study of estrogen replacement therapy and risk of breast cancer in postmenopausal women. JAMA 1990;264:2648–2653.
23. Mackarem G, Yacoub LK, Lee AKS, et al. Effects of screening on detection of lobular carcinoma in situ of the breast: non-specificity of mammography and physical examination. Breast Dis 1994;7:333–345.
24. Dupont DL, Dupont WD, Rogers LW, Rados MS. Atypical hyperplastic lesions of the breast. Cancer 1985;55:2698–2708.
25. Gail MH, Brinton LA, Byar DP, et al. Projecting individualized probabilities of developing breast cancer for white females who are being examined annually. J Natl Cancer Inst 1989;81:1879–1886.

26. Mackarem G, Roche CA, Hughes KS. The effectiveness of the Gail model in estimating risk for development of breast cancer in women under 40 years of age. Breast 2000 (in press).

27. Claus EB, Risch N, Thompson D. Autosomal dominant inheritance of early-onset breast cancer. Cancer 1994;73:643–651.

28. Berry DA, Parmigiani G, Sanchez J, Schildkraut J, Winer E. Probability of carrying a mutation of breast-ovarian cancer gene *BRCA1* based on family history. J Natl Cancer Inst 1997;89:227–238.

29. Offit K, Brown K. Quantitating familial cancer risk: a resource for clinical oncologists. J Clin Oncol 1994;12:1724–1736.

30. Lerman C, Rimer BK, Engstrom PF. Cancer risk notification: psychosocial and ethical implications. J Clin Oncol 1991;9:1275–1282.

31. Schwartz LM, Woloshin S, Black WC, Welch HG. The role of numeracy in understanding the benefit of screening mammography. Ann Intern Med 1997;127:966–972.

32. Richards MPM, Halowell N, Green JM, et al. Counseling families with hereditary breast and ovarian cancer: a psychological perspective. J Gentet Counsel 1995;4:219–233.

33. Ponder BAJ. Setting up and running a familial cancer clinic. Br Med Bul 1994;50:732–745.

34. Vogel VG, Yeomans A, Higginbotham E. Clinical management of women at increased risk for breast cancer. Breast Cancer Res Treat 1993;28:195–210.

35. Hoskins KF, Stopfer JE, Calzone KA, et al. Assessment and counseling for women with a family history of breast cancer: a guide for clinicians. JAMA 1995;273:577–585.

36. Miki Y, Swensen J, Shattuck-Eidens D, et al. A strong candidate for the breast and ovarian cancer susceptibility gene *BRCA1*. Science 1994;266:66–71.

37. Wooster R, Bignell G, Lancaster J, et al. Identification of the breast cancer susceptibility gene *BRCA2*. Nature 1995;378:789–792.

38. Couch FJ, Hartmann LC. *BRCA1* testing:advances and retreats. JAMA 1998;279:955–956.

39. Burke W, Daly M, Garber J, et al. Recommendations for follow-up care of individuals with an inherited predisposition to cancer: II *BRCA1* and *BRCA2*. JAMA 1997;277:997–1003.

40. Hughes KS, Papa M, Whitney T, McLellan R. Prophylactic surgery and inherited cancer predisposition. In: Shall GL, ed. Cancer Genetics for the Clinician. New York: Plenum Press, 1999;103–133.

41. Lopez MJ, Porter KA. The current role of prophylactic mastectomy. Surg Clin North Am 1996;76:231–242.

42. Fisher B, Costantino JP, Wickerham DL, et al. Tamoxifen for prevention of breast cancer: report of the National Surgical Breast and Bowel Project P-1 study. J Natl Cancer Inst 1998;90:1371–1388.

43. Prentice R, Sheppard L. Dietary fat and cancer. Cancer Causes Control 1990;1:81–97.

44. Willett WC, Hunter DJ, Stampfer MJ. Dietary fat and fiber in relation to risk of breast cancer. JAMA 1992;268:2037–2044.

45. Howe G, Rohan T, Decarli, A, et al. The association between alcohol and breast cancer risk: evidence from the combined analysis of six dietary case-control studies. Int J Cancer 1991;47:707–710.

46. Longnecker MP, Berlin JA, Orza MJ, Chalmers TC. A meta-analysis of alcohol consumption in relation to risk of breast cancer. JAMA 1988;260:652–656.

47. The American Cancer Society. 1996 Advisory Committee on Diet, Nutrition and Cancer Prevention. CA 1996;46:325–341.

48. Gross TP, Schlesselman JJ. The estimated effect of oral contraceptive use on the cumulative risk of epithelial ovarian cancer. Obstet Gynecol 1994;83:419–424.

49. Hankinson SE, Colditz GA, Hunteer DJ. A quantitative assessment of oral contraceptive use and risk of ovarian cancer. Obstet Gynecol 1992;80:708–714.

50. Struewing JP, Watson P, Easton DF, et al. Prophylactic oophorectomy in inherited breast/ovarian cancer families. J Natl Cancer Inst Monogr 1995;17:33–35.

51. Weber AM, Hewett WJ, Gajewski WH, Curry SL. Serous carcinoma of the peritoneum after oophorectomy. Obstet Gynecol 1992;80:558–560.

52. Lerman C, Schwartz M. Adherence and psychological adjustment among women at high risk for breast cancer. Breast Cancer Res Treat 1993;28:145–155.

53. Lerman C, Narod S, Schulman K, et al: *BRCA1* testing in families with hereditary breast-ovarian cancer: a prospective study of patient decision making and outcomes. JAMA 1996;275:1885–1892.

Additional Readings

Kelly P. Understanding Breast Cancer Risk. Philadelphia: Temple University Press, 1991.

Schneider K. Counseling about Cancer: Strategies for Genetic Counselors. Boston: Dana Farber Cancer Institute, 1994.

Appendix A. Risk Assessment Clinic Breast Center/Lahey Clinic North Pre-Consultation Questionnaire

Date of Birth:
Referred by:
Primary Care Provider :

How many times have you been pregnant? (include miscarriages & abortions)_____

How many children have you delivered?_____

If not pregnant, are you currently having periods?_____

If you are post-menopausal (no longer having periods), **how old were you when you stopped having them?**_____

Has your uterus been removed (hysterectomy)?_____ If yes, at what age?_____

Have both of your ovaries been removed?_____ If yes, at what age?_____

Have you ever taken birth control pills?_____ _____No _____ Currently taking _____ In the past

How long were you on birth control pills? _____

Have you ever been prescribed Premarin, estrogen, or hormones of any type?_____
    If yes, are you still taking it?_____

Have you ever taken fertility drugs?_____

Do you do a monthly breast self-exam?_____

When was your last pap smear?_____

When did you last have your stool checked for blood?_____

Have you ever had a sigmoidoscopy? _____ If yes, when_____

Do you smoke?___yes ___no If yes, how many years have you smoked? _____
    How many packs per day? _____
    Are you a former smoker?___yes ___no If yes, when did you quit? _____

Do you drink alcoholic beverages? __yes __no If yes, how many drinks per week? _____

What do you think is your risk of getting breast cancer?
____very low _____average _____somewhat higher than average ____much higher than average

How concerned are you about your risk of getting breast cancer?
___not at all _____rarely worry ____occasionally worry ____very worried ____worry constantly

Breast Risk Assessment Clinic

Ethnic background _____

Have you ever had cancer? _____

How old were you at your first period?__ _____

Have you ever had children? _____How old were you when your first child was born? _____

Have you ever had a breast biopsy (a surgery where a piece of breast tissue was removed through an incision)?_____
How many?_____   Did any biopsy show *atypical hyperplasia?*_____

FAMILY HISTORY

How many sisters do you have?_____   How many brothers?_____

How many sisters does your mother have?_____ How many brothers?_____

How many sisters does your father have?_____   How many brothers?_____

Has anyone in your family had cancer?_____

RELATIVE	FIRST NAME	CANCER TYPE, IF ANY	AGE DIAGNOSED	COMMENTS
You				
Son				
Son				
Daughter				
Daughter				
Brother				
Brother				
Sister				
Sister				
Father				
Mother				
Uncle (Father's Side)				
Uncle (Father's Side)				
Aunt (Father's Side)				
Aunt (Father's Side)				
Uncle (Mother's Side)				
Uncle (Mother's Side)				
Aunt (Mother's Side)				
Aunt (Mother's Side)				
Grandfather (Father's Side)				
Grandmother (Father's Side)				
Grandfather (Mother's Side)				
Grandmother (Mother's Side)				

11

Prophylactic Mastectomy

Kenneth C. Shestak, Daniel A. Medalie, and Scott L. Williams

All surgeons who deal with diseases of the breast must interact with patients who are considering or are referred for prophylactic mastectomy. In the current era of early detection and breast conservation, it seems almost paradoxical to propose a mastectomy as treatment for a noncancerous condition of the breast especially in light of the emerging interest in chemoprevention of breast cancer (1). Nevertheless, prophylactic mastectomy is still the only nonexperimental therapy currently being practiced for the primary prevention of breast cancer (2–9). Renewed interest in this procedure is due to dramatic improvements in breast reconstruction using a patient's own tissue coupled with discoveries linking genetic mutations with markedly increased risk of developing breast cancer in selected patients.

Historically, indications for the procedure included mastodynia, unreliable physical examination due to dense, fibrous breasts, multiple breast biopsies regardless of histopathology, "cancerphobia," family history, and a variety of histopathalogic diagnoses ranging from fibrocystic disease to lobular carcinoma in situ (2–8). These indications grew in parallel with the introduction of silicone gel implants, tissue expanders, and increasingly sophisticated uses of the patient's own (autogenous) tissue for breast reconstruction. In retrospect, it seems clear that the operation was being performed on an irregular basis without clearly defined indications. The resulting backlash against the procedure raised the valid question of whether prophylactic mastectomy was ever necessary (10). Indeed, at this time, some insurance companies do not cover the surgery, especially in the instance of bilateral mastectomy without a histologic diagnosis.

We currently stand at a crossroad where new understanding of risk factors and outcomes for breast cancer gives clinicians the objective data to define a subset of women at risk who might benefit from prophylactic mastectomy. The average lifetime risk of breast cancer for all women is around 12% (11), but mutations in the BRCA1 and BRCA2 genes recently have been shown to confer upon affected women a cumulative risk of breast cancer from 40% to 80% (11–15). A survey of a large number of surgeons suggests that at this latter risk level, most would recommend bilateral prophylactic mastectomy (16).

The purpose of this chapter is to review the current indications for prophylactic mastectomy. We will describe the techniques and cosmetic results of current extirpative and reconstructive procedures and attempt to define a subset of patients who might best benefit from the procedure.

Efficacy

Lopez and Porter in a recent review of prophylactic mastectomy (4) describe their own and other surgeons' criteria for successful surgical prophylaxis of disease. The procedure should effectively prevent the disease. The population at risk should be easily identifiable, and the cost-benefit analysis of the procedure should be documentable. We will address each one of these issues with an eye toward the efficacy of prophylactic mastectomy as a preventative measure for breast cancer.

Does removal of most of the breast effectively prevent breast cancer? Two main operations have been described for the removal of breast tissue, subcutaneous mastectomy and total mastectomy. In a *subcutaneous mastectomy* as much of the mammary tissue as possible, including the tail of Spence, is removed, but the nipple-areola complex with an underlying "bud" of breast tissue is preserved (17). Incision placement and technique have been modified frequently, with the most notable modification being the addition of a nipple coring procedure by some to remove potential ductal tissue from the retained nipple-areolar complex (3,18). *Total mastectomy* differs from subcutaneous mastectomy in that it attempts to remove all breast tissue *including* the nipple and areola (19). Reconstruction for both procedures most often is performed in the immediate setting (done at the time of the mastectomy), but in rare instances it can be accomplished as a delayed reconstruction (performed at a later date).

Several studies have shown that subcutaneous or even total mastectomy does not remove all the breast tissue however. Goldman and Goldwyn (20) in 1973 performed 12 subcutaneous mastectomies through an inframammary incision in 6 cadavers with no known breast pathology. Following extensive subcutaneous removal of breast tissue, multiple biopsies were taken from all borders of resection, including the axillary extension of the breast and the undersurface of the nipple-areola complex. In all cases, breast tissue was identified in the nipple complex biopsies, and 3 of 6 cadavers had breast tissue remaining bilaterally, whereas 2 others had breast tissue on one side. The conclusion was that subcutaneous mastectomy could not be considered completely prophylactic. In fact, it has been estimated that residual breast tissue varies as much as 5% to 25% following subcutaneous mastectomy (20). Similar findings relating to the "completeness" of breast tissue removal were noted by Barton and colleagues (21), who studied total mastectomy specimens. Breast tissue can be found on the underlying pectoralis muscle, in the axilla, on the undersurface of the breast flaps, and in the overlying dermis and areola (4,20). The obvious question that arises is what significance does the residual breast tissue have in terms of breast cancer prevention?

Although is seems intuitively obvious that the risk of breast cancer should decrease in proportion to the amount of breast tissue removed, the literature has many reports of breast cancer following prophylactic mastectomy (22–26). Most disconcerting, perhaps, are laboratory data in rodents that suggest that no amount of breast tissue removal is effective in preventing breast cancer (27,28). Sprague-Dawly rats were subjected to partial and total mastectomies and then exposed to DMBA, a known breast carcinogen (27). Although it took longer for rodents with mastectomies to develop tumors, there was no statistically significant difference in overall tumor incidence. The conclusion was that the risk of developing breast tumors in this rodent model was not reduced in proportion to the amount of breast tissue removed. Studies on breast tumor-forming mice reported similar findings; mammary tumor incidence at 12 months was not decreased by 50% or 100% mastectomy (28). One can conclude from these animal studies that residual breast tissue is left in all mastectomies and that this tissue has an equal chance of forming tumors.

Although there have been relatively few large studies of prophylactic mastectomy performed in humans, these studies are far more encouraging from the standpoint of derived benefit than the animal data (23). A number of the studies have been efficiently summarized by Ziegler and Kroll (23) (Table 11-1). One of the problems with all these trials is that the indications for mastectomy, the surgical technique, and the estimated quantity of breast tissue left behind were all variable (20). Pennisi and Capozzi (8) analyzed 1500 patients treated with prophylactic mastectomy performed by 165 surgeons throughout the United States. Unfortunately, 30% of the patients were lost to follow-up, and average duration of follow-up was only 9 years. Occult pathology and histology were evaluated. Of these specimens, ductal carcinoma in situ (DCIS) was present in 5.2%, lobular carcinoma in situ (LCIS) in 3.4%, and atypia in 11%. One hundred and thirty-nine patients in the series underwent prophylactic contralateral mastectomy having already been treated for cancer in the opposite breast, and of these, 3% had carcinomas in the specimen and 3.6% were

Table 11-1. Studies of prophylactic mastectomy

	Humphrey (1)	Woods (13)	Bohmert (12)	Pennisi (14)[a]
Total no. of patients	285	1,400	155	1,500
No. of high-risk patients[b]	16 (6%)	NS	90 (58%)	735 (49%)
Mastectomy	Subcutaneous	Subcutaneous	Simple	Subcutaneous
Median follow-up (years)	NS	16–20	2	9
Total no. of patients who developed cancer	3	3	NS	6
Percent high-risk patients who developed cancer	19	NS	NS	0.81

Note: NS, not stated.
[a]Table 11-4 presents our critical reevaluation of the data in this study.
[b]Includes patients with positive family history of breast cancer, histology indicative of a slightly increased risk (6), lobular carcinoma in situ, ductal carcinoma in situ, or contralateral breast cancer.
Source: Ziegler LD, Kroll SS. Primary breast cancer after prophylactic mastectomy. Am J Clin Oncol 1991;14:451–454, with permission.

Table 11-2. Criteria for enrollment in the high-risk category*

Two or more first-degree relatives with breast cancer
One first-degree relative and two or more second- or third-degree relatives with breast cancer
One first-degree relative with breast cancer before the age of 45 years and one other relative
    with breast cancer
One first-degree relative with breast cancer and one or more relatives with ovarian cancer
Two second- or third-degree relatives with breast cancer and one or more with ovarian cancer
One second- or third-degree relative with breast cancer and two or more with ovarian cancer
Three or more second- or third-degree relatives with breast cancer
One first-degree relative with bilateral breast cancer

*To be considered at high risk, women had to meet at least one of these criteria.
Source: Hartmann LC, et al. Efficacy of bilateral prophylactic mastectomy in women with a family history of breast cancer. New Engl J Med 1999;340:77–84, with permission.

found to have LCIS. Only 20% of the patients undergoing the procedure had a first-degree relative with invasive cancer. Reanalysis of the risk factors for the population and indications for the procedure suggests that 49% of the patients had a true indication for the procedure, with 51% of the patients undergoing the surgery for nonproliferative "fibrocystic" disease that is not linked to an increased risk of breast cancer (23). The original rate of cancer formation, presented as 0.6% by the authors, thus can be doubled to determine rates of cancer only in those women who were at high risk (23). Although this is twice the value reported, it is still well below the average woman's lifetime risk of developing cancer. Since the average follow-up in this study was 9 years, it is unknown how many of these women went on to develop breast carcinomas.

By far, the most compelling evidence to date supporting the efficacy of prophylactic mastectomy in reducing the risk of breast cancer development in a population of women at greatest risk is that published by Hartmann and colleagues (2) in the *New England Journal of Medicine* in 1999. The authors retrospectively reviewed the Mayo Clinic experience with prophylactic mastectomy in 1065 women over a 33-year period. Careful chart review identified 214 patients deemed to be at high risk and 425 patients felt to be at moderate risk for developing breast cancer using family history as the predictor of risk (Table 11-2) who were treated by prophylactic mastectomy with a median follow-up of 14 years. Outcome analysis demonstrated a 90% reduction in the incidence of breast cancer in the high-risk group when compared with family members who had not undergone prophylactic mastectomy (2). Similarly, the authors demonstrated an 89.5% reduction ($p < 0.0001$) in the expected number of

Table 11-3. Expected and actual numbers of breast cancers among the high-risk women who underwent prophylactic mastectomy[a]

Events in Sisters Used to Calculate Rate	Person-Years of Follow-Up		Breast Cancer		Reduction in Risk (95%CI), Percent
	Sisters	Probands	No. Expected	No. Observed	
All breast cancers (before and after prophylactic mastectomy) from age 18 to end of follow-up					
Unadjusted	13,336	2964	52.9	3	94.3 (83.5–98.8)
Adjusted[b]	12,710	2964	30.0	3	90.0 (70.8–97.9)
Breast cancer after prophylactic mastectomy to end of follow-up	3,109	2964	37.4	3	92.0 (76.6–98.3)

[a]The expected incidence of breast cancer was calculated on the basis of a number of factors analyzed in the control group consisting of sisters of the probands. CI denotes confidence interval.
[b]The method of adjustment for ascertainment bias is described in the "Methods" section.
Source: Hartmann LC, et al. Efficacy of bilateral prophylactic mastectomy in women with a family history of breast cancer. New Engl J Med 1999;340:77–84, with permission.

Table 11-4. Expected and actual numbers of deaths from breast cancer among the high-risk women who underwent prophylactic mastectomy[a]

Events in Sisters Used to Calculate Rate	Person-Years of Follow-Up		Breast Cancer		Reduction in Risk (95%CI), Percent
	Sisters	Probands	No. Expected	No. Observed	
All breast cancers (before and after prophylactic mastectomy) from age 18 to end of follow-up					
Unadjusted	14,896	2970	30.6	2	93.5 (76.4–99.2)
Adjusted[b]	13,569	2970	19.4	2	89.7 (62.8–98.9)
Deaths from breast cancer after prophylactic mastectomy to end of follow-up	3,356	2970	10.5	2	80.9 (31.4–97.7)

[a]The expected incidence of death from breast cancer was calculated on the basis of a number of factors analyzed in the control group consisting of sisters of the probands. CI denotes confidence interval.
[b]The method of adjustment for ascertainment bias is described in the "Methods" section.
Source: Hartmann LC, et al. Efficacy of bilateral prophylactic mastectomy in women with a family history of breast cancer. New Engl J Med 1999;340:77–84, with permission.

breast cancers predicted by the Gail model in the group at moderate risk (Table 11-3). There was a corresponding decrease in the number of deaths due to the breast cancer diagnosis (Table 11-4). This sophisticated epidemiologic analysis demonstrated a significant reduction in the incidence of breast cancer development following subcutaneous mastectomy in women judged to be at high risk on the basis of family history and strongly supports its role in breast cancer prophylaxis (4).

In summary, taken in the aggregate, these studies (2,4,8,23) demonstrate a significantly decreased incidence of subsequent breast carcinoma in women who have undergone prophylactic mastectomy, suggesting that the procedure can be effective in diminishing, but not eliminating, the risk of carcinoma in selected populations of high risk women. What the studies do not tell us is whether prophylactic mastectomy is superior to careful clinical and mammographic screening of women at high risk in reducing fatality from breast cancer. A prospective, randomized, controlled trial comparing careful surveillance to prophylactic mastectomy in the patient at high risk for breast cancer has yet to be done and is unlikely to take place given the current climate of breast cancer prevention and treatment.

The alternative to subcutaneous mastectomy is total simple mastectomy. As already mentioned, this does not ensure complete eradication of residual breast tissue, but by excising the nipple-areola complex as part of the specimen, it does reduce the amount of breast tissue elements left behind (22). It is known that the nipple is part of the ductal system of the breast, thus to leave it intact while performing a purported cancer prophylaxis operation seems contradictory. A subcutaneous mastectomy with nipple coring theoretically would offer a greater protection, but ductal tissue elements occasionally can be found in dermis and areola, again calling in to question the wisdom of leaving this tissue behind. This intuitive argument notwithstanding, Woods and Meland (18) report their results with 1500 subcutaneous mastectomies and describe a postmastectomy cancer in only 5 patients. Unfortunately, patient selection is not well delineated. They do, however, report an incidence of nipple-areola necrosis in 5% to 15% of all patients. It is their opinion that a superior cosmetic result is obtained from preservation of the nipple-areola complex. Others have described the cosmetic outcome of the nipple following subcutaneous mastectomy to be substandard, with a distorted, insensate nipple with decreased erectile function (26). The possibility of nipple-areola necrosis or poor cosmetic outcome following nipple and areola preservation in combination with the seemingly obvious risk of leaving behind breast tissue that may become cancerous leads us to regard subcutaneous mastectomy as an operation of second choice for cancer prophylaxis.

Our procedure of choice for breast cancer prophylaxis is total mastectomy with immediate breast reconstruction. Interestingly there were no instances of subsequent breast cancer development in any (0 of 64) of the women at moderate or high risk in the Hartmann study (2), but the

number of patients treated by this method was not large enough to demonstrate a statistically significant difference when compared with those treated by subcutaneous mastectomy.

Refinements in the techniques of both breast and nipple-areola complex reconstruction, however, make this operation of total mastectomy our strong preference for breast cancer prophylaxis (2). This procedure allows better operative exposure for elevating skin flaps and permits a more precise excision of the breast parenchyma, entails complete excision of the nipple-areola complex, and can be done with maximal skin sparing incisions that optimize cosmetic outcome regardless of the reconstruction technique used. Following nipple-areola removal, a new nipple-areola complex reconstruction usually can be carried out within 12 weeks of surgery. An intradermal tattoo procedure done shortly thereafter can restore the visual appearance of a normal areola and can look surprisingly natural, especially in the situation of bilateral breast reconstruction.

Population at Risk

In our criteria for evaluating the efficacy of surgical prophylaxis, we have indicated that the patient population at risk should be easily identifiable. This is, in essence, the crux of the issue. Until very recently there has been great difficulty in building a consensus about which patients are at high risk for the development of breast cancer. As mentioned previously, several of the large studies attempting to determine the benefits of prophylactic mastectomy failed to standardize patient selection criteria. More frustratingly, factors that in the past were believed to increase the risk of cancer subsequently have turned out to be relatively benign. This chapter is but one chapter in an entire book devoted to the management of women at high risk for breast cancer. Thus we will not attempt to review in depth each of the important advances in understanding of the pathophysiology of breast cancer. Rather we will focus on some of the most recent discoveries that lend support to or oppose the concept of prophylactic mastectomy.

Table 11-5 lists indications for prophylactic simple mastectomy as outlined by Lopez and

Table 11-5. Indications for prophylactic simple mastectomy

No prior invasive breast cancer (candidate for bilateral mastectomies with immediate reconstruction)	Bilateral, multifocal DCIS Unilateral DCIS or LCIS with contralateral ADH Bilateral ADH and a first-degree relative with premenopausal breast cancer Bilateral moderate- to high-risk proliferative breast histology[a] and two or more first-degree relatives with premenopausal or bilateral breast cancer Any of above with mutated *BRCA1* gene[b]	Bilateral ADH in premenopausal woman No family history of breast cancer Nonproliferative histology, but two or more first-degree relative with breast cancer
Prior breast cancer (candidate for contralateral mastectomy and reconstruction	DCIS, LCIS, or ADH of remaining breast One or more first-degree relatives with breast cancer Combinations of above factors	Large, pendulous remaining breast, causing shoulder or back pain due to asymmetry Multiple breast biopsies resulting in difficulty performing or interpreting diagnostic breast examinations; the patient refuses more biopsies and is desirous of bilateral reconstruction

Note: DCIS, ductal carcinoma in situ; LCIS, lobular carcinoma in situ; ADH, atypical ductal (or lobular) hyperplasia.
[a]Moderate or florid hyperplasia, papillomatosis is with fibrovascular core, atypical ductal, or lobular hyperplasia.
[b]Recommended under strict research protocols.
Source: Modified from Nemecek JR, Young VL, Lopez MJ. Indications for prophylactic mastectomy. Missouri Med 1993;90:136, with permission.

Porter (4). This table is a variant of the previously described indications by the Society for Surgical Oncology (8). All the risk factors in the "Strong" column are recognized markers for future malignancy. It should be noted that none of these risk factors are absolute indicators for prophylactic mastectomy (29). In the instance of prior breast cancer, the stage of the previous tumor is all important in determining surgical therapy for the contralateral breast. Patients who are node-positive have a higher likelihood of dying from their current disease than from any future contralateral breast cancer. Concurrent medical problems also may preclude prophylactic surgery (4).

Gail and colleagues in 1989 described a model that projected breast cancer susceptibility in white females being examined annually (30) that later was validated by Bondy and colleagues (31). These data, in combination with a better understanding of precancerous breast pathology significantly increase our ability to determine for some patients what their current and lifetime risk for developing breast cancer is (30–32). It should be noted that it is the very rare

patient whose risk of developing breast cancer ever exceeds 25% to 30% (4,33). The reader is referred to Chapter 4, which outlines quantitative risk assessment.

Are there patients who most breast cancer specialists agree, unequivocally, could benefit from prophylactic mastectomy? Houn and colleagues (16) sent a cross-sectional survey to 522 general surgeons, 80 plastic surgeons, and 801 gynecologists in the state of Maryland asking their opinions of the role of prophylactic mastectomy in the high-risk woman. Mean threshold risk at which surgeons would recommend bilateral prophylactic mastectomy was 51% for the general surgeons, 41% for the plastic surgeons and 54% for the gynecologists. All surgeons also were asked to manage a hypothetical case of a woman with a risk assessment of 25% over 30 years according to the Gail model. In all, 92% of general surgeons, 83% of plastic surgeons, and 85.6% of gynecologists recommended surveillance rather than mastectomy for this hypothetical woman. This survey suggests that, in general, practicing clinicians are quite heterogeneous but conservative in their recommendation for prophylactic mastectomy. Several authors in the literature (34,35) recommend lower risk levels in the 15% to 25% range for prophylactic mastectomy to be performed, indicating that the practice of clinicians may be more conservative than the recommendations of experts. Nevertheless, the 50% mark seems to be a significant number for most clinicians above which they would seriously consider prophylactic mastectomy for their patients.

While only 5% to 10% of all breast cancers are thought to be hereditary, patients with these germ-line mutations have a cumulative risk of developing cancer of 40% to 85% (12–14). These numbers are within the range of the clinician cut off for recommending prophylactic mastectomy (13). Family history is a widely recognized risk factor (2) for breast cancer, but it is important to distinguish between familial cancer, which is defined as one or more first- or second-degree relatives with breast cancer, and hereditary cancer (36). *Hereditary cancer* is a subset of *familial cancer* and refers to those patients who demonstrate an autosomal dominant pattern of disease incidence. The Li-Fraumeni syndrome is a rare familial syndrome linked to a germ-line mutation in the *p53* tumor suppresser gene. Patients are predisposed to brain and adrenal tumors as well as breast cancers. Mutations in the *BRCA1* and *BRCA2* genes recently have been discovered to predispose women to breast cancer (12). *BRCA1* mutation has been linked to approximately 45% of genetically transmitted breast cancer. Carriers also have an increased risk of ovarian carcinoma. *BRCA2* carriers do not have an increased risk of ovarian disease, but males in the family appear to have an increased incidence of breast cancer (13,36).

Schrag and colleagues (12) performed a decision analysis comparing prophylactic mastectomy and prophylactic oophorectomy with no surgery among women who carry *BRCA1* or *BRCA2* mutations (12). Varying estimates of risk for breast cancer and varying estimates of effectiveness of prophylactic mastectomy and oophorectomy were plugged into a hypothetical model in an attempt to determine the effects of surgical intervention on life expectancy. The authors calculated that on average, a 30-year-old woman who was positive for a *BRCA1* or *BRCA2*

mutation would gain from 2.9 to 5.3 years of added life expectancy from prophylactic mastectomy depending on her cumulative risk of cancer. This estimate takes into account the fact that women with a germ-line mutation would be undergoing more rigorous surveillance and could be expected to have tumors discovered at an earlier stage. To put these results in perspective, the authors placed the benefit of prophylactic mastectomy at the same range as or higher than the benefit derived from lowering an extraordinarily high cholesterol level to normal in the same woman. Limitations of this analysis include the fact that only surgical prevention was studied, excluding the possible effects of hormonal therapies. Without a prospective trial, there is also no effective way to prove that prophylactic mastectomy has any efficacy at all in genetically influenced breast cancer (37). As has already been mentioned, mastectomy in breast cancer prone mice showed no evidence of cancer reduction (27,28). Nevertheless, this study suggests that there is an indication for prophylactic mastectomy in the subset of patients with a proven genetic predisposition for breast cancer.

If we summarize the data presented so far, we can generate several hypothetical patients for whom prophylactic mastectomy not only would be reasonable but also would be recommended. One such patient would be a 30-year-old white, gravida 0 woman with a mother and sister who have each had bilateral premenopausal breast cancer and who tests positive for *BRCA1* or *BRCA2*. In this woman the risk of getting breast cancer has been estimated by some to be as high as 85% (36). Another patient might be a 35-year-old woman who has already undergone mastectomy and chemotherapy for a node-negative breast cancer on one side who now has a biopsy of the remaining breast revealing lobular carcinoma in situ or atypical ductal hyperplasia. In this patient's case psychological factors also may be an important consideration. Fear of repeat cancer and subsequent chemotherapy may influence such a patient to undergo early preventative surgery. In the case of a contralateral breast that is large, mastectomy and reconstruction may provide the patient with more breast symmetry than one reconstruction and one native breast.

Cost-Benefit Analysis

Three criteria were listed as being necessary for surgical prophylaxis to be a widely accepted procedure. Efficacy and patient selection have been addressed. The final criterion, documentation of cost-benefit analysis, can never be completed adequately. It is obvious that if surgical prevention of breast cancer required a cluster organ transplant, then there would be no prophylaxis. What is required is a randomized trial comparing two populations of high-risk patients. One population would receive prophylactic mastectomy, and the other would undergo current recommended screening procedures including mammography and breast examination. It is unlikely that women would agree to be randomized to such a drastic choice. Several other issues need to be addressed when considering the risks and benefits of prophylactic mastectomy. Psychological and socioeconomic factors can have a dramatic influence on both testing for and treatment of breast cancer. Additionally, new treatments and prophylactic regimens are currently being evaluated that may tip the scale away from prophylactic mastectomy. Each of these will be addressed separately.

In modern society, the breast is not just an organ of lactation but also an object of desire and allure. A woman's attitude toward her breasts reflects her overall sense of femininity, sexuality, and beauty. In 1917, an author noted that "it is the fear of having the breast mutilated that keeps patients away and allows a tumor to run a progressive course" (38). In opposition to this fear is the fear of cancer, which is perceived by many lay people to be one of the only afflictions untouched by modern medicine. Truths and myths about chemotherapy can also profoundly influence a patient's actions. A practitioner who is in consultation with a patient who is a potential candidate for prophylactic mastectomy thus has to contend with a complex array of emotions.

Mastectomy is a mutilating procedure, and there are several studies that demonstrate that women who have undergone mastectomy experience feelings of denial, anger, and loss (39–41). One study found that up to 33% of patients with mastectomies for breast cancer no longer engage in sexual intercourse (39). Short- and long-term adaptation to bilateral prophylactic subcutaneous mastectomy was studied in 25 patients (40). The conclusions were that subcutaneous mastectomy resulted in substantial mental morbidity approaching that reported for primary mastectomy in the treatment of diagnosed cancer. Depression and anxiety, sexual dysfunction, and difficulty in accepting the surgical result were all observed. This suggests that the radical prophylaxis is as disturbing an event as the actual cancer. In fact, women treated with breast-conserving therapy for breast cancer were significantly happier and more positive about their prospects than those who had undergone mastectomy (39), raising the possible scenario of a prophylactic mastectomy patient who has no diagnosed cancer ending up more depressed than a patient with diagnosed cancer who is treated with a breast-conserving regimen.

The argument for prophylaxis is made by several authors who cite "cancerphobia" as an important criterion in the selection of suitable patients (4,10). It is unclear, however, whether this should be used as a criterion only in conjunction with other obvious risk factors or as a stand alone criterion. The lack of accurate grading and definitions of "cancerphobia" make it a criterion that is important to consider but almost impossible to quantify (4). It is clear, nevertheless, that there will be some patients for whom the cost of lifelong fear of and surveillance for breast cancer outweighs the obvious cost of prophylactic mastectomy.

At the beginning of this chapter it was stated that prophylactic mastectomy is the only nonexperimental treatment for the prevention of breast cancer. This chapter, however, is being written in the midst of an explosion of new information about the causes and possible hormonal prevention of breast cancer. In April of 1998, the National Surgical Adjuvant Breast and Bowel Project (NSABP) halted their tamoxifen Breast Cancer Prevention Trial (BCPT) after 6 years of study because of a positive result as described in Chapter 12 (41a). An independent evaluation of results had revealed that there was a 45% reduction in the incidence of breast cancer among the 13,388 women enrolled in the trial. These results confirm and extend earlier work demonstrating that hormonal therapy actually can prevent breast cancer (42). Analyses of more specific patient subgroups within the larger study have been performed, but it is not known whether tamoxifen had any benefit in patients who were positive for *BRCA1* or *BRCA2* mutations. These genetic analyses are not yet completed.

Another point not widely addressed in the lay press was that the incidence of breast cancer did not necessarily correlate with mortality from breast cancer. Intensive screening of participants resulted in discovery of tumors at an earlier stage, thus resulting in more frequent cure. Overall mortality from breast cancer in the tamoxifen group was 3 patients and in the placebo group was 5 patients (43,44). However, those participants in the study who were taking tamoxifen evidenced an increased rate of endometrial cancer, deep vein thrombosis, and pulmonary embolism. One patient in the tamoxifen group died from endometrial cancer, and 2 died from pulmonary embolism. Thus the number of patients who died in the tamoxifen group from causes known to be related to the treatment (6 patients) actually was greater than the placebo group. Other hormonal agents with less adverse side effects than tamoxifen are currently being evaluated, however.

A final word should be made about the socioeconomic impact of newly available scientific methods. It is easy to make the statement that all women with a family history of breast cancer should be genetically screened for the specific mutations associated with a high risk of contracting the disease. However, screening is very expensive, and laws are not yet in place to protect the patients from the results of their screening. Ashkenazi Jews as a population have a relatively homogeneous genome that makes genetic mutations responsible for disease relatively easy to find. As a result, there is much interest in testing Jews for breast cancer genes. There has been a new wariness recently among potential subjects as implications of the results sink in. Few states have legislation in place to prevent genetic discrimination in employment and insurance, and several Jewish leaders worry about the social stigma of being the most genetically studied population in the country. In 1996, 20 Jewish families were asked about their opinion of recent breast cancer research. Half were

in favor, and half felt that they were being victimized by it (NYT, 4/22/98). It is clear that society's new ability to detect disease and effect treatment is more advanced than its ability to deal with the social implications of that detection and treatment. Before effective cost-benefit models can be created, there must be a consensus about who should be screened, who should pay for the screening, and who should know about the results.

Indications

The foregoing discussion outlines the issues pertinent to and the controversies surrounding the operation of prophylactic mastectomy. Although one must be cautious when describing subcutaneous mastectomy as a prophylactic procedure, recent evidence indicates that the risk of breast cancer following this procedure is extremely low even in the high-risk breast patient (2,3). Our preferred procedure for prophylactic mastectomy is that of simple or total mastectomy including resection of the nipple-areola complex (NAC), as opposed to subcutaneous mastectomy, and this will be discussed below.

Currently, our indications for prophylactic mastectomy depend on the patient's medical history and specifically on whether the patient has had a previous invasive breast cancer or not. Strong indications for prophylactic mastectomy in the patient *with* a prior breast cancer include:

- Biopsy-proven DCIS, LCIS, or severe atypical ductal hyperplasia in the remaining breast
- One or more first degree relatives with breast cancer

Relative indications in this subgroup of patients include:

- Multiple breast biopsies resulting in difficulty performing or interpreting diagnostic breast examinations (It should be considered in patients who refuse additional biopsies and who desire bilateral breast reconstruction.)
- A patient who presents with a large, pendulous contralateral breast that is difficult to examine

or which is causing shoulder pain or back pain due to asymmetry after a contralateral mastectomy

In the patient *without* prior breast cancer the following indications for bilateral prophylactic mastectomies with immediate reconstruction should be recognized. Strong indications include:

- Bilateral multifocal DCIS
- Unilateral DCIS or LCIS with contralateral proliferative histologic changes
- Bilateral severe atypical ductal hyperplasia and a first-degree relative with premenopausal breast cancer
- Bilateral moderate- to high-risk proliferative breast histology and two or more first-degree relatives with premenopausal or bilateral breast cancer

Relative indications for bilateral prophylactic mastectomy in the *absence* of previous breast cancer include:

- Bilateral severe atypical ductal hyperplasia in a premenopausal woman without a family history
- Nonproliferative histologic changes but two or more first-degree relatives with breast cancer

It is our feeling that prophylactic mastectomy should not be done for mastodynia or mastalgia. The etiology of breast pain is multifocal and very often unclear. For this reason, the persistence of or recurrence of breast discomfort is highly likely after subcutaneous mastectomy. Finally, we believe that this procedure should rarely, if ever, be performed for "cancerphobia" and only undertaken in this setting after appropriate psychological and psychiatric recommendations and considerations are made.

Operative Technique

As noted previously, our choice for prophylactic mastectomy is that of total mastectomy (45). This involves removal of the breast gland and the accompanying nipple-areola complex, with excision of both elements performed through a single incision. This may take the form of a periareolar incision (Fig. 11-1A) with breast resection, which results in a near total skin sparing mastectomy. Surgical exposure is more difficult, but a superior aesthetic result is often obtained in this manner. Should the surgeon be more comfortable with a longer horizontal incision (Fig. 11-1B) this is also possible. This is commonly referred to as the tennis racquet incision. The operation entails elevation of skin flaps that are developed after lifting the skin flaps at the plane of the anterior breast fascia (9). Once the periphery of the gland is identified medially, laterally, superiorly, and inferiorly, the deep surface of the breast gland is lifted off the underlying pectoralis major muscle fascia. It is *very important* to preserve this fascia in its entirety because this will facilitate the soft tissue coverage of a subpectoral tissue expander or implant. There is no oncologic reason to include the pectoralis fascia, and in fact, the dissection is more hemostatic and readily accomplished with preservation of this fascial layer.

Following removal of the breast tissue, reconstruction can be carried out. Commonly, this is performed using synthetic material in the form of either an implant or a tissue expander. These devices are placed in this subpectoral position, which allows the most natural appearance of the breast and seems to reduce the possibility of capsular contracture or undesirable breast firmness. This subpectoral space is accessed by splitting the pectoralis major muscle in the direction of its fibers approximately 2 cm medial to the lateral edge. Then, using headlight assisted dissection, the muscle is elevated off the underlying ribs, with coagulation of the small blood vessels from the intercostal system and the internal mammary system being controlled under direct vision. We strongly believe that this layer should be elevated confluently with the anterior rectus fascia and the fascia of the external oblique muscle inferiorly. After dissecting beneath these fascial layers for a distance of 1 or 2 cm, the dissection is brought more superficially, and the subcutaneous space beneath the superficial fascial system is entered allowing the positioning of the lower pole of the implant or expander in the subcutaneous tissue. This will give the most natural appearance to

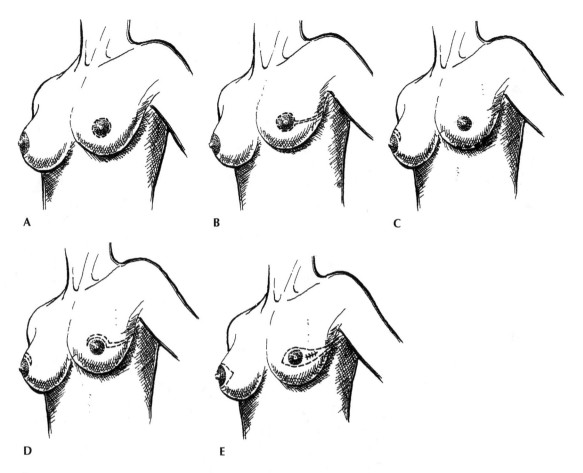

Figure 11-1. Incisions for total mastectomy. (**A**) Periareolar incision. (**B**) Transverse incision centered around the nipple used to facilitate exposure of the breast. (**C**) The inframammary incision. (**D**) A supra-areolar incision with lateral extension to preserve NAC. (**E**) A transversely oriented elliptical incision including removal of the NAC preserving maximum native breast skin.

the breast because it allows the production of a well-defined inframammary fold.

If a tissue expansion is elected, the maximum amount of fluid that can be accommodated by the expander without producing undue tension on the skin flaps is instilled at the time of the immediate reconstruction. Further fluid can be added to this device on subsequent office visits. When the appropriate amount of skin expansion has been achieved the patient undergoes exchange of the expander for a permanent synthetic implant (Fig. 11-2).

If a permanent implant is placed at the time of the immediate reconstructive procedure (Figs. 11-3A,B) the device is positioned carefully and the symmetry between the reconstructed

breasts is checked, especially noting the level of the inframammary folds and the superior breast contours. The lateral submuscular dissection involves elevation of the serratus anterior muscle in continuity with the pectoralis major muscle. Total muscle coverage is possible and desirable laterally.

Closure of the muscle layer over the implant or tissue expander is straightforward and involves the use of interrupted 3-0 polyglycolic acid or chromic suture. A single suction drain is placed routinely in the plane between the muscle and the overlying skin flaps. This is brought out through a small stab incision positioned laterally. Procedures for nipple-areola reconstruction are well established and dependable. These are

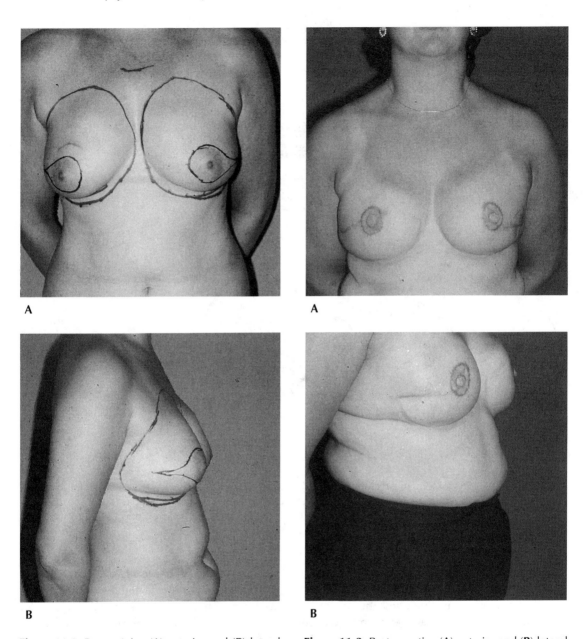

Figure 11-2. Preoperative (**A**) anterior and (**B**) lateral views of the patient who will undergo total mastectomy with implant reconstruction.

Figure 11-3. Postoperative (**A**) anterior and (**B**) lateral views following synthetic implant reconstruction with nipple-areola reconstruction.

usually done approximately 3 months following the reconstructive surgery (Figs. 11-2A,B).

If the surgeon elects to perform a traditional subcutaneous mastectomy with preservation of the nipple-areola complex, this procedure also will lend itself to an immediate reconstruction.

The operative technique for subcutaneous mastectomy originally was described by Freeman

(14), and it has been extensively employed by Woods and colleagues (3,18). The operation was designed to allow removal of the breast tissue while maintaining the patient's native nipple-areola complex as part of the skin envelope. Preservation of the nipple-areola complex with its thickened breast bud maintained on a subcutaneous vascular pedicle differentiates the procedure from a simple or total mastectomy as described earlier. Various incisional approaches are possible for the performance of a subcutaneous mastectomy. The operation was performed initially through an inframammary incision (Fig. 11-1C), which facilitated the immediate reconstruction using a submuscular implant. Our preferred incision is a laterally positioned incision that is slightly curved in a convex downward fashion, extending from the 1 o'clock position of the nipple-areola complex and running along the superior areolar margin directed laterally to an area past the lateral border of the pectoralis major muscle. This incision described by Horton (Fig. 11-1D) is ideal for maximizing surgical exposure, scar aesthetics, and vascularity of the nipple-areola complex. For a simple or total mastectomy an elliptical excision of skin including the nipple-areola complex is acceptable (Fig. 11-1E). It can be performed with either a scalpel, surgical scissors, or an electrocautery device depending on the surgeon's preference. The skin flaps should be of uniform thickness, except at the site of the nipple-areola complex where additional tissue is maintained initially. In order to treat the increased concentrations of ducts in the nipple-areola complex, a coring of the center of the nipple is performed. This maneuver is felt to be necessary by Woods (18). It does, however, carry with it an increased possibility for compromise of the vascularity of the nipple-areola complex.

Once again, we believe that it is imperative that the fascia overlying the pectoralis major muscle be preserved. This preservation of the fascial layer facilitates the secure placement and reliable soft tissue coverage of a breast implant or tissue expander because it allows an extra layer of tissue in the form of muscle coverage.

There has been a dramatic change in breast reconstruction related to the use of the patient's own tissue or autologous reconstructions. The most common donor area for such a reconstruction is tissue transfer from the lower abdomen to the chest region. This operation is commonly referred to as a transverse rectus abdominis musculocutaneous (TRAM) flap (46) because it uses a transversely oriented skin paddle overlying the rectus abdominis muscle, which is harvested to provide the circulation to the transferred tissue. The conventional method of tissue transfer involves elevation of the abdominal skin and fatty layer with subsequent passage of this tissue composite through a tunnel made between the abdominal area and the breast region, with attachments to the muscle and fascia preserved. With this pedicled-flap transfer, the circulation is provided by the superior epigastric artery and its venae comitantes. It is possible to harvest tissue on both sides of the lower abdominal midline and use each rectus muscle in the reconstruction of a bilateral subcutaneous mastectomy defect (Fig. 11-4A–D)

An alternative to this approach would be the use of a microvascular free tissue transfer (47). This involves providing circulation to the lower abdominal tissue by means of the deep inferior epigastric artery and venae comitantes. These vessels are isolated in continuity with a small segment of rectus muscle through which passes the musculocutaneous perforating blood vessels. These blood vessels are kept in continuity with the overlying skin and adipose tissue. Once isolated, the proximal muscle is divided, and the deep inferior epigastric artery and its accompanying veins are also divided at their origin from the external iliac vessels. Microvascular expertise is required for reanastomosis of these vessels to vessels at the mastectomy site, most commonly to the thoracodorsal system, but the internal mammary artery and accompanying vein is also a suitable recipient vessel.

The TRAM flap procedure provides the most natural and permanent appearing result that can be obtained following subcutaneous mastectomy. It is not necessary to elevate the pectoralis major muscle because this vascularized flap tissue is placed immediately beneath the preserved skin envelope.

Slightly increased patient morbidity is noted with this flap transfer procedure in the form of abdominal tightness and/or pain, but generally these conditions are short-lived. The patient benefits from an improved contour of the waist and lower abdomen and the fact that complications related to implants will not be encountered following an autologous tissue reconstruction.

Implant complications most frequently encountered by the patient include capsular contracture or firmness in the reconstructed breast

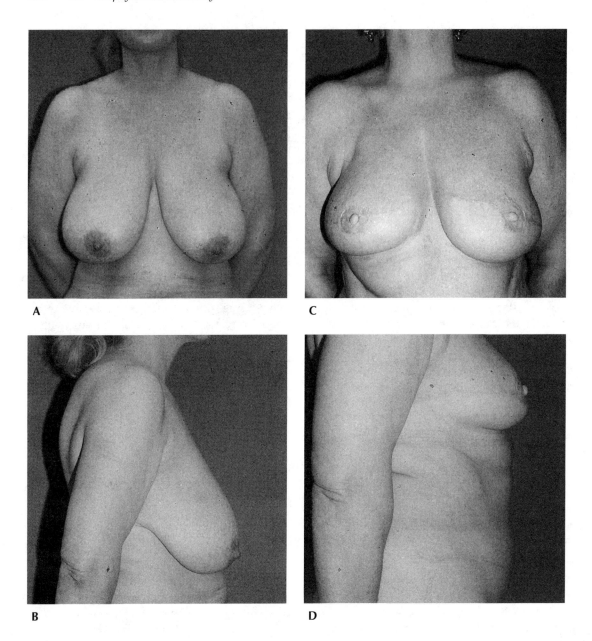

A

C

B

D

Figure 11-4. Preoperative (**A**) anterior and (**B**) lateral views prior to bilateral total mastectomy with immediate reconstruction with TRAM flaps. Mastectomies performed for LCIS and atypical hyperplasia. TRAM flap breast reconstruction and nipple-areola reconstruction have been performed (**C** and **D**).

(Fig. 11-5). The risk of capsular contracture following subcutaneous mastectomy reconstruction may be as high as 50% or greater (48). Additional complications include breast asymmetries, the presence of visible or palpable wrinkles or ripples arising from the implant that can be noted through the skin, rupture of the implant with deflation of the saline device if it has been used or silicone extrusion if a silicone implant is employed, and the unusual complication of implant infection that might necessitate removal of the implant. Such complications are a reasonable "trade-off" for a bilateral mastectomy defect, which is the result of no reconstruction at all (Fig. 11-6).

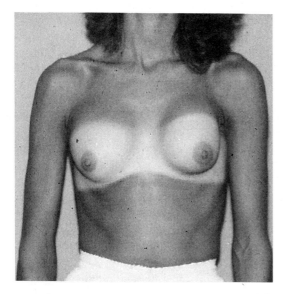

Figure 11-5. Patient demonstrating bilateral capsular contracture following subcutaneous mastectomy and implant reconstruction.

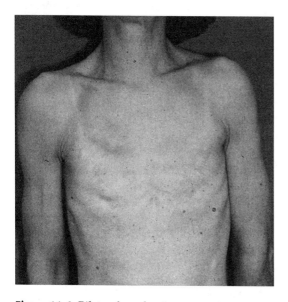

Figure 11-6. Bilateral subcutaneous mastectomy defect without reconstruction demonstrating sub-optimal cosmetic outcome.

The operation of breast reconstruction has been refined over the past decade to a point where very good facsimiles of the resected breast can be created, especially if flap tissue is used. This has opened new treatment avenues and possibilities for patients who might consider prophylactic mastectomy after careful consultation with a surgeon who is knowledgeable about and familiar with the issues described previously in this chapter.

Conclusion

Prophylactic mastectomy is an operation designed to reduce the potential risk of a particular patient developing breast cancer. Although the risk cannot be eliminated completely there is strong evidence showing a decrease in the incidence of breast cancer following prophylactic mastectomy in patients at high and moderate risk based on family history (2).

The Society of Surgical Oncology (49) has recognized the potential value of prophylactic mastectomy and has formulated a position statement regarding indications (Table 11-6). We also believe that it is a valuable therapeutic option for patients who fall into the specific increased risk categories as outlined in the foregoing Indications section.

Owing to improvements in breast reconstruction techniques using the patient's own (autologous) tissue (47,48), the operation has gained popularity with physicians caring for these patients.

Despite the fact that our ability to define which patients would most likely benefit from the surgery has improved dramatically, breast cancer risk assessment remains an inexact science. Oncologists can examine a women's risk factors and make increasingly sophisticated predictions about her chances of developing pathology. The discovery and isolation of specific genes that predispose certain women to breast cancer has further defined a subset of patients who have a high likelihood of contracting the disease and who may benefit greatly from prophylactic surgery. A 90% reduction in the risk of developing breast cancer is significant in the population

Table 11-6. Prophylactic mastectomy: Society of Surgical Oncology position statement

No Previous Breast Cancer[a]	Previous Breast Cancer[b]
Atypical (ductal or lobular hyperplasia (strong indication when multicentric)	Diffuse microcalcifications of remaining breast (especially when DCIS has been diagnosed in the ipsilateral breast)
Family history of breast cancer in first-degree relative who is premenopausal and has had bilateral breast cancer	Lobular carcinoma in situ
Patient with fibronodular, dense breasts that are mammographically and/or clinically difficult to follow (evaluate) and presents with either of the above	Large (ptotic) breast difficult to evaluate (stronger indications with qualifiers below)
	Presence of the following qualifiers: atypical hyperplasia, first-degree relative with breast cancer, younger than 40 years
	Patient observed for LCIS; if she develops invasive cancer, she is at significant risk for cancer developing in the opposite breast

[a]Indications for consideration of bilateral prophylactic mastectomy.
[b]Indication for unilateral prophylactic mastectomy.
Second surgical and pathology opinions recommended in all cases.
Source: Modified from Society of Surgical Oncology. SSO develops position statement on prophylactic mastectomies. SSO News 1993;1:10, with permission.

of women who may be at moderately increased risk for contracting the disease and may do much to assuage a woman's fears (2).

In evaluating candidates, practitioners increasingly must rely on sophisticated algorithms and a multidisciplinary approach, seeking input from medical, radiation, and surgical oncologists, plastic surgeons, geneticists and psychologists. Nevertheless the decision eventually will come down to the experienced surgeon's careful exploration of the individual patient's breast problem, fears, and desires.

It is our sincere hope that in the near future all indications for prophylactic mastectomy will be eliminated. It is our current conclusion, however, that there do still remain indications for the surgery.

References

1. Fisher B, Costantino J, Redmond C. A randomized clinical trial evaluating tamoxifen in the treatment of patients with node-negative breast cancer who have estrogen-receptor positive tumors. New Engl J Med 1989;320:479.
2. Hartmann LC, Schaid DJ, Woods JE, et al. Efficacy of bilateral prophylactic mastectomy in women with a family history of breast cancer. New Engl J Med 1999;340:77–84.
3. Woods JE. Subcutaneous mastectomy: current state of the art. Ann Plast Surg 1983;11:541–550.
4. Lopez MJ, Porter KA. The current role of prophylactic mastectomy. Surg Clin North Am 1996;76:231–242.
5. Ariyan S. Prophylactic mastectomy for precancerous and high-risk lesions of the breast. Can J Surg 1985;28:262–264.
6. Buehler PK. Patient selection for prophylactic mastectomy: who is at high risk? Plast Reconstr Surg 1983;72:324–334.
7. Pennisi VR, Capozzi A. Treatment of chronic cystic disease of the breast by subcutaneous mastectomy. Plast Reconstr Surg 1973;52: 520–524.
8. Pennisi VR, Capozzi A. Subcutaneous mastectomy data: a final statistical analysis of 1500 patients. Aesthetic Plast Surg 1989;13:15–21.
9. Freeman BS. Technique of subcutaneous mastectomy with replacement; immediate and delayed. Br J Plast Surg 1969;22:161–166.
10. Wapnir IL, Rabinowitz B, Greco RS. A reappraisal of prophylactic mastectomy. Surg Gynecol Obstet 1990;171:171–184.
11. Bilimoria MM, Morrow M. The woman at increased risk for breast cancer: evaluation and management strategies. CA 1995;45:263–278.
12. Schrag D, Kuntz KM, Garber JE, Weeks JC. Decision analysis-effects of prophylactic mastectomy and oophorectomy on life expectancy among women with *BRCA1* or *BRCA2* mutations [published erratum appears in New Engl J Med 1997;337(6):434]. New Engl J Med 1997;336:1465–1471.

13. Miki Y, Swensen J, Shattuck-Eidens D, et al. A strong condidate for the breast and ovarian cancer susceptibility gene BRCA1. Science 1994;266:66–71.

14. Easton DF, Bishop DT, Ford D, Crockford GP. Genetic linkage analysis in familial breast and ovarian cancer: results from 214 families. Am J Hum Genet 1993;52:678–701.

15. Wooster R, Neuhausen SL, Mangion J, et al. Localization of a breast cancer susceptibility gene, *BRCA2*, to chromosome 13q12-13. Science 1994;265:2088–2090.

16. Houn F, Helzlsouer KJ, Friedman NB, Stefanek ME. The practice of prophylactic mastectomy: a survey of Maryland surgeons. Am J Public Health 1995;85:801–805.

17. Freeman BS. Subcutaneous mastectomy for benign breast lesions with immediate or delayed prosthetic replacement. Plast Reconstr Surg 1962;30:676–682.

18. Woods JE, Meland NB. Conservative management in full-thickness nipple-areola necrosis after subcutaneous mastectomy. Plast Reconstr Surg 1989;84:258–264. See comments.

19. Rubin LR. Prophylactic mastectomy with immediate reconstruction for the high-risk woman. Clin Plast Surg 1984;11:369–381.

20. Goldman LD, Goldwyn RM. Some anatomical considerations of subcutaneous mastectomy. Plast Reconstr Surg 1973;51:501–505.

21. Barton FE, English JM, Kingsley WB, et al. Glandular excision in total glandular mastectomy and modified radical mastectomy: a comparison. Plast Reconstr Surg 1991;88:389.

22. Temple WJ, Lindsay RL, Magi E, Urbanski SJ. Technical considerations for prophylactic mastectomy in patients at high risk for breast cancer. Am J Surg 1991;161:413–415.

23. Ziegler LD, Kroll SS. Primary breast cancer after prophylactic mastectomy (clinical conference). Am J Clin Oncol 1991;14:451–454.

24. Goodnight JJ, Quagliana JM, Morton DL. Failure of subcutaneous mastectomy to prevent the development of breast cancer. J Surg Oncol 1984;26:198–201.

25. Eldar S, Meguid MM, Beatty JD. Cancer of the breast after prophylactic subcutaneous mastectomy. Am J Surg 1984;148:692–693.

26. Slade CL. Subcutaneous mastectomy: acute complications and long-term follow-up. Plast Reconstr Surg 1984;73:84–90.

27. Wong JH, Jackson CF, Swanson JS, et al. Analysis of the risk reduction of prophylactic partial mastectomy in Sprague-Dawley rats with 7,12-dimethylbenzanthracene-induced breast cancer. Surgery 1986;99:67–71.

28. Nelson H, Miller SH, Buck D, et al. Effectiveness of prophylactic mastectomy in the prevention of breast tumors in C3H mice. Plast Reconstr Surg 1989;83:662–669.

29. Hoffman S, Pressman PI. Prophylactic mastectomy. Mt Sinai J Med 1982;49:102–109.

30. Gail MH, Brinton LA, Byar DP, et al. Projecting individualized probabilities of developing breast cancer for white females who are being examined annually. J Natl Cancer Inst 1989;24:1879–1886.

31. Bondy ML, Lustbader ED, Halabi S, et al. Validation of a breast cancer risk assessment model in women with a positive family history. J Natl Cancer Inst 1994;86:620–625.

32. Morrow M. Identification and management of the woman at increased risk for breast cancer development. Breast Cancer Res Treat 1994;31:53–60.

33. Page DL. The woman at high risk for breast cancer: importance of hyperplasia. Surg Clin North Am 1996;76:221–230.

34. Snyderman RK. Prophylactic mastectomy: pros and cons. Cancer 1984;1:53:803–808.

35. Dowden RV, Grundfest-Broniatowski S. Prophylactic mastectomy: when and how? In: Grundfest-Broniatowski S, Esselstyn CBJ, eds. Controversies in Breast Disease: Diagnosis and Management. New York: Marcel Dekker, 1988:219–233.

36. Berchuck A, Carney M, Lancaster JM, et al. Familial breast-ovarian cancer syndromes: *BRCA1* and *BRCA2*. Clin Obstet Gynecol 1998;41:157–166.

37. Winchester DP. Putting prophylactic mastectomy in proper perspective. CA 1995;45:261–262. Editorial.

38. Bartlett W. An anatomic substitute for the female breast. Ann Surg 1917;6:208–216.

39. Bartlenik H, Van Dam F, Van Dongen J. Psychological effects of breast conserving therapy in comparison with radical mastectomy. Int J Radiat Oncol Biol Phys 1985;11:381–385.

40. Maguire GP, Lee EG, Bevington DJ. Psychiatric problems in the first year after mastectomy. Br Med J 1978;1:963–965.

41. Meyer L, Ringberg A. A prospective study of psychiatric and psychosocial sequelae of bilateral subcutaneous mastectomy. Scand J Plast Reconstr Surg 1986;20:101–107.

41a. Fisher B, Costantino JP, Wickerham DL, et al. Tamoxifen for prevention of breast cancer: Report of the National Surgical Adjuvant Breast and Bowel Project P-1 Study. J Natl Cancer Inst 1998;90:1371–1388.

42. Pennisi VR. The prevention of breast cancer by subcutaneous mastectomy. Surg Clin North Am 1977;7:1023–1034.

43. Cook LS, Weiss NS, Schwartz SM, et al. Population-based study of tamoxifen therapy and subsequent ovarian, endometrial, and breast cancers. J Natl Cancer Inst 1995;87:1359–1364.

44. New York Times, April 22, 1998. p. 47.

45. Horton CE, Adamson JE, Mladick RA, et al. Simple mastectomy with immediate reconstruction. Plast Reconstr Surg 1974;53:42.

46. Hartrampf CR Jr, Scheflan M, Black PW. Breast reconstruction with a transverse abdominal island flap. Plast Reconstr Surg 1982;69:216.

47. Grotting JC, Urist MM, Maddox WA, Vasconez LO. Conventional TRAM flap versus free microsurgical TRAM flap for immediate breast reconstruction. Plast Reconstr Surg 1989;83:828.

48. Woods JE, Irons GB, Arnold PG. The case for submuscular implantation of prostheses in reconstructive breast surgery. Ann Plast Surg 1980;5:115.

49. SSO develops position statement on prophylactic mastectomies. SSO News 1993;1:10.

12

Chemoprevention: Reducing Breast Cancer Risk

Victor G. Vogel

Chemoprevention can be defined as the use of specific natural or synthetic chemical agents to reverse, suppress, or prevent the progression of premalignant lesions to invasive carcinoma (1–3). Because the lifetime probability of developing breast cancer is large among women with known epidemiologic risk factors for breast cancer, there is considerable interest in identifying agents that can reduce this risk by employing the mechanism of prospective clinical trials. Our basic understanding of human carcinogenesis indicates that the process proceeds through multiple discernible stages of molecular and cellular alterations that provide the basis and scientific rationale for clinical cancer chemoprevention. This chapter reviews the basic science and clinical data that point us to several potentially active agents for the reduction of breast cancer risk.

The Role of Hormones

Hormones, especially estrogens, have been linked to breast cancer (4,5), and their role has been attributed to their ability to stimulate cell proliferation, which in turn leads to accumulation of random genetic errors that result in neoplasia (6). Epidemiologic studies indicate that estrogen-mediated events play a role in the development of breast cancer (7,8) and support the hypothesis that intact ovarian function is required for the development of breast cancer. Prior investigations also show that oophorectomy or radiation-induced ovarian ablation can reduce the incidence of breast cancer by up to 75%.

These observations suggest that estrogen antagonists may play a role in the primary prevention of breast cancer by reducing the rate of cell division through administration of antihormones.

Mammary Gland Development and the Biology of Prevention

The mammary gland is one of the few organs that is not fully developed at birth, and no other organ presents such dramatic changes in size, shape, and function as does the breast during growth, puberty, pregnancy, and lactation. Russo and Russo (9,10) have carefully described the developmental progression of the human breast and list four distinct types of breast lobules. Type 1 lobules are the most undifferentiated ones; they are also called *virginal lobules* because they are present in the immature female breast before menarche. Type 2 lobules evolve from the previous ones and have a more complex morphology, being composed of a higher number of ductular structures per lobule. Type 3 lobules are characterized by having an average of 80 ductules or alveoli per lobule; they are frequently seen in the breasts of women under hormonal stimulation or during pregnancy. A fourth type of lobule, the type 4 lobule, has been described as being present during the lactational period.

Study of the pathogenesis of human breast cancer indicates that the type 1 lobules are the site of origin of preneoplastic lesions such as atypical ductal hyperplasia, which evolve to ductal carcinoma in situ, progressing to invasive carcinoma. Although ductal breast cancer originates in type 1 lobules, or terminal ductal lobular units, the epidemiologic observation that nulliparous women exhibit a higher incidence of breast cancer than parous women indicates that type 1 lobules in these two groups of women may be biologically different or exhibit different susceptibility to carcinogenesis. Parous women undergo lobular differentiation, whereas nulliparous women seldom reach the type 3 lobule stage.

Type 1, 2, and 3 lobules also exhibit different cell kinetic characteristics; type 1 and 2 lobules grow faster in vitro and have higher DNA labeling index and a shorter doubling time than type 3 lobules. Correspondingly, the breasts of nulliparous women free of cancer and of nulliparous women with cancer have a similar architecture. The breasts of parous women free of cancer have the lowest percentage of type 1 lobules, and a slightly higher percentage of type 2 lobules, and parous women who develop breast cancer have breasts that contain higher numbers of type 1 lobules.

The degree of breast development is of importance in the susceptibility to carcinogenesis, and it has been suggested that parous women who develop breast cancer may exhibit a defective response to the differentiating effect of the hormones of pregnancy. Breast tissue composed almost exclusively of type 3 lobules exhibits a significantly lower number of doublings. These data also suggest that exposure of women with risk factors for breast cancer to agents that act as hormones or antihormones in the breast may modify the breast in a manner that will reduce the incidence of breast cancer.

Interaction of Estrogen and Antiestrogens with the Estrogen Receptor

Estradiol regulates reproductive tissue function by modulating gene transcription through the estrogen receptor (ER). The ER is a ligand-activated transcription factor with six structural domains of overlapping function labeled A through F. ER-mediated gene transcription is initiated by binding of the DNA domain of the receptor to a consensus palindromic DNA sequence, the *estrogen-response element* (ERE). Subsequent transcriptional activation of the target gene is mediated through two distinct transactivation domains of the receptor termed *AF-1* and *AF-2*. Binding of ligand to the latent ER induces conformational changes that favor dissociation of heat-shock proteins followed by ER dimerization and binding of cell-specific proteins to the active, dimerized complex (11). The strength of the ligand-ER-induced activating function is modulated by these cell-specific adapter proteins and perhaps by other signaling transcription factors such as AP-1. The AP-1 enhancer element requires ligand and the AP-1 transcription factors fos and jun for transcriptional activation. The prototypical antiestrogen, tamoxifen, inhibits the transcription of genes that are regulated by classic ERE, but like estradiol, tamoxifen activates the transcription of genes that are under the control of an AP-1 element.

Estrogens bind to the ER, inducing a conformational change that leads to activation of gene transcription through specific EREs of target genes (12). The ER belongs to a superfamily of ligand-inducible transcription factors. Functions of these proteins (e.g., dimerization, DNA binding, and interaction with other transcription factors) are modulated by binding of their corresponding ligands. It is controversial, however, whether various ER ligands affect the receptor's ability to bind its specific DNA element (ERE). Ligand binding dramatically influences the kinetics of ER interaction with specific DNA. Binding of estradiol induces the rapid formation of a relatively unstable ER-ERE complex. Binding of ICI 182,780 (a "pure" antiestrogen) leads to slow formation of a stable receptor-DNA complex. Therefore, binding of estradiol accelerates the frequency of receptor-DNA complex formation more than 50-fold compared with ER not bound with ligand and more than 1000-fold compared with ER bound with ICI 182,780. It is therefore possible that a correlation exists between the rate of gene transcription and the frequency of receptor-DNA complex formation (13).

Differential activation of these two domains by estrogens and antiestrogens explains the tissue selectivity of the latter. Peptide growth factors stimulate estrogen-dependent transcriptional activation of ERE and are themselves activated by the ER. Estrogens and selective estrogen-receptor modulators (SERMs) such as raloxifene may in part maintain bone mass, for example, through regulation of the gene for transforming growth factor beta (TGF-β) by means of the ER. Deletion of the ligand-binding domain of the ER abolishes both estradiol- and raloxifene-induced activation of the TGF-β promoter. However, deletion of the AF-1 domain of the ER abolishes estradiol but not raloxifene-induced TGF-β activation, and deletion of the AF-2 domain abolishes raloxifene but not estradiol-induced activation of the TGF-β promoter (14). The gene encoding TGF-β3, for example, is activated by both estrogen and raloxifene in intact bone and cultured bone cells through a promoter-mediated and ER-dependent mechanism, although raloxifene is more active than estradiol in the TGF-β3 gene system. Deletion of the ligand-binding domain of the ER abolishes both estradiol- and raloxifene-induced TGF-β3 promoter activation. Deletion of the transcription-activation function of the AF-1 domain abolishes estradiol-induced but not raloxifene-induced TGF-β3 promoter activation. Deletion of the DNA-binding domain of the ER enhances the ability of the receptor to activate the TGF-β3 promoter in response to estradiol.

Antiestrogens compete with estradiol for binding to the ER but can be either steroidal or nonsteroidal in structure. The term *antiestrogen* covers a wide range of compounds that demonstrate a spectrum of ER activity, ranging from that of "pure" estrogen antagonists to mixed estrogen agonist/antagonists (11). The term *selective estrogen-receptor modulator* (i.e., SERM) has been suggested to more precisely characterize compounds that bind to and activate the ER but which have tissue-specific effects distinct from estradiol (14a). The SERM classification includes all the compounds previously classified as antiestrogens excluding the "pure" antiestrogens such as ICI 182,780 (Faslodex) which has shown early promise in the treatment of tamoxifen-refractory advanced breast cancer. A number of synthetic compounds generally display a mixed estrogen agonist/antagonist profile.

The best known are the triphenyethylenes, examples of which include clomiphene, tamoxifen and its derivatives, and the benzothiophene raloxifene. Other compounds with mixed agonist/antagonist properties include tetrahydronaphthylenes and distinct molecules such as ormeloxifene. Representative SERM compounds currently used clinically or under investigation are shown in Figure 12-1.

Rationale for the SERM classification emerged from preclinical studies of raloxifene (the first compound to be labeled as a SERM) demonstrating that, in rodents, raloxifene prevented estrogen deficiency associated bone loss and lowered the serum cholesterol level following ovariectomy without stimulating proliferation of the endometrium. Raloxifene thus exhibited apparent estrogen agonist effects in some tissues (e.g., bone and liver) but, at the same doses, was neutral with respect to estrogenic activity in others (e.g., endometrium). Based on its pattern of tissue specificity, raloxifene was deemed representative of a second-generation SERM, the first generation being represented by tamoxifen and its derivatives, which demonstrate estrogen agonist properties in the endometrium. Tamoxifen appears to act as an estrogen agonist in bone and liver but as an estrogen antagonist in the breast.

While the estrogen antagonist properties of antiestrogens originally were ascribed to simple competition for ER binding, it is now believed that estrogen antagonism is an active process derived from manifold ER and, perhaps, non-ER-mediated events (15,16). Importantly, the relationship between the agonist and antagonist properties of antiestrogens appears to depend on the gene or cellular context in which the observation is made, giving rise to an apparent tissue-specific pattern of action unique to each compound. While ICI 164,384 (a primarily "pure" antagonist), 4-hydroxytamoxifen (a potent tamoxifen metabolite), and raloxifene all bind the ER, each affects different transcriptional profiles depending on the cell and gene promoter context in vitro. The three antiestrogens form distinct ER-ligand complexes representing different points along a continuum of potential ER activation. Consistent with this model, tamoxifen binding to the ER distinctly affects the two transcription-activation

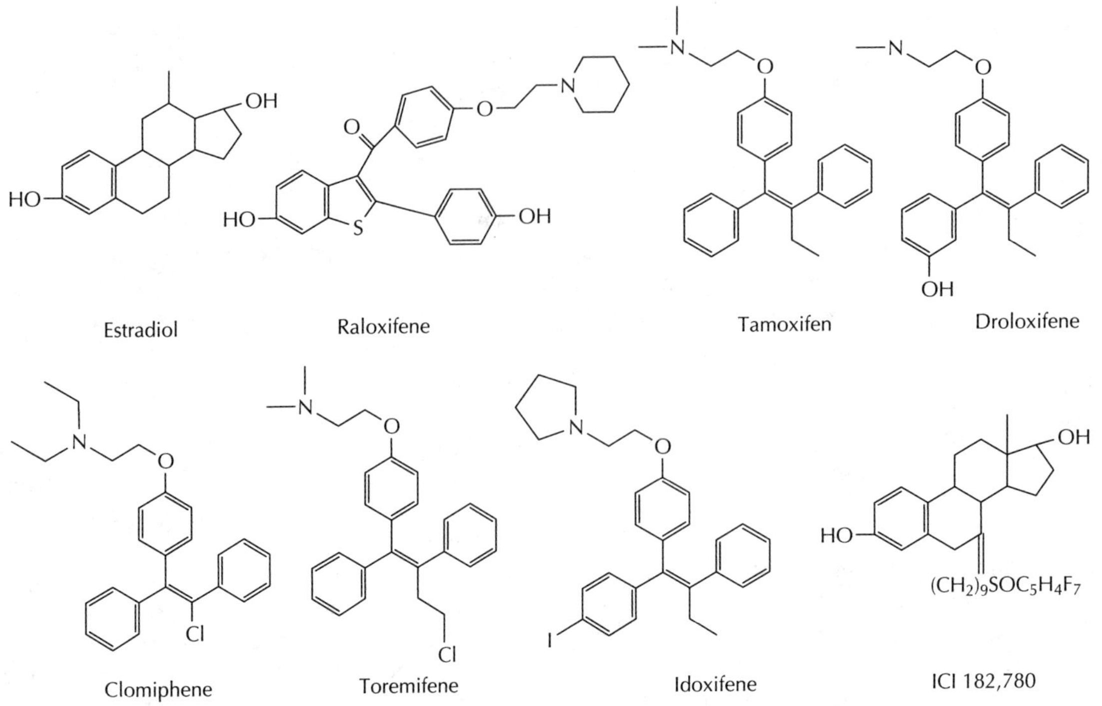

Figure 12-1. Chemical structure of estradiol and selected SERMs. (Used with permission from Discovery International.)

functions of the ER compared with estradiol such that AF-2 (the hormone-dependent transcription-activation function) is usually enhanced by estradiol binding, whereas it may be suppressed by tamoxifen in a dose- and cell-specific manner (17,18). Therefore, the estrogen agonist/antagonist profile of tamoxifen in a given tissue results from the relative strength of AF-2 inhibition versus constitutive (hormone-independent) AF-1 activation, both of which may be modulated by cell-specific adapter proteins and transcription factors.

Katzenellenbogen and colleagues (19) have proposed a model to account for the diversity in ER-mediated genomic effects. In this model, the ultimate genetic response to estrogens and antiestrogens is a result of a tripartite interaction between the ligand, receptor, and effector system. Diversity in the response is provided by the existence of gene- and/or cell-specific effectors, receptors, additional hormone-response elements, and unique ligands, including endogenous steroid hormones and their metabolites.

Two estrogen receptors, designated ERα and ERβ, have been cloned in humans (20–23). Experimental data show that ERα and ERβ respond differently to certain ligands at an AP-1 element, with raloxifene inducing transcription the least. Raloxifene induction is weaker than induction by estradiol, and raloxifene-induced transactivation results from binding to ERα. If estradiol is classified as a full activator of ERα at an AP-1 element, then raloxifene functions as a partial activator and tamoxifen functions as a full activator (24). In cells transfected with ERβ, both raloxifene and tamoxifen increase transcription, and the inhibitory effect of estradiol on transcription is overcome by higher concentrations of raloxifene. It appears, therefore, that the pharmacology of ER ligands is reversed in vitro at an AP-1 element coupled with ERβ, where the antiestrogens act as transcription activators and the estrogens act as transcription inhibitors. Two nuclear ER subtypes can respond in opposite regulatory modes to estradiol from the same DNA response element. The ligand-induced responses with ERβ at an AP-1 site provide an example of negative transcriptional regulation by estradiol and strong positive regulation by synthetic antiestrogens. The role of estradiol complexed to ERβ is to turn off the transcription of these genes, whereas raloxifene overrides this blockade and activates gene transcription. This activation has important implications in tissues such as bone, where negative regulation has a detrimental physiologic effect.

Tamoxifen

Tamoxifen is a triphenylethylene synthesized in 1966 as a potential fertility agent. Tamoxifen has been shown to be species-, tissue-, and cell-type-specific (25,26). In the pubertal rat, tamoxifen is capable of promoting full ductal development in the mammary gland. In the mature cycling animal, tamoxifen acts as an antiestrogen, causing atrophy of lobular structures. In postmenopausal women, tamoxifen treatment results in upregulation of the proportion of ductal cells expressing ER.

The parent compound and the conjugates are excreted in the bile and undergo enterohepatic circulation. This recirculation and the high volume of distribution result in a terminal elimination half-life of 4 to 7 days, and at least six different metabolites have been isolated from the bile. Demethylation to the active metabolite N-desmethyl tamoxifen is the principal metabolic pathway in humans. Maximum serum concentration of N-desmethyl tamoxifen is observed within 12 to 24 hours of dosing; its serum half-life is about 12 days.

Tamoxifen can suppress the appearance of chemically induced breast tumors in laboratory animals. Both dimethylbenzanthracene (DMBA) and nitroso-methyl urea (NMU) induce hormone-responsive mammary tumors in rats, but spayed animals or animals treated with androgens rarely develop DMBA-induced mammary carcinomas. Experimentally, chemical initiation by DMBA is followed by a period of promotion with estrogen, prolactin, and progesterone; tumors appear 3 to 4 months later. The simultaneous administration of a large dose of tamoxifen and DMBA to 50-day-old female Sprague-Dawley rats results in a dramatic

reduction (<10% of control) in the number and type of palpable mammary tumors. A second-dose regimen of tamoxifen administered 30 days after DMBA inhibits tumorigenesis for up to 120 days. In rats, ovariectomy or the injection of antiestrogens after carcinogen administration results in the appearance of very few mammary tumors.

Administration of tamoxifen does not result in a dramatic increase in the proportion of animals that remain tumor-free, but a clear-cut dose-response relationship is observed in the number of mammary tumors that develop. When tamoxifen is given to rats 1 month after DMBA administration, there is a dose-related delay in the appearance of palpable mammary tumors. Eventually, however, all the animals develop tumors, with some reduction in the tumor burden as compared with nontreated animals. In contrast, the continuous administration of tamoxifen results in more than 90% of the animals remaining tumor-free. Retreatment following DMBA administration results in further inhibition of tumorigenesis. Tamoxifen also produces a dose-related delay in the appearance of DMBA-induced tumors in animals that are not spayed, and continuous treatment with lower daily doses of tamoxifen suppresses the appearance of DMBA-induced tumors until therapy is withdrawn. Tamoxifen, therefore, does not appear to produce a tumoricidal effect in animals, but because the drug has a long biologic half-life, it produces a tumoristatic effect until the drug is cleared.

Several mechanisms of tamoxifen's ability to prevent or suppress breast carcinogenesis have been proposed. Tamoxifen may inhibit cell proliferation by the mechanisms shown in Table 12-1.

Not all effects of tamoxifen are beneficial, however. Prolonged administration shows suppression of natural killer cell activity, and this suppression may play some role in the inability of tamoxifen to prevent breast tumors with complete efficiency. Resistance to the inhibitory effects of tamoxifen is also possible through several alternative mechanisms (27):

1. Through the production and localized accumulation of an estrogenic metabolite(s) of tamoxifen

Table 12-1. Mechanisms of tamoxifen's ability to prevent or suppress breast carcinogenesis

- Modulating the production of transforming growth factors (TGFα and TGFβ) that help regulate breast cancer cell proliferation, including proliferation of estrogen-receptor–negative cell lines. Tamoxifen antagonizes estrogen-enhanced production of TGFα in estrogen receptor–positive cell lines, and it downregulates TGFα levels in estrogen receptor–positive human breast carcinoma.
- Binding to cytoplasmic antiestrogenic binding sites, increasing intracellular drug levels.
- Increasing sex-hormone–binding globulin (SHBG), which may decrease the availability of free estrogen for diffusion into tumor cells.
- Increasing levels of natural killer (NK) cells.
- Decreasing circulating insulin-like growth factor (IGF-I), which may, in turn, modify the endocrinologic regulation of breast cancer cell kinetics. Serum IGF-I levels decline in women receiving tamoxifen.

2. Through the loss of ER on precancerous or cancerous breast tissue
3. Through the production of mutated ERS that produce an estrogenic stimulus to cells when bound with estrogen
4. Through altered subcellular factors and consequently altered signal transduction

Any of these mechanisms or others not yet known could explain the failure of tamoxifen to prevent all newly emerging malignant breast clones.

The factors that determine hormone receptor status in human breast cancer are complex and far-ranging and include menopausal status, body weight, and complex endocrine interactions. Postmenopausal breast cancer patients who receive tamoxifen demonstrate increases in both ERs (201%) and progesterone receptors (163%) measured using immunohistochemical techniques on fine-needle aspiration from primary breast tumors over a period of 6 to 10 days (28,29).

Additional Benefits of Tamoxifen

There is approximately a 12% reduction in nonbreast cancer deaths associated with long-term use of tamoxifen for the adjuvant treatment of breast cancer, a 25% reduction in deaths from

vascular disease, and a 9% reduction in other causes of death. A major proportion of the reduction in noncancer deaths is due to a reduction in cardiovascular disease mortality, and these results are due, in part, to decreases in low-density lipoprotein (LDL)–cholesterol observed as early as 2 months after the initiation of tamoxifen therapy. These reductions are followed at 6 months by either no change or an increase in high-density lipoprotein (HDL)–cholesterol, a fall in LDL-cholesterol, and an increase in triglycerides. Tamoxifen's estrogenic effect on the liver may lead to increased synthesis of very low-density lipoprotein (VLDL)–cholesterol and increased triglyceride levels, decreased levels of apolipoprotein B synthesis, and increased levels of apolipoprotein A-1 synthesis, with resulting increased levels of HDL-cholesterol. Longitudinal observations of women at risk for heart disease are limited, but available data indicate that a 15% to 20% decrease in LDL-cholesterol may result in a 6% to 20% decrease in coronary heart disease.

The effect of tamoxifen on the development of atherosclerotic cardiovascular disease also may relate to its antithrombotic properties. Postmenopausal women taking tamoxifen show an average drop of only 10% in antithrombin III levels during therapy, whereas fibrinogen levels decline 16% or more (30). Population studies demonstrate a relationship between fibrinogen levels, myocardial infarction, and stroke, with lower fibrinogen levels associated with lower cardiovascular risk (31,32). Concerns about the durability of these effects arise from studies of former users of tamoxifen that show reversal of the increases in HDL-cholesterol at cessation of tamoxifen therapy (33). A final assessment of the effect of tamoxifen on the risk of morbidity and mortality from cardiovascular disease in healthy women awaits completion of ongoing studies.

In addition to these beneficial effects on risk factors for developing cardiovascular disease, tamoxifen appears to have beneficial effects on bones as well. Tamoxifen preserves bone mineral density in postmenopausal women (34,35), presumably because of its estrogenic effect on osteoclasts, which slows bone resorption. Experimental data in vitro showing that tamoxifen blocks bone resorption induced by parathyroid hormone, prostaglandin E_2, and 1,25-dihydroxy vitamin D_3 support these clinical observations of benefit (36). Of some concern is the observation that tamoxifen may reduce bone mineral density in premenopausal women by 1.9% annually while increasing bone density in postmenopausal women by 1.8% (37).

Clinical Trials of Tamoxifen as Adjuvant Therapy for Breast Cancer

The earliest evidence for the chemopreventive or chemosuppressive actions of tamoxifen in breast cancer derived from observations on the occurrence of second primary breast tumors in women participating in clinical trials of adjuvant therapy. An unexpected but important observation from these trials was the reduction in the incidence of contralateral breast cancer in the patients receiving tamoxifen. The largest of these trials is the National Surgical Adjuvant Breast and Bowel Project (NSABP) protocol B-14, which began in 1982 and randomized 2892 women to either placebo or tamoxifen twice daily for at least 5 years (38). Although distinction between secondary cancers, primary cancers, and metastatic lesions of the contralateral breast is not always possible, it has been demonstrated previously that most are second malignancies (39). Women taking tamoxifen adjuvant therapy in the B-14 trial experienced approximately one-third fewer second primary breast tumors as women taking placebo (2.4% versus 1.6%).

A comprehensive assessment of the ability of tamoxifen to prevent second primary breast tumors is found in the overview of the world's literature on tamoxifen as adjuvant therapy for breast cancer (40), where there are more than 32,000 women for whom information about contralateral second primary breast cancers is available. At the time of the publication, there were 55 reported randomized comparisons of tamoxifen and placebo. Among the women who received placebo in these trials, the risk of a contralateral second primary breast cancer was 4.7% 10 years after their first diagnosis of breast cancer compared with a 10-year rate of only 2.6% among women who received an average of 5 years of tamoxifen adjuvant therapy. This 47% relative reduction in the risk of a second primary breast cancer with the use of tamoxifen varied

with the duration of tamoxifen adjuvant therapy. Among those women who received less than 2 years of adjuvant therapy, the reduction in the odds was only 13%, compared with 26% among those women with exactly 2 years of therapy.

Clinical Trials for Reducing Breast Cancer Risk

Three prospective studies evaluating tamoxifen for reducing the risk of invasive breast cancer have been published. The findings from these studies are summarized in Table 12-2. Two of the studies are small European trials that reported negative results. The British Royal Marsden Hospital Trial was designed and initiated as a pilot feasibility trial prior to the International Breast Cancer Intervention Study (41). Results of this pilot trial are derived from an interim analysis at 70 months' median follow-up. Participants were women of younger age who had a stronger family history of breast cancer, and 26% of the subjects used hormone-replacement therapy concurrent with their tamoxifen. It is not clear why the study produced negative results, but it is possible that more of the British women were at greater risk for *BRCA1* mutations and the development of ER-negative tumors that were not influenced by tamoxifen use. The Italian study enrolled a low-risk population of women in whom 48% had bilateral prophylactic oophorectomies prior to entering the trial, and only 41 breast cancers developed at a median follow-up of 46 months (42). There was poor compliance with the study medication, and 26% of participants left the trial early, leading to premature closure to accrual. The largest of the three studies, the Breast Cancer Prevention Trial, will be reviewed in detail below.

The Breast Cancer Prevention Trial
The National Cancer Institute, in collaboration with the NSABP (a large clinical trials cooperative group), launched the Breast Cancer Prevention Trial (BCPT) in 1992 to evaluate the ability of tamoxifen to prevent breast cancer in women who were at increased risk (43). Women eligible for the trial were either older than 60 years of age at entry, were 35 years of age or older with a breast biopsy showing lobular carcinoma in situ, or were between 35 and 59 years of age with

Table 12-2. Summary of risks of breast cancer and SERM-related side effects in randomized trials of tamoxifen and raloxifene for women without breast cancer

	Breast Cancer Prevention Trial (BCPT)	Royal Marsden Hospital Chemoprevention Trial	Italian Tamoxifen Prevention Study	Multiple Outcomes Raloxifene Evaluation Trial (MORE)
Subject characteristics	High breast cancer risk (age ≥60 years or a combination of risk factors using the Gail model); 39% <50 years	Family history of breast cancer <50 years old or 2 or more affected first-degree relatives	Women with hysterectomy (48% bilateral oophorectomy); Median age: 51 years	Postmenopausal women with osteoporosis; Median age: 66.9 years
Number randomized	13,388	2471	5408	7705
Daily treatment	Tamoxifen 20 mg	Tamoxifen 20 mg	Tamoxifen 20 mg	Raloxifene 60 mg or 120 mg
Proportion who took estrogen	<10%	26%	14%	10%
Median follow-up, months	54.6	70	46	40
Breast cancer rates per 1000 woman-years and relative risks of cancer (95% CI)	Invasive Placebo: 6.8 Tamoxifen: 3.4 RR: 0.51 (0.39–0.66) Noninvasive Placebo: 2.7 Tamoxifen: 1.4 RR: 0.50 (0.33–0.77)	All cases Placebo: 5.0 Tamoxifen: 4.7 RR: 1.1 (0.7–1.7)	All cases Placebo: 2.3 Tamoxifen: 2.1	All cases Placebo: 4.3 Raloxifene: 1.5 RR: 0.35 (0.21–0.58) Invasive Placebo: 3.6 Raloxifene: 0.9 RR: 0.24 (0.13–0.44)

Number and relative risk of ER-positive breast cancer	Placebo: 130 Tamoxifen: 41 RR: 0.31 (0.22–0.45)	Not available	Placebo:10 Tamoxifen: 8	Placebo: 20 Treatment: 4 RR: 0. 10 (0.04–0.24)
Number and relative risk of endometrial cancer	Placebo: 15 Tamoxifen: 36 RR: 2.53 (1.35–4.97)	Placebo: 1 Tamoxifen: 4	Not reported (women had hysterectomy prior to entry)	Placebo: 4 Raloxifene: 6 RR: 0.8 (0.2–2.7)
Number and relative risk of pulmonary emboli and deep venous thrombosis	Pulmonary embolism Placebo: 6 Treatment: 18 RR: 3.0 (1.2–9.3) DVT Placebo: 22 Treatment: 35 RR: 1.60 (0.91–2.86)	DVT and pulmonary embolism Placebo: 4 Tamoxifen: 7	DVT and pulmonary embolism Placebo: 4 Tamoxifen: 7 Superficial phlebitis Placebo: 9 Tamoxifen: 33	DVT and pulmonary embolism Placebo: 8 Raloxifene: 49 RR: 3.1 (1.5–6.2)

Reprinted with permission from Cummings SR, Eckert S, Krueger KA, et al. The effect of raloxifene on risk of breast cancer in postmenopausal women: results from the MORE randomized trial. JAMA 1999;281:2189–2197.

an estimated annual risk for developing breast cancer equal to that of a 60-year-old woman. The 5-year predicted risk of breast cancer required to enter the trial, therefore, was at least 1.66%. Risk was estimated using the model developed by Gail and colleagues (44) that was validated by Bondy and colleagues (45) and Spiegelman and colleagues (46), as well as in an epidemiologic study of hormone use (47). The model also was validated among the women taking placebo in the BCPT (48). The Gail model considers current age, ages at menarche and first live birth, number of first-degree relatives with breast cancer, and number of breast biopsies ever done. A previous diagnosis of atypical hyperplasia doubles the estimated risk; there are interaction terms for age and the number of breast biopsies, and for family history and age at first live birth.

Hormone-replacement therapy for menopausal symptoms was not permitted during the trial, although former users of replacement therapy were eligible to participate after stopping hormones for 90 days. The design schema for BCPT is shown in Figure 12-2. Between June 1, 1992 and September 30, 1997, 13,388 women aged 35 years and older entered the trial and were randomly assigned to receive tamoxifen 20 mg daily versus placebo therapy. Characteristics of participants in the trial are shown in Table 12-3. Approximately 40% were between the ages of 35 and 49 years, 30% were aged 50 to 59 years, and

Table 12-3. Characteristics of participants in the NSABP Breast Cancer Prevention Trial

Characteristic	Placebo (n = 6599) %	Tamoxifen (n = 6576) %
Age, years		
35–39	3	2
40–49	36	37
50–59	31	31
60–69	24	24
≥70	6	6
Number of first-degree relatives with breast cancer		
0	24	23
1	57	57
2	16	16
≥3	3	3*
Lobular carcinoma in situ		
No	94	94
Yes	6	6
Atypical hyperplasia		
Yes	91	91
No	9	9

*Numbers do not total 100% due to rounding.
Data from Fisher B, Costantino JP, Wickerham DL, et al. Tamoxifen for prevention of breast cancer: report of the National Surgical Adjuvant Breast and Bowel Project P-1 study. J Natl Cancer Inst 1998;90:1371–1388.

30% were 60 years of age or older. The trial was stopped in late March 1998 and results reported because statistical significance had been achieved in a number of study end points.

Reduction in Incidence of Invasive Breast Cancer. Through July 1998, a total of 368 invasive and noninvasive breast cancers occurred among 13,175 women with evaluable end points in BCPT. Results from the trial are summarized in Table 12-4. There were a total of 175 cases of invasive breast cancer in the placebo group as compared with 89 in the tamoxifen group (risk ratio 0.51, 95% confidence interval CI 0.39–0.66, $p < 0.00001$). The annual event rate for invasive breast cancer among women taking tamoxifen was 3.4 per 1000 women compared with 6.8 per 1000 women taking placebo. An important observation was a reduced risk of developing invasive breast cancer among all age groups in the trial. Risk ratios were 0.56 for women younger than 49 years of age, 0.49

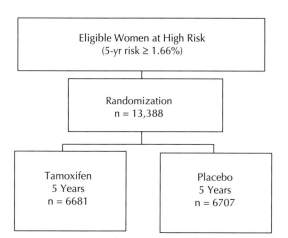

Figure 12-2. Schema for the Breast Cancer Prevention Trial (BCPT).

Table 12-4. Average annual rates for outcomes in the Breast Cancer Prevention Trial

Cancer Outcome	Rate per 1000 Women		Risk Ratio
	Tamoxifen	**Placebo**	**(95% Confidence Interval)**
Invasive breast cancer	3.4	6.8	0.51 (0.39–0.66)
Noninvasive breast cancer	1.4	2.7	0.50 (0.33–0.77)
Invasive breast cancer by patient characteristic			
Age, years			
≤49	3.8	6.7	0.56 (0.37–0.85)
50–59	3.1	6.3	0.49 (0.29–0.81)
≥60	3.3	7.3	0.45 (0.27–0.74)
History of lobular carcinoma in situ			
Yes	5.7	13.0	0.44 (0.16–1.06)
No	3.3	6.4	0.51 (0.39–0.68)
History of atypical hyperplasia			
Yes	1.4	10.1	0.14 (0.03–0.47)
No	3.6	6.4	0.56 (0.42–0.73)
Number of first-degree relatives with breast cancer			
0	3.0	6.4	0.46 (0.24–0.84)
1	3.0	6.0	0.51 (0.35–0.73)
2	4.8	8.7	0.55 (0.30–0.97)
≥3	7.0	13.7	0.51 (0.15–1.55)
Risk of breast cancer within 5 years (%)			
≤2	2.1	5.5	0.37 (0.18–0.72)
2.01–3.0	3.5	5.2	0.68 (0.41–1.11)
3.01–5.0	3.9	5.9	0.66 (0.39–1.09)
≥5.01	4.5	13.3	0.34 (0.19–0.58)
Invasive endometrial cancer			
Age, years			
≤49	1.3	1.1	1.21 (0.41–3.60)
≥50	3.0	0.8	4.01 (1.70–10.90)
Fractures			
Hip	0.5	0.8	0.55 (0.25–1.15)
All sites	4.3	5.3	0.81 (0.63–1.05)
Cardiovascular events			
Stroke	1.4	0.9	1.59 (0.93–2.77)
Transient ischemic attack	0.7	1.0	0.76 (0.40–1.44)
Pulmonary embolism	0.7	0.2	3.01 (1.15–9.27)
Deep vein thrombosis	1.3	0.8	1.60 (0.91–2.86)

Data from Fisher B, Costantino JP, Wickerham DL, et al. Tamoxifen for prevention of breast cancer: report of the National Surgical Adjuvant Breast and Bowel Project P-1 study. J Natl Cancer Inst 1998;90:1371–1388.

for women 50 to 59 years of age, and 0.45 for women 60 years of age or older. All the 95% CIs for these observations excluded 1.0 and were statistically significant. Figure 12-3 shows that a benefit also was seen for women with a history of lobular carcinoma in situ (risk ratio 0.44, 95% CI 0.16–1.06); for women with a history of atypical lobular or ductal hyperplasia, the risk ratio was markedly diminished at 0.14 (95% CI 0.03–0.47). Reduced risk ratios were seen at all projected levels of risk and among women with one, two, or three or more

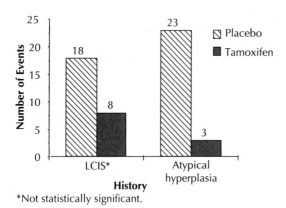

*Not statistically significant.

Figure 12-3. Reduction in the risk of invasive breast cancer for women entering the BCPT with a previous biopsy showing either lobular carcinoma in situ or atypical hyperplasia. [Data from Fisher et al. (43).]

first-degree relatives with a history of invasive breast cancer.

The reduction in the risk of invasive breast cancer was seen within the first year of the trial, and lower incidence rates for women taking tamoxifen compared with those taking placebo were seen for each subsequent year of the trial throughout 6 years of maximum follow-up at the time the results were reported (Fig. 12-4). The distribution of primary tumor size and pathologic involvement of the axillary lymph nodes was

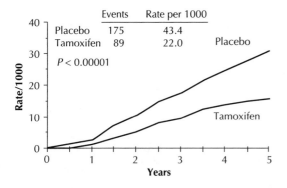

Figure 12-4. Cumulative rates of invasive breast cancers occurring among participants in the NSABP BCPT. The total number of events in the placebo group was 175 compared with 89 in the tamoxifen group. The corresponding event rates per 1000 women were 43.4 and 22.0, respectively ($p < 0.00001$). [Data from Fisher et al. (43).]

not markedly different among women taking tamoxifen when compared with women taking placebo. There was a substantial difference, however, when comparing the proportion of ER-positive tumors that occurred among women taking tamoxifen. Not surprisingly, the incidence rate of ER-positive breast cancers was 5 per 1000 women in the placebo group compared with only 1.6 per 1000 women in the tamoxifen group, a 69% reduction. Concordant with this observation, rates of ER-negative tumors were not significantly different in the two treatment groups (1.46 per 1000 women in the tamoxifen group compared with 1.20 per 1000 women in the placebo group).

Ischemic Heart Disease. Because only 30% of the participants in BCPT were age 60 years or older, and because the median duration of follow-up at the time of the report of the trial was only approximately 4 years, few ischemic heart disease events occurred within the trial population. The total number of events was 133, and the event rate was similar among women taking tamoxifen or placebo. The limited number of events makes it impossible to reach definitive conclusions about the effect of tamoxifen on ischemic heart disease event rates despite the fact that this observation has been made in at least one adjuvant treatment trial (49).

Fracture Rates. At the time of the BCPT report, 955 women had experienced bone fractures. The incidence of osteoporotic fracture events involving the hip, spine, or lower radius was reduced 19% among women receiving tamoxifen (111 events versus 137 events in the placebo group). Most notable was a 45% reduction in fractures of the hip that missed reaching statistical significance because of the small total number of events reported (n = 34) in a population whose median age at enrollment was 52 years (and only 30% were age 60 years or older). It is likely that tamoxifen does have a significant effect on fractures in postmenopausal women, but additional data are required to confirm this initial observation.

Incidence of Invasive Endometrial Cancer. As discussed previously, tamoxifen is a drug with both estrogen agonist and antagonist properties

(50). Women who received tamoxifen in the BCPT had a 2.5 times greater risk of developing invasive endometrial cancer than did women who received placebo; the average annual rate was 2.3 per 1000 women in the former group and 0.9 per 1000 women in the latter group. This is similar to the rate of endometrial carcinoma occurring among women receiving tamoxifen as adjuvant therapy for breast cancer in the NSABP protocol B-14 (51). All 36 invasive endometrial cancers that occurred among women receiving tamoxifen in the BCPT were FIGO stages 0 or I and had excellent clinical prognoses, although it is too early to make definitive statements about the long-term outcome of these tumors.

Other Unfavorable Events. There was an increase in the number of thromboembolic vascular events among women taking tamoxifen in the BCPT. While only the event rate for pulmonary embolism reached statistical significance, there is cause for concern when looking at the increased event rates for stroke, transient ischemic attack, and deep vein thrombosis, particularly among women 50 years of age and older.

In addition to these toxicities, there was a statistically marginal increase of approximately 14% in the rate of cataract development among women who were free of cataracts at the time of entry into the BCPT. Event rates for cataract surgery also were increased for women taking tamoxifen when compared with those taking the placebo. Bothersome hot flashes were reported by 46% of women in the tamoxifen group compared with only 29% in the placebo group. Similarly, vaginal discharge reported as moderately bothersome or worse was seen in 29% of the tamoxifen group as compared with 13% of the placebo group.

Appropriate Candidates for Reduction of Breast Cancer Risk with Tamoxifen

The BCPT is regarded as one of the sentinel events in the history of cancer management in the 20th century (52). The use of tamoxifen for the reduction of breast cancer risk requires consideration of a woman's absolute risk of breast cancer as determined by quantitative modeling (described in Chapters 2 and 4) or the presence

of risk factors themselves known to increase the risk of breast cancer substantially (e.g., lobular carcinoma in situ). It is also necessary to evaluate risk-benefit considerations that include the absolute reduction in the risk of breast cancer that is expected to accrue with the use of tamoxifen. The absolute risk reduction can be approximated by assuming that the calculated risk of breast cancer will be reduced by one-half in women using tamoxifen. For example, a women for whom the estimated 5-year risk of developing invasive breast cancer is 4% can anticipate a 2% absolute reduction in her risk of breast cancer with 5 years of tamoxifen therapy. Additional benefits include the reduction in incidence of both noninvasive breast cancer and osteoporotic fractures. The risks associated with tamoxifen are well described by the BCPT and include endometrial cancer, thrombosis and embolism, postmenopausal symptoms such as hot flashes, and an increased risk of developing cataracts or requiring surgery for their management. Each of these risks, in part, depends on age, as do the benefits to osteoporosis that accrue only to postmenopausal women.

A strategy to weigh risks and benefits of tamoxifen therapy in the setting of breast cancer risk reduction in a semiquantitative manner was developed at a national conference of breast cancer experts, and the methods and recommendations have been published (53). Risk of developing breast cancer is the primary determinant of net benefit, with greater net benefits accruing to women at the highest risk of breast cancer. Weighing the relative risks and benefits associated with tamoxifen has a modest effect on calculated net benefits. If, for example, endometrial cancer is regarded as less serious than breast cancer for women with a uterus, the potential adverse impact of an incident endometrial cancer will be lessened, and a woman and her clinician may then decide to accept this risk of tamoxifen therapy. Increasingly greater risks of thromboembolic events are seen with increasing age, and net benefit is likely to be negative in older women. An increase in the rates of either thrombosis or endometrial cancer was not seen among premenopausal women in the BCPT. Thus, both age and the presence of factors that increase the risk of toxicity have the

Table 12-5. Using tamoxifen for the reduction of breast cancer risk

Women in whom tamoxifen should be considered

- History of lobular carcinoma in situ (LCIS)
- History of ductal carcinoma in situ (DCIS)
- History of atypical ductal or lobular hyperplasia
- Women aged 60 years or older
- Premenopausal women with mutations in either the *BRCA1* or *BRCA2* genes or other predisposing genetic mutations
- Premenopausal women with 5-year probability of breast cancer ⩾1.66% as determined using multivariable risk model predictions

Women in whom caution should be used when considering the use of tamoxifen

- History of stroke, transient ischemic attack, deep vein thrombosis, pulmonary embolus
- History of cataracts or cataract surgery
- Current use of hormone replacement therapy

Women who may consider the use of tamoxifen

- Remote history of invasive breast cancer with no history of adjuvant tamoxifen therapy
- Postmenopausal women with osteoporosis

---

greatest effect on the net benefit associated with tamoxifen.

Indications and contraindications for the use of tamoxifen for reduction of breast cancer risk are listed in Table 12-5. Absolute contraindications to the use of tamoxifen for risk reduction include a history of deep venous thrombosis or pulmonary embolism, a history of stroke or transient ischemic attack, a history of uncontrolled diabetes or hypertension, and/or a history of uncontrolled atrial fibrillation. Those women currently taking estrogen, progesterone, androgens, or birth control pills should discontinue these medications prior to initiating tamoxifen therapy. Tamoxifen also should be avoided by women who may be pregnant or become pregnant.

Considerations for Use Based on Calculated Risk of Breast Cancer

Based on the results of the BCPT, the Food and Drug Administration (FDA) approved tamoxifen for reduction of breast cancer risk in women whose risk of developing breast cancer is equal to the minimum eligibility for the trial, that is, 1.66% or greater in 5 years, as determined by the Gail

model. Additional candidates for consideration of tamoxifen for primary risk reduction are discussed below.

Lobular Carcinoma in Situ and Atypical Hyperplasia

Women with a history of lobular carcinoma in situ (LCIS) experienced an annual risk for invasive breast cancer of 1.3% per year in the BCPT, and tamoxifen reduced this risk by approximately 50%. In addition, women with atypical ductal or lobular hyperplasia experience an increased risk of subsequent invasive breast cancer. Women with either LCIS or atypical hyperplasia should be considered candidates for primary prevention with tamoxifen if there are no absolute contraindications to its use.

Ductal Carcinoma in Situ (DCIS)

The NSABP conducted a double-blind, randomized, controlled trial to determine whether a regimen of lumpectomy, radiation therapy, and tamoxifen was of more benefit than lumpectomy and radiation therapy alone for DCIS (54). A total of 1804 women with DCIS, including those whose resected sample margins were involved with tumor, were randomly assigned lumpectomy, radiation therapy (50 Gy), and placebo (n = 902). An equal number were assigned lumpectomy, radiation therapy, and tamoxifen 20 mg daily for 5 years. With a median follow-up of 74 months, the investigators compared annual event rates and cumulative probability of invasive or noninvasive ipsilateral and contralateral tumors over the 5-year period following randomization. Women in the tamoxifen group had fewer breast cancer events at 5 years than did those on placebo (8.2% versus 13.4%, $p = 0.0009$). The cumulative incidence of all invasive breast cancer events in the tamoxifen group was 4.1% at 5 years: 2.1% in the ipsilateral breast, 1.8% in the contralateral breast, and 0.2% at regional or distant sites. The risk of ipsilateral breast cancer was reduced 30% by tamoxifen therapy, and this reduction was comprised of a 44% decrease in invasive breast cancer ($p = 0.03$) and a nonsignificant 18% reduction in recurrent DCIS. The risk of contralateral breast cancer was reduced 52% by tamoxifen, including a 37% decrease in invasive breast cancer and a 68% reduction in noninvasive disease ($p = 0.02$).

Supporting these data are observations from NSABP protocol B-17 in which women with DCIS were treated with either lumpectomy alone or lumpectomy plus radiation (55). Women treated with lumpectomy alone had a 5-year risk of invasive breast cancer of 14.7%, and the risk of contralateral invasive breast cancer was 1.9%. The 5-year cumulative risk of invasive breast cancer for women treated with lumpectomy and radiation was 6.9% in NSABP protocol B-17, and the 5-year cumulative risks of contralateral invasive cancer was 2.1%. Thus the risk of contralateral disease alone in these studies is comparable with the 5-year risk of all invasive breast cancers seen in the placebo arm of the BCPT, and the 5-year risk for all invasive breast cancers for women with DCIS is at least as high as that for average BCPT participants. Based on these high 5-year risks, even in women treated with lumpectomy and radiation, the data suggest a potential benefit of tamoxifen for some women with DCIS even though such women were excluded from the BCPT.

Recent Small Invasive Breast Cancers
Women with a history of invasive breast cancer have a risk of developing a second, contralateral primary breast tumor of about 0.6% per year (40). This corresponds to a 5-year risk of about 3%, which is greater than the risk of invasive breast cancer of 2.2% over 5 years that occurs among high-risk women experiencing incidence rates equal to those in the BCPT placebo arm. Consensus opinion suggests that adjuvant therapy with tamoxifen is not indicated for women with invasive breast tumors less than 1 cm in size with negative axillary lymph nodes (56). However, these opinions were based on studies of tamoxifen as treatment for primary cancer rather than as a preventive agent against a second new breast cancer. Because the risk of a second, contralateral invasive breast malignancy approaches 20% during the remaining years of life of a woman diagnosed with a first breast cancer at age 40 and is similar to the risk for women in the BCPT, the use of tamoxifen for primary prevention may be a reasonable option, particularly for younger women. There are no data available from studies designed to examine this question, but a review of data from the

NSABP treatment trials and other trials showed that tamoxifen reduces the incidence of second, contralateral primary breast cancers by roughly the same proportion as observed for primary breast malignancies in the BCPT (57). Preventive use of tamoxifen for women with small, node-negative invasive breast cancers may be justified, therefore, in some cases where there is doubt about its use as adjuvant therapy.

It is not known whether some breast cancers arise without expressing ER at any point in their genesis or whether all invasive breast cancers pass through a developmental phase in which they produce ER protein. The data from the BCPT indicate that the breast cancers arising among women taking placebo were more likely to express ERs than were tumors arising in women taking tamoxifen. This suggests that tamoxifen suppressed developing lesions that expressed ERs but had little or no effect on tumors that did not express ERs. An alternative explanation is that there are breast tumors that arise without expressing ERs at any time in their natural history. If the latter hypothesis is true, and if subsequent breast cancers in women whose first cancer did not express ERs are also ER-negative, tamoxifen would offer them little benefit. Alternatively, if all breast tumors pass through a phase of ER expression, then tamoxifen may offer benefit even to those women whose first primary breast cancer was ER-negative. More basic and clinical research is necessary to resolve this question. Limited data available from the meta-analysis of adjuvant therapy by the Early Breast Cancer Trialists' Cooperative Group(40) among women with ER-negative primary breast cancer suggest reduction in the risk of second, contralateral primary breast malignancies that is equivalent to that seen in women with ER-positive primary tumors.

BRCA1/2 Mutation Carriers
Both prospective and retrospective genetic epidemiologic studies have demonstrated that women who carry mutations in either the *BRCA1* or the *BRCA2* genes are at very high risk of developing both breast and ovarian cancer (58–60). These women appear to be ideal candidates for the use of tamoxifen as primary prevention of breast cancer, but no data are yet available that relate directly to them. While the mechanisms

whereby tamoxifen may prevent breast cancer in *BRCA1* and *BRCA2* mutation carriers are not fully understood, there is no reason to suppose a priori that tamoxifen necessarily would be less effective in mutation carriers, other than the observation that *BRCA1* carriers are more likely to develop ER-negative tumors (61,62). The idea that a SERM may be effective in lowering the incidence of primary invasive breast cancer among mutation carriers is supported by the observation that prophylactic oophorectomy reduces the risk of breast cancer by approximately 30% in women who carry mutations in either the *BRCA1* or *BRCA2* gene (63).

In the BCPT, 23% of participants had no first-degree relatives with breast cancer, 57% had only one affected relative, and 20% had two or more affected relatives. Because all these women have heritable risk for developing breast cancer, and some have high probabilities of harboring mutations in breast cancer–susceptibility genes, a study of anonymized specimens is being performed in all cases of breast cancer and in selected controls to determine the efficacy of tamoxifen in reducing breast cancer risk in carriers of mutations in either the *BRCA1* or *BRCA2* genes. Results from this testing will be available sometime in the year 2001 or thereafter. Additional laboratory modeling of the effects of tamoxifen in vitro is necessary to address this question, as are prospective data from primary prevention trials that use tamoxifen in mutation carriers. Until these studies are completed, the use of tamoxifen in such women should be accompanied by disclosure beforehand that tamoxifen may not be effective.

Clinical Monitoring of Women Taking Tamoxifen

Experience with appropriate clinical management and follow-up of women taking tamoxifen for primary prevention is limited to only a few studies, principally the BCPT. Surprisingly little published information is available from clinical trials that used tamoxifen to treat breast cancer. Hyperplasia and endometrial cancer were more frequent among women taking tamoxifen than among women taking placebo in the BCPT, but there was no statistically significant evidence of elevated risk from tamoxifen in women under age 50 (relative risk 1.21, 95% CI 0.41–3.60). While there is insufficient evidence for or against the use of transvaginal ultrasound or endometrial sampling for the early detection of endometrial cancer, women on tamoxifen should have annual gynecologic examinations with Pap smears and pelvic examinations. Any abnormal bleeding should be evaluated with appropriate diagnostic testing. Women should be counseled as to the risk of benign and malignant conditions associated with tamoxifen. Screening procedures or diagnostic tests should be at the discretion of the treating physicians, and options should be discussed with women who are considering taking tamoxifen.

Routine screening with hematologic or chemical blood tests is not indicated because no hematologic or hepatic toxicities attributable to tamoxifen were demonstrated in the BCPT or in clinical trials using tamoxifen as adjuvant therapy.

Because of the modest increase in risk of cataracts (relative risk 1.14) and cataract surgery among women on tamoxifen compared with women taking placebo, women taking tamoxifen should be questioned about symptoms of cataracts during follow-up and should discuss with their health care provider the value of periodic eye examinations.

Making Decisions About the Use of Tamoxifen for Reducing the Risk of Breast Cancer

Clinicians who counsel women about tamoxifen should strive to ensure that the patient makes a fully informed decision that incorporates her personal values and preferences (53). The counseling process should be interactive and sensitive to the patient's educational level and cultural background. Women who are actively involved in decision making about hormone-replacement therapy are more satisfied with their decisions and more informed (64). Because an individual's preferences and risk status can change substantially over time, it also is important that decisions about tamoxifen not be regarded as either urgent or irreversible.

Any discussion of tamoxifen should occur within the context of a broader discussion of health promotion and breast cancer risk. A quantitative assessment of the patient's risk should be included. The patient's perception of her own risk should be elicited so that it can be compared with an objective risk estimate. This discussion may include her personal experience of breast cancer in family members and her beliefs and fears concerning cancer etiology and treatment. Although perceived risk of breast cancer can be highly inaccurate, it is correlated with health behaviors such as use of mammography (65). Clinicians should strive, therefore, to ensure that the patient understands her objective risk and its implications for making a decision about the use of tamoxifen.

At a minimum, a risk-assessment encounter should include a clear description of the benefits and risks of taking tamoxifen for the individual woman, including a description of the side effects experienced by BCPT participants. Experience in the BCPT indicates that tools to communicate the risks and benefits of tamoxifen must be simple and short. Written materials alone are likely to be insufficient, and verbal explanations and comparisons with other risks may be needed to explain the risks and benefits of tamoxifen and to put them into perspective. Some women may be better able to understand the risks from tamoxifen by comparing them with the risks from estrogen-replacement therapy (ERT). The increased risk of venous thromboembolism associated with tamoxifen is similar to that found for ERT. A pooled analysis of studies of the risk of venous thromboembolism with ERT revealed a risk ratio of 1.7 for prospective studies and 2.4 for case-control studies (53), similar to the risk ratio of 1.7 observed for deep vein thrombosis in the BCPT for women aged 50 and older. The risk of pulmonary embolism with current use of ERT is 2.1 (95% CI 1.2–3.8). Again, this is similar to the risk observed with tamoxifen in the BCPT. The absolute risk of deep vein thrombosis and pulmonary embolism is low for both tamoxifen and ERT in women under age 50.

Ethical Considerations in the Use of Tamoxifen for Reduction of Breast Cancer Risk

There are a number of features that are unique to the clinical discipline of primary cancer prevention (66). First is the issue of a *target population*. Cancer is a rare disease among individuals who are at usual risk. It is clear, however, that individuals with a family history of the disease, with or without an identified predisposing genetic mutation, constitute a unique target population for primary preventive interventions. It is difficult, though, to determine whether these individuals should be considered "patients," "subjects," or "participants." Labeling healthy individuals as patients carries the potentially negative connotations of illness in all the behavioral metaphors associated with illness. The creation of new classes of the asymptomatic sick (e.g., considering gene carriers as ill) and the "medicalization" of conditions for which there may not be a medical solution have important implications for the predisposed individual's sense of self-identity, health beliefs and behaviors and specific social institutions such as health insurance and employment.

Second is the issue of allowable toxicity from a putative chemopreventive agent. While cancer patients and their physicians may tolerate significant toxicity, or even death, as a result of therapy, it is unlikely that patients who do not yet have malignancy, even if they are at substantially increased risk of developing cancer, will find serious toxicity acceptable. The challenge, then, in chemoprevention clinical trials is to find agents that are both effective and safe.

Finally, the duration of treatment must be considered. Our current understanding of carcinogenesis is that it is a chronic process that must be suppressed with chronic drug administration. It is not possible at the present time to administer a single dose of a preventive agent and permanently reverse the tendency for development of malignancy. Each chronic suppressive approach requires daily administration of an active agent and creates the need for the healthy individual to remain in contact with the health care system throughout prolonged periods of drug administration. This can be a difficult burden for active, mobile, healthy subjects who are employed and dealing with other demanding life issues, as well as cancer prevention. The effectiveness of tamoxifen for prevention of primary breast cancer beyond 5 years of treatment is uncertain.

Raloxifene

Raloxifene is a nonsteroidal benzothiophene that inhibits the growth of ER-dependent, DMBA-induced mammary tumors and reduces the occurrence of NMU-induced mammary tumors in rats (67). Raloxifene was investigated initially as a therapy for breast cancer. In preclinical studies, raloxifene inhibited binding of estradiol to the ER and estradiol-dependent proliferation of MCF-7 breast cancer cells (68). Consistent with these observations, in vivo studies demonstrated antitumor activity in carcinogen-induced tumors in rodents of a magnitude similar to what had been observed previously with tamoxifen (69).

Preclinical Data with Raloxifene

After absorption, raloxifene undergoes glucuronidation and an extensive enterohepatic circulation (70). Pharmacokinetics are variable, but the dose-response curve is linear at doses up to and including 60 mg orally. The terminal half-life is approximately 28 hours, and 2% of the parent drug is bioavailable. Raloxifene blocks the effects of estrogen on some tissues, such as the breast and uterus, while mimicking estrogen in other tissues, such as bone. In human breast cancer cells, the glucuronide conjugates show little affinity for the ER and are more than two orders of magnitude less potent at inhibiting cell proliferation than raloxifene itself. In nontraditional estrogen target tissue such as bone, these metabolites are also less effective than the parent at inhibiting cytokine-stimulated bone-resorbing activity in rat osteoclasts or producing TGF-β3. In animal models, tissue distribution studies with radiolabeled metabolite indicate that conversion to raloxifene occurs readily in a variety of tissues, including the liver, lung, spleen, kidney, bone, and uterus. Differential conversion of metabolites in target organs such as bone and the uterus is not observed, indicating that the origin of raloxifene's pharmacology does not result from tissue-selective deconjugation of a metabolite to the parent drug.

The pharmacology of SERMs is complex. While these agents are "antiestrogenic" in the sense that they 1) compete with estrogen for ER, 2) produce partial uterine atrophy in intact animals, and 3) cause regression in certain estrogen-dependent tumors, tamoxifen, for example, also displays estrogen agonist-like effects on certain tissues (71). Raloxifene, however, is a more "pure" antagonist of estrogenic effects in the uterus, lacking appreciable agonist activity at that site (72). Thus raloxifene is a unique agent that apparently possesses sufficient intrinsic activity to act like an agonist in bone and liver but is a relatively pure antagonist in uterine tissue. In rats, both raloxifene and ethynyl estradiol cause statistically significant increases in uterine weight relative to controls. This effect of raloxifene, however, is only about one-third of that observed in intact controls or in estrogen-treated animals. Raloxifene's minimal stimulatory effect on endometrial epithelium suggests a lower cancer risk compared with chronic administration of estrogen. The precise mechanism for raloxifene's beneficial effect on bone and lipids in the rat, as well as for its relative tissue specificity (i.e., lack of agonistic effect on uterine epithelia), remains uncertain.

In animal studies, 5 weeks of oral dosing confirmed that ethynyl estradiol, tamoxifen, and raloxifene are all potent inhibitors of the loss in volumetric bone mineral density (BMD) induced by ovariectomy, as measured by computed tomography (73). In the metaphysis of distal femora from ovariectomized rats, analysis showed a significant 12% to 20% decrease ($p < 0.01$) in BMD. In the uterus, raloxifene has minimal effects on the endometrium and smaller effects on uterine eosinophil peroxidase activity than nafoxidine, tamoxifen, and estrogen, respectively. Estrogen is the most potent in reducing cholesterol levels in ovariectomized rats, whereas tamoxifen and nafoxidine are more effective than raloxifene in blocking gain in body weight. These data show that raloxifene has potentially important advantages over estrogen, tamoxifen, and nafoxidine in the uterus.

Reduction in BMD generated by ovariectomy in rats is associated with reduction in TGF-β3 messenger RNA expression in the femur. Administration of 17-β-estradiol or raloxifene to ovariectomized rats restores both BMD and TGF-β3 messenger RNA expression in the femur to levels measured in intact animals (74). In transient transfection assays, the promoter sequence from

−38 to +110 of the human TGF-β3 gene, which contains no palindromic ERE, is sufficient to mediate 17-β-estradiol- or raloxifene-induced reporter gene expression in the presence of the ER. Raloxifene activates TGF-β3 promoter as a full agonist at nanomolar concentrations. In the same cellular system, raloxifene inhibits the ERE-containing vitellogenin promoter expression as a pure estrogen antagonist. In addition, in two well-characterized osteoclast differentiation models, TGF-β3 significantly inhibits the differentiation and bone-resorptive activities of murine and avian osteoclasts. These findings suggest that regulation of TGF-β3 gene expression by raloxifene or estrogen in bone may be an important target to mediate bone maintenance.

The tissue-specific beneficial effect of SERMs is supported by the observation that the human TGF-β3 gene is activated by ER in the presence of estrogen metabolites or estrogen antagonists. Activation is mediated by a polypurine sequence, termed the *raloxifene-response element* (RRE), and does not require the DNA-binding domain of the ER. Interaction of the ER with the RRE appears to require a cellular adapter protein. The observation that individual estrogens modulate multiple DNA response elements may explain the tissue-selective estrogen agonist or antagonist activity of compounds such as raloxifene (74). Certain key estrogen regulatory events in bone, for example, appear to be mediated through pathways independent of EREs in which the antiestrogens function as agonists.

The RRE shows no similarity to either the palindromic ERE or the AP-1 binding site. In vitro experiments with the RRE show that it is a factor in but is not sufficient by itself to mediate full hormonal regulation of the TGF-β3 gene. A high concentration of cyclohexamide blocks raloxifene-induced but not estradiol-induced increase in the amount of TGF-β3 transcripts; raloxifene additionally inhibits estradiol-induced increases in the expression of the ERE-containing progesterone receptor (PR) gene. These observations indicate that two ER regulatory pathways mediated by the ERE and RRE appear to control endogenous gene expression in cultured cells by distinct mechanisms. The ER also may contribute to one of the RRE-protein complexes, but an endogenous ligand that mediates RRE activation

has not been found. The observation that the ER, in combination with different estrogen entities, regulates more than one DNA response element (ERE and RRE) may explain the wide range of estrogen effects in nonreproductive tissues.

Clinical Data with Raloxifene

Raloxifene has been shown to have beneficial effects in selected organ systems in postmenopausal women These effects have been summarized previously (75) and will be reviewed briefly here.

Effects on Bone, Lipids, and Endometrium

In a randomized, double-blind, placebo-controlled multicenter 8-week study that evaluated short-term effects of raloxifene on bone turnover, serum lipids, and endometrium in healthy postmenopausal women (76), a total of 251 women received either placebo, raloxifene 200 or 600 mg/day, or conjugated estrogens (Premarin, 0.625 mg/day). Bone turnover (i.e., serum alkaline phosphatase, serum osteocalcin, urinary pyridinoline crosslinks, urinary calcium excretion, urinary hydroxyproline) and serum lipids (i.e., total serum cholesterol, HDL- and LDL-cholesterol) were evaluated. Endometrial biopsies also were performed. Treatment groups were compared for each parameter for baseline-to-end-point changes. The estrogen and raloxifene groups experienced similar decreases in serum alkaline phosphatase (range 10% to 11%), serum osteocalcin (range 21% to 26%), urinary pyridinoline crosslinks (range 20% to 25%), and urinary calcium excretion (range 45% to 72%). These decreases differed significantly compared with placebo-treated subjects for all markers except serum osteocalcin in the raloxifene HCl 200 mg group. LDL-cholesterol decreased significantly in the estrogen and both raloxifene groups (range 5% to 9%) compared with placebo-treated subjects. HDL-cholesterol increased significantly in the estrogen group (16%) but was unchanged in the raloxifene groups. Ratios of HDL-cholesterol to LDL-cholesterol increased significantly in the estrogen and raloxifene groups (range 9% to 29%). Serum cholesterol decreased significantly in both raloxifene groups (range 4% to 8%) but was unchanged in the estrogen group. Uterine biopsies of raloxifene-treated subjects showed no change in the endometrium during this short-term treatment. Biopsies of the estrogen group showed significant endometrial stimulation. The only adverse event possibly related to raloxifene was vasodilatation (hot flashes), which was most common in the group that received 600 mg of raloxifene.

Osteoporosis Trials

The initial studies of the effect of raloxifene on osteoporosis were two randomized, double-blind, placebo-controlled clinical trials. Both trials used 3 years of drug administration followed by 2 years of observation on a total of 1145 postmenopausal women (Joan Glussman, M.D., Eli Lilly Company, personal communication, 1998). Within these and other noncontrolled trials, there was an accumulated experience of approximately 14,800 women-years of raloxifene exposure and 6750 women-years of placebo exposure at the time of initial reporting. The mean age of the participants was 45 years, and they were an average of 4 years after menopause at the time of enrollment into the trials. Participants were permitted to take 400–600 mg of calcium daily by mouth during participation. At the 2-year interim analysis, raloxifene increased BMD by 2%, as measured by dual-energy x-ray absorptiometry (DEXA) of the spine and hip, compared with a bone mineral loss of 2% per year in women taking placebo. Raloxifene decreased urinary excretion of C-telopeptide and preserved total-body calcium.

Results from these trials have been published. Delmas and colleagues (77) studied the effect of chronic raloxifene administration on BMD, serum lipid concentrations, and endometrial thickness in 601 postmenopausal women. The women were randomly assigned to receive 30, 60, or 150 mg raloxifene or placebo daily for 24 months. The women receiving each dose of raloxifene had significant increases from baseline values in BMD of the lumbar spine, hip, and total body, whereas those receiving placebo had decreases in BMD. At 24 months, the mean difference in the change in BMD between the women receiving 60 mg raloxifene per day and those receiving placebo was 2.4% $\pm$ 0.4% for the lumbar spine, 2.4% $\pm$ 0.4% for the total hip,

and 2.0% $\pm$ 0.4% for the total body ($p < 0.001$ for all comparisons). In the placebo group, serum concentrations of bone-specific alkaline phosphatase and osteocalcin and the ratio of urinary type I collagen C-telopeptide to creatinine decreased slightly over 24 months. As compared with the placebo group, each of the raloxifene groups had a statistically significant decrease in the concentrations of the three markers of bone turnover. The serum osteocalcin concentrations and the ratio of urinary type I collagen C-telopeptide to creatinine decreased during the first 6 to 9 months of treatment and remained stable thereafter. Serum concentrations of bone-specific alkaline phosphatase decreased during the first 12 months and did not change thereafter. The median base-line serum concentrations of osteocalcin and bone-specific alkaline phosphatase and the median ratio of urinary type I collagen C-telopeptide to creatinine were similar to published values for healthy postmenopausal women. After 24 months, the median serum concentrations of bone-specific alkaline phosphatase and osteocalcin and the median ratio of urinary type I collagen C-telopeptide to creatinine had declined by 23.1%, 15.0%, and 34.0%, respectively, in the group that received 60 mg raloxifene per day. At that time, the median serum concentrations of bone-specific alkaline phosphatase and osteocalcin and the median ratio of urinary type I collagen C-telopeptide to creatinine were similar to the values in premenopausal women. Serum concentrations of total cholesterol and LDL-cholesterol decreased in all the raloxifene groups, whereas serum concentrations of HDL-cholesterol and triglycerides did not change. Endometrial thickness was similar in the raloxifene and placebo groups at all times during the study.

The effects of raloxifene on calcium metabolism have been examined quantitatively and preliminarily reported. Heaney and Draper (78) demonstrated that bone remodeling declined significantly and similarly in estrogen/progesterone- and raloxifene-treated subjects. The acute effect of raloxifene on calcium kinetics and bone remodeling was similar to that of hormone-replacement therapy in early postmenopausal women. Raloxifene has a unique

SERM profile that is distinct from both estrogens and tamoxifen. Short-term treatment with raloxifene revealed estrogenic effects on the skeleton and serum lipids without concomitant stimulation of endometrial proliferation.

The Multiple Outcomes of Raloxifene Evaluation (MORE) trial was designed to test whether 3 years of raloxifene therapy reduced the risk of fracture in postmenopausal women with osteoporosis (79). The study was a multicenter, randomized, double-blind trial in which women taking raloxifene or placebo were followed from 1994 through 1998 at 180 clinical centers composed of community settings and medical practices in 25 countries, including the United States and Europe. A total of 7705 postmenopausal women with osteoporosis, younger than age 81, whose mean age was 66.5 years were enrolled. Osteoporosis was defined by the presence of vertebral fractures or a femoral neck or spine BMD T-score of at least 2.5 standard deviations below the mean for young, healthy women. Incident vertebral fracture was determined radiographically at baseline and at scheduled 24- and 36-month visits. Nonvertebral fracture was ascertained by interview at 6-month interim visits. BMD was determined annually by dual-energy x-ray absorptiometry. Women who had a history of breast cancer or who were taking estrogen were excluded. Participants were assigned to receive raloxifene 120 mg daily, raloxifene 60 mg daily, or placebo.

After 36 months of observation or treatment, 7.4% of subjects had at least one new vertebral fracture, including 10.1% of women receiving placebo, 6.6% of those receiving 60 mg of raloxifene daily, and 5.4% of those receiving 120 mg raloxifene daily. Risk of vertebral fracture was reduced in both study groups receiving raloxifene (by 30% for the group receiving 60 mg/day and by 50% for the group receiving 120 mg/day). The frequency of vertebral fracture was reduced in both women who did and those who did not have a prevalent fracture. The risk of nonvertebral fracture for raloxifene versus placebo did not differ significantly. Compared with placebo, raloxifene increased BMD in the femoral neck by 2.1% (in the 60-mg group) and by 2.4% (in the 120-mg group) and in the spine by 2.6% (60 mg) and 2.7% (120 mg) ($p < 0.001$ for all

comparisons). Women receiving raloxifene had increased risk of venous thromboembolus versus placebo (RR 3.1, 95% CI 1.5–6.2). Raloxifene did not cause vaginal bleeding or breast pain and was associated with a lower incidence of breast cancer (79).

Effect on the Incidence of Primary Breast Cancer

No prospective studies have yet been done to examine specifically the effect of raloxifene on the incidence of breast cancer. Data are available, however, from the studies of raloxifene for osteoporosis (i.e., the MORE trial described above) on the effect of raloxifene on the subsequent development of breast cancer (80). Following publication of the results of the BCPT, the MORE investigators sought to determine whether women taking raloxifene have a lower risk of invasive breast cancer (see Table 12-2). New cases of breast cancer were confirmed by histopathology, and transvaginal ultrasonography was used to assess the endometrial effects of raloxifene in 1781 of the women. The occurrence of deep vein thrombosis or pulmonary embolism was determined by chart review. After a median follow-up of 40 months, 13 cases of breast cancer were confirmed among the 5129 women assigned to raloxifene group versus 27 among the 2576 women assigned to placebo. The relative risk of breast cancer was 0.24 (95% CI 0.13–0.44, $p < 0.001$). To prevent 1 case of breast cancer, 126 women would have needed treatment. Raloxifene decreased the risk of ER-positive breast cancer by 90% but not ER-negative invasive breast cancer.

Raloxifene increased the risk of venous thromboembolic disease threefold (RR 3.1, 95% CI 1.5–6.2) but did not increase the risk of endometrial cancer (RR 0.8, 95% CI 0.2–2.7). This finding was based, however, on only 10 total cases of invasive endometrial cancer (6 among those taking either 60 or 120 mg raloxifene and 4 among those taking placebo) and requires additional years of observation. Endometrial cancer was a rare event occurring at a rate of only 2 to 3 cases per 1000 person-years, and these results are based on only 25,000 total person-years of observation. It is possible that additional cases will occur in the future and alter these estimates of the risk of endometrial cancer associated with raloxifene. Raloxifene at either 60 or 120 mg daily also was associated with statistically significant increases in the incidence of influenza-like symptoms, hot flashes, leg cramps, and endometrial cavity fluid.

Other Effects of Raloxifene

In rats, raloxifene inhibits atherogenesis. It lowers LDLs and increases LDL oxidation. It inhibits endothelial thickening and decreases smooth muscle cell migration. In limited studies in humans, raloxifene decreased LDL levels by approximately 0.3 mmol/liter, or 10%, without a significant reduction in HDL levels. It decreases both triglycerides and fibrinogen and reduces lipooxygenase a levels.

In the uterus, raloxifene can block both estradiol- and tamoxifen-induced proliferation of the endometrium. Among 3809 women taking raloxifene and having transvaginal uterine ultrasonography, the effect of raloxifene 60 mg daily by mouth on the uterus was no greater than that of placebo. In a separate study of 43 patients with endometrial atrophy taking 150 mg raloxifene daily, all patients maintained the atrophic condition after an observation period of 24 months. Among women taking 60 mg raloxifene daily in studies of osteoporosis, there was no reported difference in the rates of uterine bleeding among treated women compared with those taking placebo.

In postmenopausal women taking raloxifene, the risk of venous thromboembolism is increased approximately three-fold. This is virtually identical to the risk of thromboembolism seen with estrogen-replacement therapy in postmenopausal women. Most of the thrombotic events reported with raloxifene are from the MORE study, where the mean age of participants was 67 years. When patients with risk factors for thrombosis (e.g., immobilization, prior history of thrombotic event, etc.) are removed from this analysis, the risk drops to 1.7-fold.

Among women taking 60 mg raloxifene daily, 24% reported hot flashes compared with 18% among women taking placebo, and the severity of the hot flashes was identical in the two groups. Approximately 2% of postmenopausal women taking raloxifene report severe hot flashes, but the rate of discontinuation of the drug in these women was not greater than that in the women who did not have severe hot flashes.

The NSABP STAR Trial

Neither the MORE trial nor any other completed study of raloxifene was designed to evaluate invasive breast cancer as a primary end point. In addition, women in the MORE trial were at significantly lower risk of breast cancer when compared with the women in the BCPT. In both trials, raloxifene and tamoxifen were associated with an approximately three-fold increase in the risk of venous thromboembolism. While raloxifene was not associated with a significant increase in the risk of endometrial cancer, tamoxifen has been shown in several studies to cause a two- to four-fold increase in this side effect. All the cases of endometrial carcinoma associated with tamoxifen have been stage I disease.

Given these preliminary data, there are sufficient reasons to propose a direct comparison of tamoxifen and raloxifene in a trial designed primarily to assess reduction in the risk of invasive breast cancer. With the support of the National Cancer Institute, Astra-Zeneca Pharmaceuticals, and Eli Lilly Company, the NSABP will conduct the Study of Tamoxifen and Raloxifene (STAR). STAR will be conducted in 22,000 postmenopausal women because the preliminary raloxifene data are from this population, and there is a lack of adequate long-term safety testing in premenopausal women. The primary aim of the STAR trial is to determine which of the following three statements is true:

1. Compared with tamoxifen, raloxifene significantly reduces the incidence rate of invasive breast cancer.
2. Compared with raloxifene, tamoxifen significantly reduces the incidence rate of invasive breast cancer.
3. The statistical superiority of one of the treatments cannot be demonstrated, and the choice of therapy should be based on risk-benefit considerations.

In addition to evaluating breast cancer end points, the STAR trial will evaluate the effect of raloxifene and tamoxifen on the following end points:

- Lobular carcinoma in situ and ductal carcinoma in situ
- Endometrial cancer
- Ischemic heart disease
- Fractures
- Quality of life

The trial design for STAR is shown in Figure 12-5. The trial will be restricted to post-menopausal women whose projected 5-year risk of developing invasive breast cancer is 1.66% or higher. *Postmenopause* is defined as being 12 or more months without spontaneous menstrual bleeding or having a prior documented hysterectomy and bilateral oophorectomy; or being greater than 55 years of age with a prior hysterectomy, with or without oophorectomy; or being less than 55 years of age with a history of prior hysterectomy and an elevated serum follicle-stimulating hormone (FSH) level.

Women 60 years of age or older are members of the risk-eligible group due to their high age-specific incidence of breast cancer, as are women with lobular carcinoma in situ, which was associated with an annual incidence of invasive breast cancer of 1.3% in the BCPT. Women aged 35 years or older who are postmenopausal will

have their risk of breast cancer evaluated using the Gail model, which uses age, age at menarche, age at first live birth (or nulliparity), number of first-degree relatives with breast cancer, number of breast biopsies, presence of atypical lobular or ductal hyperplasia, and race to determine risk. Eligible women will be stratified by age, relative risk, race, and history of lobular carcinoma in situ. They will be randomly assigned to receive tamoxifen 20 mg orally daily or raloxifene 60 mg orally daily for 5 years. Because of the difference in the shapes of raloxifene and tamoxifen, each subject will receive two tablets, one containing tamoxifen or its placebo and the other containing raloxifene or its placebo; hence each subject will receive only one active compound. There will be no "placebo group" in the STAR trial because of the positive and dramatic findings in the BCPT that now make a placebo control unethical in a trial of SERMs for reduction in breast cancer incidence. It is also important to determine the chronic effects of selective ER modulators because breast cancers have been shown to develop resistance to tamoxifen after long-term exposure (81–84).

Women ineligible to participate in the STAR trial include those with a prior history of invasive breast cancer, a history of ductal carcinoma in situ, a history of deep venous thrombosis or pulmonary embolism, a history of stroke or transient ischemic attack, and/or a history of uncontrolled atrial fibrillation. Those women currently taking estrogen, progesterone, androgens, or birth control pills are also ineligible, but risk-eligible subjects may enter the trial if they discontinue hormonal medications for 3 months prior to randomization.

Participants must have a breast examination that shows no malignancy prior to entry, along with a normal mammogram, normal complete blood count and serum chemistries, and a pelvic examination that shows no pathology. The breast examination will be repeated at 6-month intervals, and the entry examinations will be repeated yearly. Paraffin blocks of pathology tissue specimens will be submitted for cancer events, and one paraffin tissue block also will be submitted for those subjects entering the trial with a prior history of lobular carcinoma in situ or atypical hyperplasia. A number of ancillary

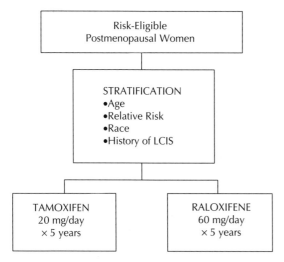

Figure 12-5. Schema for the NSABP STAR trial.

studies are being considered for inclusion in the trial.

References

1. Sporn MB, Dunlop NM, Newton DL, et al. Prevention of chemical carcinogenesis by vitamin A and its synthetic analogues (retinoids). Fed Proc 1976;35:1332–1338.
2. Lippman SM, Benner SE, Hong WK. Cancer chemoprevention. J Clin Oncol 1994;12:851–873.
3. Lippman SM, Hong WK, Benner SE. The chemoprevention of cancer. In: Greenwald P, Kramer BS, Weed DL, eds. Cancer Prevention and Control. New York: Marcel Dekker, 1995:329–352.
4. Henderson BE, Ross RK, Pike MC, et al. Endogenous hormones as a major factor in human cancer. Cancer Res 1982;42:3232–3239.
5. Russo J, Russo IH. Toward a physiological approach to breast cancer prevention. Cancer Epidemiol Biomark Prev 1994;3:353–364.
6. Henderson BE, Ross RK, Pike MC. Hormonal chemoprevention of cancer in women. Science 1993;259:633–638.
7. Kelsey JL, Gammon MD. Epidemiology of breast cancer. Epidemiol Rev 1990;12:228–240.
8. Kelsey JL, Gammon MD, John EM. Reproductive factors and breast cancer. Epidemiol Rev 1993;15:36–47.
9. Russo IH, Russo J. Chorionic gonadotropin: a tumoristatic and preventive agent in breast cancer. In: Teicher BA, ed. Drug Resistance in Oncology. New York, Marcel Dekker, Inc, 1992;537–560.
10. Russo J, Russo IH. Toward a physiological approach to breast cancer prevention. Cancer Epidemiol Biomark Prev 1994;3:353–364.
11. Mitlak, BH, Cohen FJ. In search of optimal long-term female hormone replacement: the potential of selective estrogen receptor modulators. Horm Res 1997;48:155–163.
12. Fuleihan GE-H. Tissue-specific estrogens: the promise for the future. New Engl J Med 1997;337:1686–1687.
13. Cheskis BJ, Karathanasis S, Lyttle CR. Estrogen receptor ligands modulate its interaction with DNA. J Biol Chem 1997;272:11384–11391.
14. Yang NN, Venugopalan M, Hardikar S, et al. Identification of an estrogen response element activated by metabolites of 17β-estradiol and raloxifene. Science 1996;273:1222–1225.
14a. Sato M, Glasebrook AL, Bryant HU. Raloxifene: a selective estrogen receptor modulator. J Bone Miner Metab 1994;12(Suppl):S9–S20.
15. Colletta AA, Benson JR, Baum M. Alternative mechanisms of action of anti-oestrogens. Breast Cancer Res Treat 1994;31:5–9.
16. Katzenellenbogen BS. Antiestrogens: mechanisms of action in target cells. J Steroid Biochem Mol Biol 1995;53:387–393.
17. Berry M, Metzger D, Chambon P. Role of the two activating domains of the oestrogen receptor in the cell type and promotor-context dependent agonist activity of the anti-oestrogen 4-hydroxytamoxifen. EMBO J 1990;9:2811–2818.
18. Danielian PS, White R, Lees JA, et al. Identification of a conserved region required for hormone dependent transcriptional activation by steroid hormone receptors. EMBO J 1992;11:1025–1033.
19. Katzenellenbogen JA, O'Malley BW, Katzenellenbogen BS. Tripartite steroid hormone receptor pharmacology: interaction with multiple effector sites as a basis for cell- and promoter-specific action of these hormones. Mol Endocrinol 1996;10:119–131.
20. Ferguson AT, Davidson NE. Regulation of estrogen receptor alpha function in breast cancer. Crit Rev Oncogen 1997;8:29–46.
21. Murphy LC, Dotzlaw H, Leygue E, et al. Estrogen receptor variants and variations. J Steroid Biochem Mol Biol 1997;62:363–372.
22. Sasano H, Suzuki, Matsuzaki Y, et al. Messenger ribonucleic acid in situ hybridization of estrogen receptors alpha and beta in human breast carcinoma. J Clin Endocrinol Metab 1999;84:781–785.
23. Speirs V, Parkes AT, Kerin MJ, et al. Coexpression of estrogen receptor alpha and beta: poor prognostic factors in human breast cancer? Cancer Res 1999;59:525–528.
24. Paech K, Webb P, Kuiper GGJM, et al. Differential ligand activation of estrogen receptors ERα and ERβ at AP1 sites. Science 1997;277:1508–1510.
25. Vogel VG. Evaluation of risk and preventive approaches to breast cancer. In: Kavanagh J, Singletary SE, Einhorn N, DePetrillo AD, eds. Cancer in Women. Boston: Blackwell Science, 1998:58–91.
26. Vogel VG. Primary prevention of breast cancer. In: Bland KI, Copeland EM, eds. The Breast: Comprehensive Management of Benign and Malignant Disease. Vol 1. Philadelphia: WB Saunders, 1998:352–369.
27. Morrow M, Jordan VC. Molecular mechanisms of resistance to tamoxifen therapy in breast cancer. Arch Surg 1993;128:1187–1191.

28. Giuffrida D, Lupo L, La Porta GA, et al. Relation between steroid receptor status and body weight in breast cancer patients. Eur J Cancer 1992;28:112–115.

29. Noguchi S, Motomura K, Inaji H, et al. Down regulation of transforming growth factor-α by tamoxifen in human breast cancer. Cancer 1993;72:131–136.

30. Love RR, Wiebe DA, Newcomb PA, et al. Effects of tamoxifen on cardiovascular risk factors in postmenopausal women. Ann Intern Med 1991;115:860–864.

31. Kannel WB, Wolf PA, Castelli WP, et al. Fibrinogen and risk of cardiovascular disease. JAMA 1987;258:1183–1186.

32. Hoffman CJ, Miller RH, Lawson WE, et al. Elevation of factor VII activity and mass in young adults at risk of ischemic heart disease. J Am Coll Cardiol 1989;14:941–946.

33. Cuzick J, Allen D, Baum M, et al. Long-term effects of tamoxifen: Biological Effects of Tamoxifen Working Party. Eur J Cancer 1993;29:15–21.

34. Love RR, Mazess RB, Borden HS, et al. Effects of tamoxifen on bone mineral density in postmenopausal women with breast cancer. New Engl J Med 1992;326:852–856.

35. Kristensen B, Ejlertsen B, Dalgaard P, et al. Tamoxifen and bone metabolism in postmenopausal low-risk breast cancer patients: a randomized study. J Clin Oncol 1994;12:992–997.

36. Stewart PJ, Stern PH. Effects of the antiestrogens tamoxifen and clomiphene on bone resorption in vitro. Endocrinology 1986;118:125–131.

37. Powles TJ, Hickish TF, Kanis JA, et al. Effect of tamoxifen on bone mineral density measured by dual-energy x-ray absorptiometry in healthy premenopausal and postmenopausal women. J Clin Oncol 1996;14:78–84.

38. Fisher B, Costantino J, Redmond C, et al. A randomized clinical trial evaluating tamoxifen in the treatment of patients with node-negative breast cancer who have estrogen receptor-positive tumors. New Engl J Med 1989;320:479–484.

39. Fisher ER, Fisher B, Sass R, et al. Pathological findings from the National Surgical Adjuvant Breast Project (protocol no. 4): bilateral breast cancer. Cancer 1984;54:3002–3011.

40. Early Breast Cancer Trialists' Collaborative Group. Tamoxifen for early breast cancer: an overview of the randomized trials. Lancet 1998;351:1451–1467.

41. Powles T, Ecles R, Ashley S, et al. Interim analysis of the incidence of breast cancer in the Royal Marsden Hospital tamoxifen randomised chemoprevention trial. Lancet 1998;352:98–101.

42. Veronesi U, Maissonneuve P, Costa C, et al. Prevention of breast cancer with tamoxifen: preliminary findings from the Italian randomised trial among hysterectomised women. Italian Tamoxifen Prevention Study. Lancet 1998;352:98–101.

43. Fisher B, Costantino JP, Wickerham DL, et al. Tamoxifen for prevention of breast cancer: report of the National Surgical Adjuvant Breast and Bowel Project P-1 study. J Natl Cancer Inst 1998;90:1371–1388.

44. Gail MH, Brinton LA, Byar DP, et al. Projecting individualized probabilities of developing breast cancer for white females who are being examined annually. J Natl Cancer Inst 1989;81:1879–1886.

45. Bondy ML, Lustbader ED, Halabi S, et al. Validation of a breast cancer risk assessment model in women with a positive family history. J Natl Cancer Inst 1994;86:620–625.

46. Spiegelman D, Colditz GA, Hunter D, et al. Validation of the Gail et al. model predicting individual breast cancer risk. J Natl Cancer Inst 1994;86:600–607.

47. Wingo PA, Ory HW, Layde PM, Lee NC. The evaluation of the data collection process for a multi-center, population-based, case-control design. Am J Epidemiol 1988;128:206–217.

48. Costantino JP, Gail MH, Pee D, et al. Validation studies for models projecting the risk of invasive and total breast cancer incidence. J Natl Cancer Inst 1999;91:1541–1548.

49. McDonald CC. Fatal myocardial infarction in the Scottish adjuvant tamoxifen trial. Br Med J 1991;303:435–437.

50. Vogel VG. Tamoxifen for the prevention of breast cancer. In: DeVita VT Jr, Helman S, Rosenberg SA, eds. Important Advances in Oncology — 1995. Philadelphia: JB Lippincott, 1995:187–200.

51. Fisher B, Costantino JP, Redmond CK, et al. Endometrial cancer in tamoxifen-treated breast cancer patients: findings from the National Surgical Adjuvant Breast and Bowel Project (NSABP) B-14. J Natl Cancer Inst 1994;86:527–537.

52. Lippman SM, Brown PH. Tamoxifen prevention of breast cancer: an instance of the fingerpost. J Natl Cancer Inst 1999;91:1809–1819.

53. Gail MH, Costantino JP, Bryant J, et al. Weighing the risks and benefits of tamoxifen treatment for preventing breast cancer. J Natl Cancer Inst 1999;91:1829–1846.

54. Fisher B, Dignam J, Wolmark N, et al. Tamoxifen in treatment of intraductal breast cancer: National Surgical Adjuvant Breast and Bowel Project B-24 randomized controlled trial. Lancet 1999;353:1993–2000.

55. Fisher B, Dignam J, Wolmark N, et al. Lumpectomy and radiation for the treatment of intraductal cancer: findings of the National Surgical Adjuvant Breast and Bowel Project B-17. J Clin Oncol 1998;16:441–452.

56. Goldhirsch A, Wood WC, Senn HJ, et al. Fifth International Conference on Adjuvant Therapy of Breast Cancer, St. Galen, March 1995: international consensus panel on the primary treatment of breast cancer. Eur J Cancer 1995;31A:1754–1759.

57. Fisher B, Redmond C. New perspective on cancer of the contralateral breast: a marker for assessing tamoxifen as a preventive agent. J Natl Cancer Inst 1991;83:1278–1280.

58. Strewing JP, Hartge P, Wacholder S, et al. The risk of cancer associated with specific mutations of *BRCA1* and *BRCA2* among Ashkenazi Jews. New Engl J Med 1997;337:1401–1408.

59. Easton DF, Ford D, Bishop DT. Breast and ovarian cancer incidence in *BRCA1*-mutation carriers: The Breast Cancer Linkage Consortium. Am J Hum Genet 1995;56:265–271.

60. Thorlacius S, Strewing JP, Hartge P, et al. Population-based study of risk of breast cancer in carriers of *BRCA2* mutation. Lancet 1998;352:1337–1339.

61. Karp SE, Tonin PN, Begin LR, et al. Influence of *BRCA1* mutations on nuclear grade and estrogen receptor status of breast carcinoma in Ashkenazi Jewish women. Cancer 1997;80:435–441.

62. Loman N, Johannsson O, Bendahl PO, et al. Steroid receptors in hereditary breast carcinomas associated with *BRCA1* or *BRCA2* mutations or unknown susceptibility genes. Cancer 1998;83:310–319.

63. Rebbeck TR, Levin AM, Eisen A, et al. Breast cancer risk after bilateral oophorectomy in *BRCA1* mutation carriers. J Natl Cancer Inst 1999;91:1475–1479.

64. O'Connor AM, Tugwell P, Wells GA, et al. Randomized trial of a portable, self-administered decision aid for postmenopausal women considering long-term preventive hormone therapy. Med Decision Making 1998;18:295–303.

65. McCaul KD, Branstetter AD, Schroeder DM, Glasgow RE. What is the relationship between breast cancer risk and mammography? A meta-analytic review. Health Psychol 1996;15:423–429.

66. Vogel VG, Parker LP. Ethical issues of chemoprevention clinical trials. Cancer Contr 1997;4:142–149.

67. Anzano MA, Peer CW, Smith JM, et al. Chemoprevention of mammary carcinogenesis in the rat: combined use of raloxifene and 9-*cis*-retinoic acid. J Natl Cancer Inst 1996;88:123–125.

68. Wakeling AE, Valcaccia B, Newboult E, et al. Non-steroidal antioestrogens: receptor binding and biological response in rat uterus, rat mammary carcinoma and human breast cancer cells. J Steroid Biochem 1984;20:111–120.

69. Clemens JA, Bennett DR, Black LJ, et al. Effects of a new antiestrogen keoxifene (LY156758) on growth of carcinogen-induced mammary tumors and on LH and prolactin levels. Life Sci 1983;32:2869–2875.

70. Dodge JA, Lugar CW, Cho S, et al. Evaluation of the major metabolites of raloxifene as modulators of tissue selectivity. J Steroid Biochem Mol Biol 1997;61:97–106.

71. Jordan VC, Allen KE, Dix CJ. Pharmacology of tamoxifen in laboratory animals. Cancer Treat Rep 1980;64:745–749.

72. Black LJ, Jones D, Falcone JF. Antagonism of estrogen action with a new benzothiophene derived antiestrogen. Life Sci 1983;32:1031–1036.

73. Sato M, Rippy MK, Bryant HU. Raloxifene, tamoxifene, nafoxidene, or estrogen effects on reproductive and nonreproductive tissues in ovariectomized rats. FASEB J 1996;10:905–912.

74. Yang NN, Venugopalan M, Hardikar S, et al. Identification of an estrogen response element activated by metabolites of 17β-estradiol and raloxifene. Science 1996;273:1222–1225.

75. Khovidhunkit W, Shoback DM. Clinical effects of raloxifene hydrochloride in women. Ann Intern Med 1999;130:431–439.

76. Draper MW, Flowers DE, Huster WJ, et al. A controlled trial of raloxifene (LY139481) HCl: impact on bone turnover and serum lipid profile in healthy postmenopausal women. J Bone Miner Res 1996;11:835–842.

77. Delmas P, Bjarnason NH, Mitlak BH, et al. Effects of raloxifene on bone mineral density, serum cholesterol concentrations, and uterine endometrium in postmenopausal women. New Engl J Med 1997;337:1641–1647.

78. Heaney RP, Draper MW. Raloxifene and estrogen: comparative bone remodeling kinetics. Clin Endocrinol Metab 1997;82:2425–2429.
79. Ettinger B, Black DM, Mitlak BH, et al. Reduction of vertebral fracture risk in postmenopausal women with osteoporosis treated with raloxifene: results from a 3-year randomized clinical trial. JAMA 1999;282:637–645.
80. Cummings SR, Eckert S, Krueger KA, et al. The effect of raloxifene on risk of breast cancer in postmenopausal women: results from the MORE randomized trial. JAMA 1999;281:2189–2197.
81. Gottardis MM, Jordan VC. Development of tamoxifen-stimulated growth of MCF-7 tumors in athymic mice after long-term antiestrogen administration. Cancer Res. 1988;48:5183–5187.
82. Osborne CK, Coronado E, Allred DC, et al. Acquired tamoxifen resistance: correlation with reduced breast tumor levels of tamoxifen and isomerization of *trans*-4-hydroxytamoxifen. J Natl Cancer Inst 1991;83:1477–1482.
83. Howell A, Dodwell DJ, Anderson H, Redford J. Response after withdrawal of tamoxifen and progestogens in advanced breast cancer. Ann Oncol. 1992;3:611–617.
84. Norris JD, Paige LA, Christensen DJ, et al. Peptide antagonists of the human estrogen receptor. Science 1999;285:744–746.

13

Psychological Management of Women at Risk for Breast Cancer

Donna M. Posluszny and Andrew Baum

Identification of risk for a disease is a two-edged sword. Accurate estimation of risk is an important component of disease prevention and early detection, but it also may be a source of stress and worry. Evaluation of risk and investigation of factors that put people at risk permit selective application of chemoprevention and aggressive surveillance programs. Discovering and understanding risk factors often suggest ways to prevent disease by altering modifiable risk. In addition, even if prevention efforts are ineffective or poorly implemented, identifying people who are at high risk facilitates detection of early, more readily treated disease. However, risk status is also a powerful psychological stimulus, and how people respond to learning of their risk status can affect subsequent health and well-being. It can cause stress and can be associated with dramatic increases in feelings of anxiety and depression soon after learning of one's status. Inaccurate or misleading perceptions of risk, unwarranted alarm, defensive behavior that leads people to avoid any consideration of potential disease, and the nature of one's emotional response to this stimulus are important components of response to cancer risk.

These issues are particularly relevant for breast cancer. Prevention, evaluation of risk, and participation in surveillance activities are important aspects of the effort to reduce breast cancer morbidity and mortality. Chemoprevention—primarily application of antiestrogens—appears to substantially reduce some women's risk of breast cancer (1), and surveillance efforts are important in successful treatment of the

disease (2,3). Surveillance activities traditionally have included mammography, clinical breast examination (CBE), and breast self-examination (BSE), and appropriate practice of these activities is thought to increase early detection of more successfully treated disease (4). However, learning that one is at risk for breast cancer and participating in routine or aggressive surveillance programs have costs of their own. Many women do not follow these recommendations because avoiding reminders of their risk is a part of their efforts to manage emotional reactions to their risk status.

In general, the ways in which women appraise their risk for breast cancer affect their reactions to it. Perceptions of risk can lead to worry and distress about developing cancer that may increase or decrease participation in screening activities. Risk perceptions are motivating in that they increase people's awareness of and desire to act in some way that will reduce the danger of breast cancer. However, if women react to being at risk by becoming upset or worried, they may focus on this distress instead of the real danger. In other words, their distress rather than breast cancer becomes their primary objective, and coping is directed at reducing distress rather than reducing the likelihood of disease. As a result, some women react to high-risk status by avoiding it.

Other factors, including beliefs about the severity of breast cancer, personality style, and social support, also affect the way women approach their risk for breast cancer. This chapter describes how women form perceptions of breast cancer risk, how these risk perceptions may affect them and cause stress, how distress in turn affects surveillance behaviors, and how personality factors and situational characteristics such as having a relative with breast cancer further affect these outcomes. Implications of these issues for the management of distress are also discussed.

Bases of Perceived Risk

The most basic element in people's reactions to risk-status notification is their perception of that risk. People vary in how seriously they take risk estimates and how information about risk is used, resulting in variable perceptions of risk in similar or identical situations. If people do not believe that the evaluated risk is accurate, or if they incorrectly interpret information as suggesting low risk, they are likely to behave as if they are not at risk. By the same reasoning, exaggerated estimates of risk may cause distress. Perceptions of risk for cancer are susceptible to a number of sources of bias, making accurate risk perceptions elusive.

Cancer is a highly feared disease (5), and many people still believe that it is inevitably fatal. As a result, high-risk status can be a highly threatening situation. One's well-being and survival depend on the ability to detect and avoid danger (6). When people believe they are threatened or at risk, they become motivated to somehow decrease this risk, either by altering the environment or by changing their behavior (7). If the situation or behavior cannot be changed, or if fear is so intrusive that it demands attention, people may try to deny or distract themselves from the threat to decrease discomfort due to these threatening perceptions (8). The intensity and duration of distress due to one's risk status for cancer are variably related to a host of factors and are difficult to estimate without knowledge of an individual's coping style, tolerance for uncertainty, perceptions of the disease, and general outlook. Regardless of how coping unfolds, perception of threat typically motivates increased coping efforts (7,9).

There has been considerable interest in health belief models that have been developed to explain and predict people's health behavior (10,11). Four components have been considered, including perceived risk, perceived severity of health problem or disease, and perceived costs and benefits of a preventive or surveillance behavior. Of the four components, perception of risk has shown the most value in understanding breast cancer surveillance, although results have been modest (12,13), and there are opposite findings (14).

Research on perceptions of health threats suggest that people engage in unrealistic optimism, rating themselves as less likely than others to develop most threatening diseases (15,16). One exception to this is cancer, for which people tend to overestimate risk and increase distress and worry. In general, women are not very accurate in estimating their risk of breast cancer (17,18). Objective risk estimates are now routine, based on family history, hormonal and reproductive history, previous breast problems, and other factors (19). Compared with individual risk calculations, studies suggest that 30% to 40% correctly estimate their risk, with the rest over- and underestimating their risk (20,21). Women may wrongly attribute lower perceived risk to personal action, including mammography screening (22). Reasons for overestimates are not clear, but there is substantial evidence that women overestimate their risk (18,23,24). To the extent that overestimated risk is a cause of distress or maladaptive responses such as avoidance, increasing the accuracy of risk perceptions will minimize some negative aspects of risk evaluation. Women's risk perceptions can be affected by how they process information about the event, whether or not they have accurate knowledge about the event, past exposure to the event, and personality characteristics.

Cognitive Factors

When forming a risk estimate, women must integrate many bits of information. There is a great deal of information about the probabilities of breast cancer development and specific risk reduction, but it is often confusing and difficult for women to select data that are relevant for them (25). Often there is too much information; women may be getting risk information from friends and family, the media, and their physician and may not be sure how to make sense of it all. In addition, risk estimates are sensitive to biased media coverage and the opinions of friends and family (6). Difficulty in understanding risk probabilities is compounded by a poor knowledge base about cancer; for example, many people do not know the risk factors or standard warning signs of cancer (5,26). Most who seek diagnosis for cancer present with a symptom other than one of these standard warning signs (5). In addition, women may not be familiar with all the specific risk factors for breast cancer (21,27) and may believe that factors such as bumps and bruises cause cancer (27,28).

Other factors in one's appraisal of risk include characteristics of events or of one's relationship to them. People report lower perceived vulnerability to negative events that appear to be controllable and are less optimistic about events thought to be caused by unmodifiable factors such as heredity or the environment (16,29). When people were asked to estimate their chances of experiencing health problems such as heart disease or lung and skin cancer, they gave optimistically biased estimates for all events except the unspecified category of cancer (16). This minimization bias was not apparent for cancer; ratings of risk for cancer were overestimates. Similar work by Kulik and Mahler (30) found that although people were optimistic about all health problems, they tended to be less optimistic about unspecified cancer.

The magnitude of this optimistic bias increased with the perceived preventability of the event (16). Some cancers, including lung and skin cancer, have clearly identifiable causes, and many people are aware of findings indicating that cigarette smoking can cause lung cancer (5,26) or that sun exposure increases the risk of skin cancer (31). It is possible that greater optimistic bias accompanies this sense of control precisely because it suggests that this disease would be "of their own making." People perceive general cancer to be preventable through their own behaviors, although approximately 20% thought that very little could be done (26).

Risk perception is also affected by the way information about an event is presented (32). For example, people give different risk estimates and choose different treatment options depending on how the information is framed. Information presented in terms of one's chances of living is associated with lower risk perceptions than if presented in terms of one's chances of dying, even though the information is the same (33). Laypeople and physicians can differ in how they evaluate health information. Laypeople tend to judge health information more seriously than do physicians and want full disclosure of health risks (34). Laypeople's estimates of risk are related to actual risk but are likely to be influenced by other factors, including the potential severity of the problem, the degree of controllability, and the impact on others such as their family (32).

Once risk estimates are formed, they may be difficult to change. New information is typically considered in light of already established perceptions of risk. If this new information is consistent with prevailing perceptions, it will seem to be true and will be readily accepted. New information that does not agree with prevailing risk beliefs may be ignored because it is considered false or irrelevant (32). For patients who have held strong beliefs about their health and believe that they are at low risk for serious illness, learning that they are at high risk may disturb their basic assumptions about themselves and cause distress unless the information can be disregarded or modified. Similarly, it is often difficult to reassure a patient who believes that he or she is at very high risk when he or she actually is at much lower risk.

Experience and Family History

Risk perception is also affected by one's past exposure to a particular threat. People's previous encounters with health threats make them more likely to see themselves as being vulnerable to that threat (29,35). Exposure may be gained through direct experience or by observing and hearing about others dealing with the aversive event. Having lived with a mother who had breast cancer or having cared for a friend who had it should sensitize people to the threat of breast cancer and could contribute to overestimates of risk. Conversely, low levels of experience are associated with underestimates of actual risk (15,36).

Family history is the most widely recognized index of risk for breast cancer. It is readily identifiable and reflects both inherited and environmental sources of variance. Family history is a common source of information about risk among women at risk for disease and may form the core of mental representations of that risk. Many women know that their relative risk of developing breast cancer increases with the number of first-degree relatives who have had the disease (37,38), although some evidence suggests that family history does not affect risk perceptions (18). If in addition one has endured the trials of a close relative's encounter with breast cancer, these representations may be stronger and more evocative.

Emotional Response to Risk Status

The threat of cancer can arouse feelings of vulnerability and fear (5,38). Women at risk may be apprehensive about when and if they may develop cancer, how cancer will affect their lives, how they will manage the disease, and whether they will survive the illness. These disease-related beliefs about the future also may contribute to worry and distress.

Several studies have suggested that women who are at higher risk for breast cancer experience more distress than do women who are at lower risk for the disease (40–42). One study found that 27% of the sample of women at high objective risk for breast cancer reported clinically significant distress (43). Women also report elevated anxiety about developing breast cancer and experience intrusive thoughts about their worries (44). Younger women at risk may be more vulnerable to distress (40). Intrusive thoughts about breast cancer also were reported by women undergoing genetic counseling for breast cancer (45). However, Wellisch and colleagues (46) found no increases in psychological symptoms in daughters of breast cancer patients.

This distress is a product of individual risk evaluation and one's perceptions of this status, and any of a number of associated events. For example, receiving abnormal mammogram results often precedes a diagnosis of cancer. When a mammogram looks suspicious, women typically are called back for a second screening,

and this can be very anxiety-provoking. Women who have received suspicious abnormal results and are returning for a follow-up mammogram are more distressed than women undergoing routine screening (47). Women who were recalled continued to report anxiety about results of future mammograms and continued to worry about breast cancer after receiving results indicating that no disease was present (48). This distress did not appear to affect surveillance, since these women still maintained their usual rate of screening over the next year. Other evidence suggests that although women became anxious at the time of recall, their anxiety levels subsided over the following 3 months (49). Women with a family history of breast cancer were less anxious than those without such a history when followed up at 3 months (49).

Several theories address emotional and cognitive aspects of people's response to threat, some focusing on the threatening stimulus, others on the reaction to the stimulus, and others on both (50–53). When faced with threat, people experience heightened arousal characterized by changes in emotional, physiological, and behavioral processes. This emotional reaction is generally experienced as discomfort, tension, or negative affect, and people are motivated to reduce or eliminate it (54).

Perception of threat also has consequences for physiologic processes and health behavior. Immune system functioning can be affected by acute or chronic distress (55,56) and may contribute to increased vulnerability to illness (57). Other bodily effects include increased blood pressure, heart rate, and sympathetic nervous system arousal, and other physiologic processes are affected as well. People may try to decrease negative mood by engaging in behaviors that reduce tension but ultimately can be health damaging, such as smoking or drinking. People also may stop or decrease health enhancing behaviors such as exercise (58) and forgo the physical and psychological benefits of exercise (59,60). Stress-related increases in consumption of fattening foods and decreased exercise may lead to weight gain, which appears to increase women's risk for breast cancer (61).

There are some data that suggest that the threat of breast cancer has implications for physiologic functioning. Women with a family history of cancer have been observed to have lower levels of natural killer cell cytotoxic activity than women with no family history (62). In addition, women with higher levels of distress had lower natural cytotoxic activity, independent of family history. These findings suggest that higher-risk women who are also experiencing distress may be at an even greater risk for developing immune-related illness.

Factors Affecting Surveillance Behavior

Screening mammography significantly reduces breast cancer mortality (3), yet many women do not participate (26,63). One study of women at high risk for breast cancer found that about half the women had ever had a mammogram, and only 14% reported undergoing annual mammography (64). Risk perception has some value in predicting prevention and surveillance behavior, but it is not perfect. It is likely that one's emotional reactions to being at risk are important mediating factors in this variable relationship. One can argue, for example, that increasing risk will (should) be associated with increasing surveillance, but data suggest that this relationship may not be linear. Several of the factors that are implicated in risk perception also have been studied as determinants of adherence to surveillance recommendations.

Family History

Common sense would suggest that women with a family history of breast cancer would more readily engage in surveillance because of its relevance to their health. However, the results of investigations of this relationship have been mixed. Family history is positively related to mammography in some studies (65,66), unrelated in some investigations (22,67,64), and negatively related in others (68,69). Meta-analysis of mammography screening studies concluded that despite divergent findings, there is a small to moderate positive relationship between family history and mammography screening (70). However, most of the variance in mammography and BSE frequency is unexplained. This suggests that other

factors are important in women's decisions to engage in surveillance.

Health Beliefs

It is important to communicate to women that screening can be valuable, to provide accurate information, and to address their concerns about radiation. Beliefs that mammography is effective and that detecting breast cancer early is valuable are associated with better surveillance (66,71–73). Lack of perceived need was negatively related to surveillance (71). Thinking that surveillance, such as BSE, is not effective or not believing in one's ability to perform the behavior can lead to hopelessness as well as inaction (9,74). Poor knowledge of risk factors is related to less screening (75).

Other factors affecting surveillance include poor understanding of breast cancer or cancer surveillance and fears about pain, embarrassment, or discomfort. Women who believed that having a mammogram would alleviate their fears also were more likely to undergo mammography (76), but misconceptions that bumps and bruises may cause cancer were related to inadequate cancer screening (28). Some women do not participate in mammography screening because of embarrassment about the procedure and concerns about cost and radiation (65). Fears about pain or radiation exposure were important barriers in other studies as well (71,77; for review, see 78).

Distress

It is not clear how distress affects surveillance behaviors, and the answer is most likely complex (79). Negative emotions generally interfere with health behaviors, and fear may cause people to abandon attempts to detect or prevent disease so that attention to the disease is reduced (8,80). In addition, participation in some screening and surveillance activities is anxiety-producing (81,82). Anxiety about screening can interfere with the repeat routine screening as well (65). This anxiety may be due to the nature of the behavior: Looking for a breast abnormality increases the chance of finding something wrong (83).

If a woman does find something suspicious, she may become distressed and reluctant to seek medical care out of fear of what might be found. Over a third of a sample of middle-aged women reported being afraid of performing BSE because they feared finding a lump (84). Although not "rational," the belief that "if it has not been diagnosed, it is not real" may characterize such behavior. Women may spend several weeks or more appraising the symptom before calling for a medical appointment (85), and a third or more may wait 3 or more months (for a review, see 86). When healthy women were asked to imagine that they detected a breast abnormality, those with a family history of breast cancer reported that they would be less likely to seek care and were more pessimistic about the usefulness of care seeking than those without a family history (87). Some women may be worried that if they seek care for a lump that proves to be nonexistent after screening, their physician will think they are overreacting (84).

One of the first studies to examine distress and surveillance found that although women at higher risk for breast cancer were more knowledgeable about BSE than women at lower risk, they performed BSE less often and were more fearful of doing BSE because of fear of finding a lump (88). In addition, frequency of BSE was negatively correlated with perceived severity of breast cancer for women with a family history of breast cancer, although the correlation was positive for women without a family history (88). Since then, some studies have suggested that distress increases motivation and surveillance (89), but as noted earlier, research is inconsistent on this matter. Studies also suggest the opposite, that distress decreases surveillance activities (43,90,91). In some studies risk and distress are associated with overadherence to surveillance programs (92), whereas in others distress is not related to surveillance at all (93).

One possible explanation for these findings is that there is a curvilinear relationship between family history of breast cancer and mammography, mediated by anxiety or fear (94). This suggests that a moderate level of anxiety is optimal for motivating women to participate in surveillance behaviors. At low levels of anxiety, women are unmotivated for surveillance, and at very high levels of anxiety, women may be too upset and be "paralyzed" by this fear and avoid

the threat. This is consistent with research and theory on the impact of fear-arousing situations (8,95,96).

Some support for this curvilinear hypothesis comes from a study of breast cancer worry, mood, and daily functioning (82). Women who reported that their daily functioning was affected by their breast cancer concerns were more likely to practice monthly BSE than were women with the highest or lowest levels of impact. Mulvihill and colleagues (97) reported a case study of a distraught young woman with a family history of breast cancer who believed her death from breast cancer was inevitable. After undergoing three benign biopsies, she avoided medical follow-up for 15 years. A meta-analysis of six available studies at the time indicated that greater worry was linearly related to better levels of mammography screening (70). However, the average weighted effect size was small, and not all studies showed a positive relationship. Incorporating subsequent studies may help clarify the role of distress in surveillance.

Individual Differences

How a woman sees the world can affect her well-being and coping and health behaviors. Optimism is a personality characteristic reflecting people's expectations about positive outcomes in the world (98). There is some evidence that women who engage in surveillance are more optimistic and problem-solving oriented (99). Optimism has been linked to less delay in seeking care for cancer symptoms (100). Neuroticism, the tendency to experience negative and distressing emotions (101), has been negatively related to mammography attendance (102). Personality constructs such as extroversion and assertiveness also have been examined (103). Although predictive of mammography screening, these factors were no longer significant predictors after adjusting for traditional correlates of mammography such as perceived risk, family history, and insurance coverage (103).

Individual differences in attending to and processing threat-relevant information can determine whether or what kind of action is taken (104). Some individuals have a tendency to scan for and focus on health threats, and others tend to blunt or tune out such information (105).

Health threats that cannot be extinguished readily, such as the threat of breast cancer, may pose a greater challenge to those who are highly attentive to health information (106). These individuals may become distressed due to the severity of the threat and from the lack of a strategy for immediate resolution. Individual differences in how one takes up health-relevant information, the emotional reactions to this information, thoughts about it, and other dispositional characteristics all affect health-protective behavior (for a discussion of BSE, see 107).

Women's health also may be affected by their family and friends. *Social support* can be defined as the belief that one is a valued member of a group and that one is cared for and loved (108). There is considerable evidence that social support is linked to psychological and physical health outcomes (109). Prospective epidemiologic studies have shown that social support is associated with decreased mortality (110,111), lower levels of stress, and reduction of psychological distress during times of threat or demand (109,112,113).

People who have more extensive social relationships are more likely to avoid health-damaging behavior. Broman (114) found that married people had lower levels of smoking and drinking and that a large number of social relationships predicted such health behaviors as wearing a seat belt and engaging in less smoking and drinking. Loss of a social relationship was associated with increases in health-damaging behaviors, and gains in support were related to increases in health-protective behaviors (114). In a study of daughters of breast cancer patients, the frequency of BSE increased with the frequency of talking with their mothers about breast cancer (91). Increased BSE may have been affected by this display of support and caring.

Descriptive and demographic factors are also related to surveillance. Women who are older are less likely to engage in cancer screening (64,66,115) and are more likely to have never had a mammogram despite their increased risk of breast cancer (71). Part of this may be due to not receiving adequate surveillance information; for example, older women were less likely than younger women to be instructed in BSE by health professionals despite a similar number of health visits (84). Those with insurance, more education, and a higher income were more likely to participate in screening (63,115), and women who live in rural areas were less likely to do so (63,64). Women were more likely to engage in screening if they used estrogen, if they thought they were very healthy (71), and if they practiced other preventive health behaviors (for a review, see 116).

Reducing Distress and Increasing Surveillance

It is clear that a sizable group of women at high risk for breast cancer have inaccurate risk perceptions and are worried about developing breast cancer. Several interventions have been developed to make risk perceptions more accurate and to ameliorate distress associated with risk. Ultimately, these interventions are directed at increasing surveillance behaviors. One focus has been on reminding and encouraging women to attend mammography screening through letters, phone calls, or visits from a nurse, and these have achieved varying levels of success. Mailed reminders to set up an appointment and convey information can be effective in increasing adherence of women at high risk for cancer (117). In addition to the mailed reminder, a phone call to remind, counsel, and schedule an appointment can increase the likelihood of a woman obtaining a mammogram (118). A mailed reminder also can encourage women to keep scheduled appointments. Margolis and Menart (119) compared a mailed reminder with counseling from a nurse, finding that the mailed reminder improved appointment keeping by about 5% over the 25% failure to show rate, while nurse counseling added very little.

Another approach has been to address specific sources of distress that may affect surveillance. Receiving abnormal mammogram results and having to return for repeated screening is stress-producing, and many women do not follow up. In one effort to increase repeat mammography, women who received abnormal mammogram results were mailed a booklet containing information about abnormal mammograms, discussing the importance of continued screening and providing suggestions for managing anxiety about mammography (120). This booklet showed modest utility in helping women adhere to surveillance recommendations. Compared with women who did not receive the information, women who received the information were more likely to obtain a mammogram the following year (120). Alternatively, one can decrease anxiety associated with abnormal mammography results by providing more immediate results. When asked, women thought that their anxiety could have been reduced by shortening the waiting period for results of follow-up of abnormal results (47).

More complex interventions also have been evaluated. Accurate risk perception appears to be an important component of one's emotional and behavioral reaction to risk. An intervention designed for women with a family history of breast cancer tested the notion that modification of risk estimates to more accurate levels lead to reductions in distress (121). Women received individualized risk counseling based on the Gail model as well as information about screening recommendations and instruction in BSE techniques. Despite this counseling, almost two-thirds of the women continued to overestimate their level of risk. Analyses indicated that distress levels were not mediated by perceived risk; that is, more accurate risk estimates did not lead to decreased distress. However, women with a high-school education or less reported reductions in distress about breast cancer at 3 months after the intervention. The authors speculated that other factors may be involved in the reduction of distress, such as improvements in knowledge about breast cancer and prevention or self-efficacy (121).

Another intervention designed to make risk estimates more accurate and to decrease distress associated with risk was evaluated in a group of women with a family history of breast cancer who obtained risk counseling at a breast cancer family clinic (122). The intervention showed some promising immediate results, in that women became more accurate in estimating their risk. In addition, women who overestimated their risk initially exhibited less anxiety after counseling, but observed changes were short-lived.

Three months after the intervention, anxiety had returned to initial levels (122).

Kash and colleagues (123) reported a pilot test of a group intervention consisting of six group meetings of women at high risk. All women had two or more first-degree relatives with breast cancer and were participating in a breast cancer surveillance program. The women were given information about their risk status, taught coping skills and BSE, and as a group discussed the importance of adhering to screening guidelines. Emotional support also was provided by the group, and several booster sessions helped to reinforce the intervention. Immediately after the intervention, women reported more accurate risk estimates and more knowledge of breast cancer and risk factors, and they showed better adherence to screening. At the 3-year follow-up, gains in adherence to screening were maintained. More work is needed on ways to improve adherence to effective surveillance regimens.

Issues for Women

Women at risk for breast cancer vary in their perceptions of risk, how much they worry about their risk, and how they cope with the situation. Some women with elevated risk may worry about breast cancer to such a degree that it interferes with surveillance and disrupts everyday life (82). These worries may be so distressing that they become a barrier, preventing the women from doing the very things that provide some health benefit. Early detection and chemoprevention are among the best weapons we have against premature death from breast cancer. Avoiding surveillance or other actions may decrease short-term distress, but it maintains and may exacerbate distress over the long term and can have serious health consequences.

Women who have a relative with current or past breast cancer or a relative who died from breast cancer, may face very upsetting issues. In addition to the distress caused by having a seriously ill relative, a relative's diagnosis may remind women at risk of the reality of their own situation. Women may reevaluate their risk level and increase their perceptions of personal risk (124). Women also may feel guilty for being disease-free while a family member suffers and perhaps for passing on an inherited genetic predisposition to their daughters (123). There is little action that can be taken to reverse a relative's diagnosis or a daughter's genetic constitution, perhaps leading to feelings of anger and hopelessness. A relative's diagnosis also may affect a woman's sexuality. Although no differences were found in general distress levels, adult daughters of breast cancer patients reported less frequent sexual intercourse and lower sexual satisfaction than women without a mother with breast cancer (46).

An important aspect of coping with health threats for some people is the opportunity to discuss, compare, and interact with others about their fears or worries. However, women at elevated risk for breast cancer may feel isolated in their worries and may not feel comfortable discussing their risk or worries with friends or family. Cancer is a topic that conjures up threatening images for many people, and others may not be receptive to talking about it because it makes them anxious or uncomfortable. The threat of cancer does not lend itself to many problem-solving strategies, and people may feel frustrated that there is no solution and that management strategies are limited.

At a time when social support is very important, problems may develop in this domain as well. Some people may not be able to understand why a woman would worry about a problem that has not yet occurred and believe that she is wasting her time and energy or acting foolish. Women may feel particularly inhibited talking about their worries with a friend or relative who already has breast cancer (123). It can be difficult discussing one's fear of cancer with someone who is living with it because one's worries can seem to pale in comparison with the situation of an afflicted friend or family member. The afflicted friend or family member is likely to be caught up in her own problems of adjusting to cancer and may not be the best choice for an empathic listener. Having the support and understanding of others who are in a similar situation was part of the reasoning behind the group intervention designed by Kash and colleagues (123), and some success was achieved

as women became less distressed and more likely to maintain surveillance.

Lack of emotional support can be detrimental to one's well-being and have implications for behavior as well. Women who report having few people with whom they can discuss worries about their health or have a friend or relative who discourages them from having a mammogram are more likely to have negative attitudes about mammography (125). Negative attitudes about surveillance, together with distress about developing breast cancer, can lead to inaction and can exacerbate distress. Support from friends and family, including encouraging one's new health behaviors, giving comforting words, reassuring them about providing help in case of a future cancer diagnosis, and accompanying them on medical appointments, can help women to manage their high-risk status and to believe that they will be able to cope with a potential cancer diagnosis.

Issues for Physicians

The physician plays a key role in helping women manage their risk status and adhere to surveillance recommendations (126–128). Referral by one's physician is often cited by women as the most important reason for mammography screening (129), and lack of referral is frequently cited as a reason for not seeking screening (67). Adherence with screening guidelines requires that women are aware of screening recommendations (28,130). Guidelines for assessing genetic risk and for advising women about how to manage their risk have been discussed elsewhere (see Chap. 4) (131).

Management of women at higher risk for breast cancer involves several tasks: 1) obtaining relevant background information and informing women of their risk for breast cancer, 2) educating and correcting misconceptions about breast cancer, 3) making recommendations for screening, genetic testing, chemoprevention, or prophylactic surgery, and 4) following up on these recommendations. It is likely that women's distress levels are heightened during a breast cancer checkup and that this distress can interfere with her understanding of information, decision making, and adherence to medical advice. The main goal of effective management of women at risk is to maximize positive health behaviors such as regular mammography screening, exercise, and low-fat diet while minimizing emotional distress and increasing quality of life.

Risk Assessment

Physicians can assess risk factors and provide women with accurate estimates of risk for developing breast cancer. Risk evaluation helps both the patient and the medical staff to be vigilant, maintain surveillance for early signs of disease, and allow for modification of the patient's lifestyle to lessen risk if possible. It also permits selective application of chemoprevention. Detailed discussion of "actual" risk and of ways to obtain even more precise estimates may help dispel misconceptions and reduce risk overestimation. Discussion of risk should be done with awareness of the tendency to distort and most likely overestimate risk and should ensure that accurate perceptions are maintained. Educating women about risk and surveillance recommendations is important. Some first-degree relatives of breast cancer patients report that they never have been asked about their family history of breast cancer by their physicians or provided with familial risk information (27,132). Although risk counseling has been shown to be only partially successful, women may form perceptions of risk from inaccurate sources when no information is provided (123). Faulty estimates that may be overblown can lead to exacerbation of distress. One clear and understandable way to communicate the degree of risk is to state the risk in terms of the woman's probability of developing breast cancer in a certain number of years (126,127). A second approach is to frame the risk in terms of the chance of not developing breast cancer in that time period (123). Communicating risk estimates in a nonthreatening manner can minimize distress and improve understanding of risk information. The physician's emotional tone when talking with a woman about her risk also may make a difference. Women recall less information and inflate the severity of their risk when they perceive that the physician is anxious (133).

Management Strategies

There are several strategies for medical management of high-risk patients, including close surveillance, referral for genetic testing, bilateral prophylactic mastectomy, and referral to a research protocol testing a chemopreventive agent (eg., tamoxifen; see Chap. 12). Each strategy has it own sources of stress that may negatively affect women's emotional functioning, their relationship with their physician, and health behaviors. Surveillance is the option chosen most often by women and their physicians, and the psychological implications of surveillance are the best understood. Although bilateral prophylactic mastectomy has been offered for at least 20 years, relatively few women have chosen this option, and less is known about its psychological consequences. Psychological factors in genetic testing have been examined only recently, and less is known about chemoprevention.

Surveillance

Close surveillance involves either annual or semiannual mammography, CBE every 4 to 6 months, and proficient monthly BSE. Younger women with a family history of breast cancer may be advised to have their first mammogram about 10 years earlier than the age at which their relative was diagnosed if it was less than age 45 (134). However, women may not be performing BSE correctly (84) or may have difficulty adhering to close surveillance guidelines (97). Close surveillance requires repeated visits to the doctor that can be distressing to women, reminding them of their risk and activating the fear of learning of a cancer diagnosis, as well as reminding them of friends and family who already have cancer or may have died from breast cancer (123). These repeated follow-up visits and monthly BSEs may result in a continuously elevated level of distress.

Women may begin close surveillance with good intentions but may quickly become overcome with anxiety about discovering breast cancer. Depending on a woman's personality, coping style, and other stressors in her life, she may or may not continue to adhere to appropriate surveillance. Some women may decide to lessen their anxiety by avoiding medical visits and BSEs, whereas others may go in the opposite direction and repeatedly call and visit their physician with vague symptoms or worries about cancer and engage in excessive BSEs. Patients who overuse medical services are difficult to manage and can engender feelings of frustration in medical staff. Reassurance and support from the medical staff can make breast cancer check ups easier for women and increase the likelihood that they will appropriately adhere to the surveillance recommendations (135).

Genetic Testing

Genetic testing for the *BRCA1* and *BRCA2* mutations can provide women with information about their risk for breast cancer and reduce uncertainty about whether they are a mutation carrier. Both these benefits may help to decrease stress and anxiety associated with being at risk. They also can help women and physicians make decisions about surveillance and prophylactic surgeries. However, the uncertainty reduction associated with testing may be overwhelmed by distress associated with high-risk outcomes.

Women at high risk for breast cancer generally are interested in genetic testing. In one study, approximately three-quarters of the women with one or more first-degree relatives with breast cancer planned to seek genetic testing (136). In another, over half the sample of women with a family history of breast cancer who underwent testing chose to know their genetic testing results. Those who chose to learn the results were more likely to be experiencing cancer-specific distress (137).

There is some evidence that testing and getting results can generate anxiety and fear that may subside for noncarriers but which persists for those identified as carriers (138). Lerman and colleagues (121) found that at 1 month after disclosure of test results, evaluation of risk was associated with a significant reduction in depressive symptoms and functional impairment among noncarriers of *BRCA1* compared with carriers and nontested individuals. Of the carriers, 17% intended to have a mastectomy, and 33% planned to have oophorectomies (121).

Baum and colleagues (139) have proposed a model of emotional reactions to genetic testing that suggests that psychological response to testing will vary according to the nature of the test, uncertainty, outcome of the results, and psychosocial resources of the individual, such as social support and coping style. Being identified as a carrier will be more threatening if there are no preventive measures that can be taken and the nature of the disease and/or its treatment is severe. Ideally, those who are carriers should be motivated to increase surveillance for early signs of disease. However, stress experienced because of increased risk may interfere with appropriate surveillance activities and may reduce compliance with prevention regimens.

Although finding out that one is not a carrier of a breast cancer gene may be reassuring, it only eliminates known heritable components of breast cancer risk that account for only 5% to 10% of all cases. Noncarriers may still be at high risk for breast cancer and may need to continue close surveillance. A different problem is related to the fact that several family members undergo testing at approximately the same time. A woman who finds out she is a noncarrier may experience mixed emotions of relief and guilt if other family members are identified as carriers. Alternatively, finding out that one is a carrier may bring up feelings of anger toward family members who are noncarriers and feelings of sadness for potentially passing the gene to one's offspring.

Bilateral Prophylactic Mastectomy

Bilateral prophylactic mastectomy involves the removal of noncancerous breast tissues in both breasts in order to prevent breast cancer. In general, it appears that prophylactic mastectomy may reduce but not eliminate the risk of breast cancer (140). Perhaps the most likely candidates for this procedure are younger women who are carriers of the *BRCA1* or *BRCA2* gene (141). Gains in life expectancy decrease with age, and the benefits for a 60-year-old woman are minimal (141). In a study of high-risk women, a third of the women who were interested in genetic testing said they would seek prophylactic mastectomy if they tested positive (27).

At present, there is no established recommendation for or against this procedure in women with the *BRCA1* or *BRCA2* mutations (142). The lack of clear guidelines leaves the decision largely up to the woman and her physician. Surgeons vary on the level of absolute lifetime risk for breast cancer at which they would recommend a woman undergo prophylactic mastectomy, reporting risk estimates ranging from 0% to 100%, with an average threshold risk of 48% given by surgeons who had ever recommended the procedure (143). Of the 700 surgeons polled for this study, a minority of them cited the patient's wishes and desires as a factor influencing the decision to recommend bilateral prophylactic mastectomy (143).

Uncertainty and lack of information may make it more difficult for a women to decide whether to have the surgery or not. Before a decision is made to undergo this surgery, patients need to be aware that a bilateral prophylactic mastectomy does not guarantee that they will be cancer-free for their lifetime. Furthermore, the cosmetic outcome of the surgery, even with reconstruction, may be more disfiguring than a lumpectomy for early-stage disease (126). Women should be provided with a realistic description of the possible cosmetic results. Anxiety and perceptions of risk are also likely to influence this decision (97). In a study of women at increased risk of breast cancer, women with a history of biopsies and high perceived risk of and worry about breast cancer were the most interested in learning more about bilateral prophylactic mastectomy (144). Women who were the most worried underwent the surgery.

The psychological impact of bilateral prophylactic mastectomy has not been well studied, and little is known. In the study by Stefanek and colleagues (144), the 14 women who elected surgery were followed for 6 to 30 months and in general reported being satisfied with their decision to have the surgery. These women also reported that they received strong support for their decision from their partner, family, and friends. This indicates that an important component of the decision-making process may include inquiring about support from others in this decision. Clearly, more work needs to be done to understand how women are affected by this surgery (see also 145).

Conclusion

Ongoing identification of risk factors for breast cancer has allowed women and medical personnel to assess risk, to closely monitor health status of those most at risk, and to modify sources of risk. There are steps that women at high risk can take to facilitate early detection and ultimately better prognosis, yet many women do not take action. Reasons for this inaction are complex, but risk perception and the emotional reaction to risk perception are two main factors. Inflated risk estimates can increase distress and worry about breast cancer that negatively affect quality of life and can compromise adherence to surveillance guidelines. The continuous threats associated with risk for breast cancer and repeated routine screening suggest that this distress may be persistent and come to characterize increasingly major aspects of one's daily life. Women face several options for care, including close surveillance, genetic testing, chemoprevention, and prophylactic surgery, all of which paradoxically may increase distress in some cases and alleviate fear and uncertainty in others. A woman's physician is one of the strongest sources of motivation for screening and can play a central role in educating them about breast cancer and helping them to manage their distress. Physicians can help women by clearly communicating risk estimates, providing information about breast cancer risk factors and management options, encouraging routine screening, and offering support.

References

1. Fisher B, Costantino JP, Wickerham DL, et al. Tamoxifen for prevention of breast cancer: Report of the National Surgical Adjuvant Breast and Bowel Project P-1 Study. J Natl Cancer Inst 1998;90:1371–1388.
2. Huguley C, Brown R, Greenberg R, Clark W. Breast self-examination and survival from breast cancer. Cancer 1988;62:1389–1396.
3. Kerlikowske K, Grady D, Rubin S, et al. Efficacy of screening mammography: a meta-analysis. JAMA 1995;273:149–154.
4. Breast Cancer Facts and Figures 1997. New York: American Cancer Society, Inc. 1997.
5. Berman SH, Wandersman A. Fear of cancer and knowledge of cancer: a review and proposed relevance to hazardous waste sites. Soc Sci Med 1990;1:81–90.
6. Slovic P. Perceptions of risk. Science 1997;236:280–285.
7. Rogers R. Cognitive and physiological processes in attitude change: a revised theory

of protection motivation. Soc Psychophysiol 1983;34:562–566.

8. Leventhal H. Toward a comprehensive theory of emotion. Adv Exp Soc Psychol 1980;13: 139–207.

9. Rippetoe, P, & Rogers, R. Effects of components of protection-motivation theory on adaptive and maladaptive coping with a health threat. J Pers Soc Psychol 1987;52:596–604.

10. Janz N, Becker M. The health belief model: a decade later. Health Educ Q 1984;11:1–47.

11. Rosenstock I. The health belief model: origins and correlates. Health Edu Monogr 1974;2:336–353.

12. Aiken LS, West SG, Woodward CK, Reno RR. Health beliefs and compliance with mammography-screening recommendations in a-symptomatic women. Health Psychol 1994; 13:122–129.

13. Champion V. Compliance with guidelines for mammography screening. Cancer Detect Prev 1992;16:253–258.

14. Seydel E, Taal E, Wiegman O. Risk-appraisal, outcome, and self-efficacy expectancies: cognitive factors in preventive behavior related to cancer. Psychol Health 1990;4:99–109.

15. Lek Y, Bishop G. Perceived vulnerability to illness threats: the role of disease type, risk factor perception and attributions. Psychol Health 1995;10:205–217.

16. Weinstein N. Unrealistic optimism about susceptibility to health problems: conclusions from a community-wide sample. J Behav Med 1987;10:481–500.

17. Daly M, Lerman C, Ross E, et al. Gail model breast cancer risk components are poor predictors of risk perception and screening behavior. Breast Cancer Res Treat 1996;41:59–70.

18. Smith B, Gadd M, Lawler C, et al. Perceptions of breast cancer risk among women in breast center and primary care settings: correlation with age and family history of breast cancer. Surgery 1996;120:297–303.

19. Gail MH, Brinton LA, Byar DP, et al. Projecting individualized probabilities of developing breast cancer for white females who are being screening annually. J Natl Cancer Inst 1989;81:1877–1886.

20. Anderson E, Steel C, Smyth E, Cull A. Knowledge, attitudes, health-related behavior and emotional status of women with a family history of breast cancer. Psychooncology 1994;3:139. Meeting abstract.

21. Dolan N, Lee A, McDermott M. Age-related differences in breast carcinoma knowledge,

beliefs, and perceived risk among women visiting an academic general medicine practice. Cancer 1997;80:413–420.

22. Aiken LS, Fenaughty AM, West SG, et al. Perceived determinants of risk for breast cancer and the relations among objective risk, perceived risk, and screening behavior over time. Womens Health 1995;1:27–50.

23. Lerman C, Lustbader E, Rimer B, et al. Effects of individualized breast cancer risk counseling: a randomized trial. J Natl Cancer Inst 1995;87:286–292.

24. Black W, Nease R, Tosteson A. Perceptions of breast cancer risk and screening effectiveness in women younger than 50 years of age. J Natl Cancer Inst 1995;87:720–731.

25. Schwartz L, Woloshin S, Black W, Welch H. The role of numeracy in understanding the benefit of screening mammography. Ann Intern Med 1997;127:966–972.

26. Bostick R, Sprafka J, Virnig B, Potter J. Knowledge, attitudes, and personal practices regarding prevention and early detection of cancer. Prev Med 1993;22:65–85.

27. Royak-Schaler R, Cheuvront B, Wilson K, Williams C. Addressing women's breast cancer risk and perceptions of control in medical settings. J Clin Psychol Med Set 1996;3(3): 185–199.

28. Morgan C, Park E, Cortes D. Beliefs, knowledge, and behavior about cancer among urban Hispanic women. J Natl Cancer Inst. Monogr 1995;18:57–63.

29. Weinstein N. Why it won't happen to me: perceptions of risk factors and susceptibility. Health Psychol 1984;3:431–457.

30. Kulik J, Mahler H. Health status, perceptions of risk and prevention interest for health and nonhealth problems. Health Psychol 1987;6:15–27.

31. Baum A, Cohen L. Successful behavioral interventions to prevent cancer: the example of skin cancer. Annu Rev Public Health 1998;19: 319–333.

32. Slovic P, Fischhoff B, Lichtenstein S. Behavioral decision theory perspectives on risk and safety. Acta Psychol 1984;56:183–203.

33. McNeil B, Pauker S, Sox H, Tversky A. On the elicitation of preferences for alternative therapies. New Engl J Med 1982;306:1259–1262.

34. Keown C, Slovic P, Lichtenstein S. Attitudes of physicians, pharmacists, and laypersons toward seriousness and need for disclosure of prescription drug side effects. Health Psychol 1984;3:1–11.

35. Tversky A, Kahneman D. Availability: a heuristic for judging frequency and probability. Cogn Psychol 1973;5:207–232.

36. Weinstein N. Optimistic biases about personal risks. Science 1989;246:1232–1233.

37. Nayfield SG, Karp JE, Ford LG, et al. Potential role of tamoxifen in prevention of breast cancer. J Natl Cancer Inst 1991;83:1450–1459.

38. Vernon SW, Vogel VG, Halabi S, Bondy ML. Factors associated with perceived risk of breast cancer among women attending a screening program. Breast Cancer Res Treat 1993;28:137–144.

39. Wortman CB, Dunkel-Schetter C. Interpersonal relationships and cancer: a theoretical analysis. J Soc Issues 1979;35:120–155.

40. Lerman C, Kash K, Stefanek M. Younger women at increased risk for breast cancer: perceived risk, psychological well-being, and surveillance behavior. J Natl Cancer Inst Monogr 1994;16:171–176.

41. Valdimarsdottir H, Bovbjerg D, Kash K, et al. Psychological distress in women with a familial risk of breast cancer. Psychooncology 1995;4:133–141.

42. Gilbar O. Women with high risk for breast cancer: psychological symptoms. Psychol Rep 1997;80:800–802.

43. Kash KM, Holland JC, Halper MS, Miller DG. Psychological distress and surveillance behaviors of women with a family history of breast cancer. J Natl Cancer Inst 1992;84:24–30.

44. Lerman C, Daly M, Sands C, et al. Mammography adherence and psychological distress among women at risk for breast cancer. J Natl Cancer Inst 1993;85:1074–1080.

45. Lloyd S, Watson M, Waites B, et al. Familial breast cancer: a controlled study of risk perception, psychological morbidity and health beliefs in women attending for genetic counselling. Br J Cancer 1996;74:482–487.

46. Wellisch D, Gritz E, Schain W, et al. Psychological functioning of daughters of breast cancer patients: I. Daughters and comparison subjects. Psychosom Dis 1991;32(3):324–336.

47. Ellman R, Angeli N, Christians A, et al. Psychiatric morbidity associated with screening for breast cancer. Br J Cancer 1989;60:781–784.

48. Lerman C, Trock B, Rimer B, et al. Psychological and behavioral implications of abnormal mammograms. Ann Intern Med 1991;114:657–661.

49. Gilbert F, Cordiner C, Afleck I, et al. How anxiogenic is recall following breast screening and does a family history of breast cancer make a difference? Psychooncology 1995;4:88. Meeting abstract.

50. Cannon W. Bodily Changes in Pain, Hunger, Fear, and Rage. Boston: Branford, 1929.

51. Selye H. The Stress of Life. New York: McGraw-Hill, 1976.

52. Mason J. A historical view of the stress field. J Hum Stress 1975;1:22–36.

53. Lazarus R. Psychological Stress and the Coping Process. New York: Springer, 1996.

54. Baum A. Stress, intrusive imagery, and chronic distress. Health Psychol 1990;9:653–675.

55. Kiecolt-Glaser J, Malarkey W, Cacioppo J, Glaser R. Stressful personal relationships: immune and endocrine factors. In: Glaser R, Kiecolt-Glaser J, eds. Handbook of Human Stress and Immunity. San Diego: Academic Press, 1994:321–340.

56. Delahanty D, Dougall A, Hawken L, et al. Time course of natural killer cell activity and lymphocyte proliferation in responses to two acute stressors in healthy men. Health Psychol 1996;15:48–55.

57. Kiecolt-Glaser J, Stephens R, Lipetz P, et al. Distress and DNA repair in human lymphocytes. J Behav Med 1985;8:311–320.

58. Steptoe A, Wardle J, Pollard T, Canaan L. Stress, social support and health-related behavior: a study of smoking, alcohol consumption and physical exercise. J Psychosom Res 1996;41:171–180.

59. Leith L, Taylor A. Psychological aspects of exercise: a decade literature review. Sport Behav 1990;13:219–239.

60. Plante T, Rodin J. Physical fitness and enhanced psychological health. Curr Psychol Res Rev 1990;9:3–24.

61. Huang Z, Hankinson S, Colditz G, et al. Dual effects of weight and weight gain on breast cancer risk. JAMA 1997;278(17):1407–1411.

62. Bovjberg D, Valdimarsdottir H. Familial cancer, emotional distress, and low natural cytotoxic activity in healthy women. Ann Oncol 1993;4:745–752.

63. Calle EE, Flanders WD, Thun MJ, Martin LM. Demographic predictors of mammography and pap smear screening in U.S. women. Am J Public Health 1993;83:3–60.

64. Kaplan K, Weinberg G, Small A, Herndon J. Breast cancer screening among relatives of women with breast cancer. Am J Public Health 1991;81(9):1174–1179.

65. Lerman C, Rimer B, Trock B, et al. Factors associated with repeat adherence to breast cancer screening. Prev Med 1990;19:279–290.

66. Polednak A, Lane D, Burg M. Risk perception, family history, and use of breast cancer screening tests. Cancer Detect Prev 1991;15:257–263.

67. Vogel V, Graves D, Vernon S, et al. Mammographic screening of women with increased risk of breast cancer. Cancer 1990;66:1613–1620.

68. Laville E, Vernon S, Jackson G, Hughes J. Comparison of participants and nonparticipants in a work site cancer awareness and screening program. J Occup Med 1989;31:221–232.

69. Hyman R, Baker S, Ephraigm R, et al. Health belief model variables as predictors of screening mamography utilization. J Behav Med 1994;17(4):391–406.

70. McCaul K, Branstetter A, Schroeder D, Glasgow R. What is the relationship between breast cancer risk and mammography screening? A meta-analytic review. Health Psychol 1996;15(6):423–429.

71. Fullerton J, Kritz-Silverstein D, Sadler G, Barret-Connor E. Mammography usage in a community-based sample of older women. Ann Behav Med 1996;18:67–72.

72. Cole S, Bryant C, McDermott R, et al. Beliefs and mammography screening. Am J Prev Med 1997;13:439–443.

73. Rodriguez C, Plasencia A, Schroeder D. Predictive factors of enrollment and adherence in a breast cancer screening program in Barcelona (Spain). Soc Sci Med 1995;40:1155–1160.

74. Fletcher SW, Morgan TM, O'Malley MS, et al. Is breast self-examination predicted by knowledge, attitudes, beliefs, or sociodemographic characteristics? Am J Prev Med 1989;5:207–215.

75. Costanza M, Stoddard A, Gaw V, Zapka J. The risk factors of age and family history and their relationship to screening mammography utilization. J Am Geriatr Soc 1992;40:774–778.

76. Thomas L, Fox S, Leake B, Roetzheim R. The effects of health beliefs on screening mammography utilization among a diverse sample of older women. Womens Health 1996;24:77–94.

77. Bastani R, Marcus A, Maxwell A, et al. Evaluation of an intervention to increase mammography screening in Los Angeles. Prev Med 1994;23:83–90.

78. Keefe F, Hauck E, Egert J, et al. Mammography pain and discomfort: a cognitive-behavioral perspective. Pain 1994;56:247–260.

79. Lerman C, Schwartz M. Adherence and psychological adjustment among women at high risk for breast cancer. Breast Cancer Res Treat 1993;28:145–155.

80. Krantz D, Grunberg N, Baum A. Health psychology. Annu Rev Psychol 1985;36:349–383.

81. Dean C, Roberts M, French K, Robinson S. Psychiatric morbidity after screening for breast cancer. J Epidemiol Commun Health 1986;40:71–75.

82. Lerman C, Trock B, Rimer B, et al. Psychological side effects of breast cancer screening. Health Psychol 1991;10:259–267.

83. Mayer J, Solomon L. Breast self-examination skill and frequency: a review. Ann Behav Med 1992;14:189–196.

84. Dunbar J, Begg L, Yasko J, Belle S. Breast self-examination compliance among older high risk women. Patient Educ Couns 1991;18:223–230.

85. Andersen B, Cacioppo J, Roberts D. Delay in seeking a cancer diagnosis: delay stages and psychophysiological comparison processes. Br J Soc Psychol 1995;34:33–52.

86. Facione N. Delay versus help seeking for breast cancer symptoms: a critical review of the literature on patient and provider delay. Soc Sci Med 1993;36:1521–1534.

87. Lauver D, Change A. Testing theoretical explanations of intention to seek care for a breast cancer symptom. J Appl Psychol 1991;21:1440–1458.

88. Alagna SW, Morokoff PJ, Bevett JM, Reddy DM. Performance of breast self-examination by women at high risk for breast cancer. Womens Health 1987;12:29–46.

89. McCaul K, Schroeder D, Reid P. Breast cancer worry and screening: some prospective data. Health Psychol 1996;15:430–433.

90. Rimer BK, Kentz MK, Kessler HG, et al. Why women resist screening mammography: patient-related barriers. Radiology 1996;172:243–246.

91. Benedict S, Goon G, Hoomani J, Holder P. Breast cancer detection by daughters of women with breast cancer. Cancer Pract 1997;5:213–219.

92. Epstein S, Lin T, Audrain J, et al., and The High-Risk Breast Cancer Consortium. Excessive breast self-examination among first-degree relatives of newly diagnosed breast cancer patients. Psychosomatics 1997;38(3):253–261.

93. Sutton S, Saidi G, Bickler G, Hunter J. Does routine screening for breast cancer raise anxiety? Results from a three wave prospective study in England. J Epidemiol Commun Health 1995;49:413–418.

94. Hailey B. Family history of breast cancer and screening behavior: an inverted U-shaped curve? Med Hypoth 1991;36397–36403.

95. Janis IL, Feshbach S. Effects of fear-arousing communications. Abnorm Soc Psychol 1953;48: 78–92.

96. Janis IL. Psychological Stress: Psychological and Behavioral Studies of Surgical Patients. New York: Academic Press, 1958.

97. Mulvihill J, Safyer A, Bening J. Prevention in familial breast cancer: counseling and prophylactic mastectomy. Prev Med 1982;11: 500–511.

98. Scheier M, Carver C. Effects of optimism on psychological and physical well-being: theoretical overview and empirical update. Cognit Ther Res 1992;16:201–228.

99. Kreitler S, Chaitchik S, Kreitler H, Weissler K. Who will attend tests for the early detection of breast cancer? Psychol Health 1994;9:463–483.

100. Lauver D, Tak Y. Optimism and coping with a breast cancer symptom. Nurs Res 1995;44: 202–207.

101. Costa P, McCrae R. Role of neuroticism in the perception and presentation of chest pain symptoms and coronary artery disease. In: Elias J, Marshall P, eds. Cardiovascualr Disease and Behavior. Series in Health Psychol and Behavioral Medicine. Washington: Hemisphere, 1987:39–66.

102. Kreitler S, Chaitchik S, Kreitler H. The psychological profile of women attending breast-screening test. Soc Sci Med 1990;31:1177–1185.

103. Siegler I, Feananes J, Rimer B. Predictors of adoption of mammography in women under age 50. Health Psychol 1995;14:274–278.

104. Krohne H. The concept of coping modes: relating cognitive person variables to actual coping behavior. Adv Behav Res Ther 1989;11:235–248.

105. Miller S. Monitoring and blunting: validation of a questionnaire to assess styles of information seeking under threat. J Pers Soc Psychol 1987;52:345–353.

106. Miller S. Monitoring versus blunting styles of coping influence the information patients want and need about cancer: implications for cancer screening and management. Cancer 1995;76:167–177.

107. Miller S, Shoda Y, Hurley K. Applying cognitive-social theory to health-protective behavior: breast self-examination in cancer screening. Psychol Bull 1996;119:70–94.

108. Cobb S. Social support as a moderator of life stress. Psychosom Med 1976;38:300–314.

109. Cohen S, Wills T. Stress, social support and the buffering hypothesis. Psychol Bull 1985;98: 310–357.

110. Berkman L, Syme S. Social networks, host resistance and mortality: a nine year follow-up study of Alemeda County resident. Am J Epidemiol 1979;109:186–204.

111. House J, Robbins C, Metzner H. The association of social relationship and activities with mortality: prospective evidence from the Tecumseh Community Health Study. Am J Epidemiol 1982;116:123–140.

112. Billings A, Moos R. Social support and functioning among community and clinical groups: a path model. J Behav Med 1982;5:295–312.

113. Fleming R, Baum A, Gisriel M, Gatchel R. Mediating influences of social support on stress at Three Mile Island. J Hum Stress 1982;8:14–22.

114. Broman C. Social relationships and health-related behavior. J Behav Med 1993;16:335–350.

115. Rimer B, Conaway M, Lyna P, et al. Cancer screening practicies among women in a community health center population. Am J Prev Med 1996;12:351–357.

116. Vernon SW, Laville EA, Jackson GL. Participation on breast cancer screening programs: a review. Soc Sci Med 1990;30:1107–1118.

117. Richardson J, Mondrus G, Danley K, et al. Impact of a mailed intervention on annual mammography and physician breast examiniations among women at high risk of breast cancer. Cancer Epidemiol Biomark Prev 1996;5:71–76.

118. Davis N, Nash E, Bailey C, et al. Evaluation of three methods for improving mammograhy rates in a managed care plan. Am J Prev Med 1997;13:298–302.

119. Margolis K, Menart T. A test of two interventions to improve compliance with scheduled mammography appointments. J Gen Intern Med 1996;11:539–541.

120. Lerman C, Ross E, Boyce A, et al. The impact of mailing psychoeducational materials to women with abnormal mammograms. Am J Public Health 1992;82:729–730.

121. Lerman C, Schwartz M, Miller S, et al. A randomized trial of breast cancer risk counseling: interacting effects of counseling, educational level, and coping style. Health Psychol 1996;15:75–83.

122. Cull A, Anderson E, Mackay J, et al. The effect of attending a breast cancer family clinic on women's estimates of risk and levels of psychological distress. Conference proceedings: British Psychosocial Oncology Group 11th Annual Conference, December 1994. Psychooncolgy 1995;4:83–99. Abstract.

123. Kash K, Holland J, Osborne M, Miller D. Psychological counseling strategies for women at risk for breast cancer. J Natl Cancer Inst Monogr 1995;17:73–79.

124. Hughes C, Lerman C, Lustbader E. Ethnic differences in risk perception among women at increased risk for breast cancer. Breast Cancer Res Treat 1996;40:25–35.

125. Pearlman D, Rakowski W, Clark M, et al. Why do women's attitudes toward mammography change over time? Implications for physician-patient communication. Cancer Epidemiol Biomark Prev 1997;6:451–457.

126. Vogel V, Yeomans A, Higginbotham E. Clinical management of women at increased risk for breast cancer. Breast Cancer Res Treat 1993;28:195–210.

127. Morrow M. Identification and management of the woman at increased risk for breast cancer development. Breast Cancer Res Treat 1994;31:53–60.

128. Bilimoria M, Morrow M. The woman at increased risk for breast cancer: evaluation and management strategies. CA 1995;45(5):263–278.

129. Rimer BK. Understanding the acceptance of mammography by women. Ann Behav Med 1992;14:197–203.

130. Jepson C, Rimer B. Determinants of mammography intentions among prior screenees and nonscreenee. J App Social Psychol 1993;23:40–51.

131. Hoskins K, Stopfer J, Calzone K, et al. Assessment and counseling for women with a family history of breast cancer: a guide for clinicians. JAMA 1995;273(7):577–585.

132. Stefanek M, Wilcox P. First degree relatives of breast cancer patients: screening practices and provision of risk information. Cancer Detect Prev 1991;5(5):379–384.

133. Shapiro D, Boggs S, Melamed B, Graham-Pole J. The effect of varied physician affect on recall, anxiety, and perceptions in women at risk for breast cancer: an analogue study. Health Psychol 1992;11:61–66.

134. Sclafani L. Management of the high-risk patient. Semin Surg Oncol 1991;7:261–266.

135. Wender R. Cancer screening and prevention in primary care. Cancer Suppl, 1993:(72)1093–1099.

136. Jacobsen P, Valdimarsdottier H, Brown K, Offit K. Decision-making about genetic testing among women at familial risk for breast cancer. Psychosom Med 1997;59:459–466.

137. Lerman C, Schwartz M, Lin T, et al. The influence of psychological distress on use of genetic testing for cancer risk. J Consult Clin Psychol 1997;65:414–420.

138. Croyle R, Smith K, Botkin J, et al. Psychological responses to *BRCA1* mutation testing: preliminary findings. Health Psychol 1997;16:63–72.

139. Baum A, Friedman A, Zakowski S. Stress and genetic testing for disease risk. Health Psychol 1997;16:8–19.

140. Pennisi V, Capozzi A. Subcutaneous mastectomy data: a final statistical analysis of 1500 patients. Aesthetic Plast Surg 1989;13:15–21.

141. Stefanek M. Bilateral prophylactic mastectomy: issues and concerns. J Natl Cancer Inst 1995;17:37–42.

142. Schrag D, Kuntz K, Garber J, Weeks J. Decision analysis: effects of prophylactic mastectomy and oophorectomy on life expectancy among women with *BRCA1* or *BRCA2* mutations. New Engl J Med 1997;336:1465–1471.

143. Burke W, Daly M, Garber J, et al. Recommendations for follow-up care of individuals with an inherited predisposition to cancer: II. *BRCA1* and *BRCA2*. Cancer Genetics Studies Consortium. JAMA 1997;277:997–1003.

144. Houn F, Helzlsouer K, Friedman N, Stefanek M. The practice of prophylactic mastectomy: a survey of Maryland surgeons. Am J Public Health 1995;85:801–805.

145. Stefanek M, Helzlsouer K, Wilcox P, Houn F. Predictors of and satisfaction with bilateral prophylactic mastectomy. Prev Med 1995;24:412–419.

14

Legal and Ethical Issues in Risk Assessment, Management, and Testing

Lisa S. Parker, Alan Meisel, and Melissa J. Hogan

With isolation and identification of the *BRCA1* and *BRCA2* genes, women may seek genetic testing to determine whether they have one of these genetic mutations and, therefore, an increased lifetime risk of breast and ovarian cancer (1). With a family history of breast cancer, the presence of a *BRCA1* or *BRCA2* mutation may signify a lifetime risk of 82% for breast cancer (2) and 44% for ovarian cancer (3). In contrast, the baseline risk, or the risk of breast cancer for the average woman in the United States, is 12.6%, or 1 in 8 women (4–6). Ovarian cancer has a baseline risk of only 1.4% (7).

Genetic testing affords the opportunity and motivation for increased surveillance and prophylactic interventions; however, it also presents increased risks of undesirable negative physical, psychological, social, and economic sequelae. The availability of genetic testing for cancer risk also raises ethical and legal concerns for clinicians. Testing for breast and ovarian cancer presents particular concerns because of the lack of truly good options for cancer surveillance and prevention and because of the social and psychological significance that many women attach to their breasts and reproductive capabilities. (Although women are affected primarily by breast disease and thus by *BRCA1/2* testing,

6% of men also develop breast cancer associated with *BRCA1/2* mutations.) Clear guidelines and a standard of care for offering genetic testing for breast and ovarian cancer have not yet emerged. Nonetheless, clinicians must carefully consider these incipient ethical and legal dimensions of genetic testing. In order to meet the demands of informed consent, clinicians must educate themselves about the risks and benefits of testing, including anxiety and the psychosocial and economic risks of discrimination, and about the options for cancer prevention. They must be aware of the requirements of confidentiality and the interests of their patients' family members and possibly other third parties (such as employers and insurers), and they must know how to strike a balance among these sometimes conflicting concerns. Some clinicians may choose simply to refer their patients to specialists for risk analysis, possible testing, and posttest counseling. Nevertheless, primary care clinicians must know when to refer. This threshold question, too, has ethical and legal dimensions.

The first part of this chapter addresses whether clinicians have a legal duty to inform patients of the availability of genetic testing and to offer or refer them for such testing. The second part discusses the process of informed consent to genetic testing and recommends an expanded notion of informed consent in this context. The third part analyzes clinicians' ethical and legal duties in communicating genetic test results to patients and counseling them about their risk of developing breast or ovarian cancer (both genetically related and not). The fourth part addresses the cancer surveillance and prevention options available for patients who are found to have *BRCA1* or *BRCA2* mutations and the responsibility of clinicians to counsel those who are discovered not to have any known mutations. The fifth part considers the interests of family members and the ethical and legal implications of a clinician breaching confidentiality in order to inform relatives of genetic information that they may find material to their health decision making. Other interested third parties (e.g., insurers and employers) are the focus of the next two parts. The risk of discrimination by these third parties against those found to have *BRCA1/2* mutations creates economic and psychological risks for patients who consider genetic testing and imposes an ethical, and possibly a legal, duty on clinicians to inform patients of these risks.

Duties to Inform and to Offer Testing

Physicians may interact with patients concerning genetic testing in several different ways, ranging from offering individualized genetic counseling and testing to playing a largely educational role, informing patients about the availability of testing, and referring interested patients to a specialist (e.g., a genetic counselor). Physicians have an ethical and a legal duty to obtain such information from patients for whom they are the primary health care provider, as well as when such information is pertinent to the specialty care or specific intervention being provided (8,9). As the familial nature of some diseases has emerged, taking a family medical history has become an even more important part of taking a complete medical history. The meaningfulness of *BRCA1/2* testing for women who wish to estimate their risk of breast or ovarian cancer depends in part on their personal and family medical histories and on demographic information, including their

ethnicity. Therefore, a patient's accurate personal and family medical history provides her clinician with critical information for evaluating with her the potential usefulness of genetic testing. [If a clinician's failure to take a medical history were causally related to the patient's later injury, a relationship that admittedly may be quite difficult to establish in the case of healthy women who later develop breast or ovarian cancer, the clinician might be held liable (8).]

A key question regarding *BRCA1/2* testing is for whom such testing is appropriate and thus to whom it should be offered. Because the offer of genetic testing creates some anxiety, and because offering a test may be construed as endorsement of it or as subtle pressure to accept the offer, the apparently simple solution of offering testing to everyone and leaving the decision to individual patients is not without attendant risks. Moreover, testing is expensive, and many health insurance plans will not cover genetic testing, especially without clear indication of its likely benefit (e.g., family history of disease).

Currently, offering or recommending testing for increased susceptibility to breast and ovarian cancer to every patient is likely not within the standard of care. Policy or consensus statements by professional societies do not of themselves establish the standard of care; it rests on actual professional practice and, when questions of legal liability arise, on judicial determinations. Nevertheless, such statements do provide some guidance to clinicians, particularly as new technologies emerge from research studies into clinical practice. According to the American Society of Clinical Oncology (ASCO):

> ... cancer predisposition testing [should] be offered only when: 1) the person has a strong family history of cancer or very early age of onset of disease; 2) the test can be adequately interpreted; 3) the results will influence the medical management of the patient or family member [10, p. 1732].

The American Society of Human Genetics (ASHG) concurs with the ASCO in not recommending general population screening. The ASHG states:

It is premature to offer population screening, until the risks associated with specific *BRCA1* mutations are determined and the best strategies for monitoring and prevention are accurately assessed.... Until we know the probability that a particular mutation will occur in cancer, the efficacy and safety of follow-up interventions, and the reliability of the test, mass screening for *BRCA1* mutations is not recommended [11, pp. I–ii].

Proper interpretation of the results of a patient's *BRCA1/2* test—the *relevance* of the absence or presence of particular genetic mutations for determining an individual's cancer risk—depends, in part, on her ethnicity and family and personal medical histories.

In addition, even an informative test result may not be *beneficial* to a particular patient. She could, for example, lack the financial means, desire, or motivation to pursue preventive interventions even if she received an informative positive test result. Or a negative test result could afford a woman a false sense of security regarding her personal risk of developing disease. Thus characteristics both of the test, including its specificity and sensitivity, and of those tested, including how they will use the genetic information, influence the risk-benefit ratio of genetic testing for the individual patient. In light of psychological and economic factors, it is far from clear that offering *BRCA1/2* testing to all patients would be (even potentially) beneficial to them. As ASCO concludes, "[d]espite the rapid pace of research in cancer genetics, none of the cancer susceptibility tests currently available are appropriate for screening of asymptomatic individuals in the general population" (10, pp. 1732).

Therefore, although it seems that clinicians should not offer testing to all patients, it does seem ethically and legally incumbent on them to identify those who would most likely benefit from testing. Once the clinician has taken personal and family medical histories, he or she can determine whether the patient has certain indications that increase the likelihood that she may have one of the genetic mutations and that the presence of the mutation will be informative of her risk of developing disease. ASCO recommends the following criteria for identifying families that have a high probability for having a *BRCA1* mutation:

- Family with more than two breast cancer cases and one or more cases of ovarian cancer diagnosed at any age
- Family with more than three breast cancer cases diagnosed before age 50
- Sister pairs with two of the following cancers diagnosed before age 50: two breast cancers, two ovarian cancers, or a breast and ovarian cancer
- Relatives of individuals with breast cancer diagnosed before the age of 30 (10, p. 1733).

Other commentators note similar criteria:

- More than two relatives with breast, ovarian, or other cancers
- Two or more generations affected
- Bilateral cancer
- Multiple primary tumors, breast or other
- Early-onset cancer (age <45 years)
- Sarcomas, adrenocortical carcinomas, or other rare cancers in relatives
- *Ataxia telangiectasia* in relatives
- Premalignant condition or biopsy and family history
- Relative with known susceptibility gene mutation
- Women considering prophylactic surgery (12, p. 205)

Faced with a patient who meets these criteria, a clinician should discuss and offer genetic testing (11). If the clinician knows about a patient's family history of breast and/or ovarian cancer and fails to recommend or discuss genetic testing, the clinician may be held liable for malpractice if the patient subsequently develops a cancer, the risk of which may have been predicted by the testing.

Given current limitations on the meaningfulness of test results, clinicians do not have a legal duty to recommend testing to everyone, specifically those who do not fall within any of the familial high-risk categories. Under medical malpractice standards, clinicians are judged according to a professional standard. If professional medical associations such as ASCO and ASHG do not recommend testing for those without family history indications (7), it is unlikely that a court would impose a legal duty on a clinician to refer a patient for testing who does not meet specific medical criteria.

How should a clinician respond to a patient who does not meet criteria for referral but who nevertheless requests (or even demands) testing? Fear of liability and the "defensive medicine" stance it breeds may suggest that the clinician should simply comply with the patient's request. From an ethical perspective, however, it is crucial that the clinician stress the limitations of such testing, including the risk of both false-positive and false-negative results, as well as the possibility that cancer will develop despite the absence of the genetic mutations tested for. After doing so, if the patient still requests (or demands) testing, the clinician probably should refer her for testing, even though it does not appear to be "medically indicated" according to prevailing standards.

Why? First, genetic testing should involve continued counseling about the meaningfulness of test results. The professional to whom the patient is referred may be better able to explain the tests' limitations, which may dissuade the patient from undergoing testing. Second, the risks and benefits of testing are in part psychological and thus dependent on the individual patient's values and personality. Although it is important to guard against creating a false sense of security insofar as possible, it is wrong to withhold testing from an informed individual simply because the medical and social consensus does not support her reasons for seeking the information. Third, patients who are truly committed to undergoing genetic testing may avail themselves of testing through avenues that do not afford the benefit of counseling. Compelling patients to undertake such options by refusing to test and counsel them within the context of an ongoing professional-patient relationship may expose them to still more serious psychological risks. One problem with proceeding to perform testing for patients who do not fit the testing criteria is that unwarranted credibility thereby may be given to the test results (and the credibility of the testing criteria is undermined). Nevertheless, the tradeoff of possible

harms seems to favor referring for counseling and testing the patient who insists. Legally, however, it is unlikely that a clinician is obligated to refer the insistent patient for testing that is not deemed medically indicated.

Moreover, it is not even clear that clinicians currently have a positive legal duty to recommend testing to those patients who do fall within the aforementioned criteria or even to inform them of its availability. General practitioners may not be expected to be at the forefront of cancer genetics and to be familiar with professional society recommendations that are targeted at specialists. The legal standard of care depends on prevailing professional practice, and that practice is constantly evolving. Professional practice is likely first to conform to recommended guidelines and then perhaps to move toward testing those who fall outside recommended criteria in response to patient demand and commercial interests. Should research show that factors other than ethnicity and personal and family medical histories are reliable indicators of an increased likelihood of carrying the mutations, clinicians should begin to offer testing to those with such indications. Although it is desirable that prevailing practices be driven by sound research results, patient demand and commercial interests may push that practice ahead of any research findings that justify it.

Prenatal Testing and Testing of Minor Children

Questions about when to offer or refer for testing also must be resolved in the contexts of prenatal testing and testing of minor children. Commentators and genetic counselors object to prenatal testing for *BRCA1* and *BRCA2* because it may lead to pregnancy termination based on the increased risk of breast and ovarian cancers, which, although serious, are diseases of adulthood with chances of both early detection and treatment (13–15). Prenatal testing for adult-onset genetically related conditions, even those which are currently untreatable or for which the penetrance has been thought to be 100%, such as Huntington disease, has been resisted by the counseling community and by many groups of patients living with such diseases. It is thought that adult-onset diseases nevertheless leave individuals with the anticipation of a relatively healthy childhood and perhaps several decades of healthy adult years. Mutations such as *BRCA1/2* that merely increase lifetime risk of disease stand in sharp contrast with the conditions classically diagnosed by prenatal testing, such as trisomy 13 or Tay Sachs disease, which may admit of some phenotypic variation but confer a certainty of a severely affected childhood.

Nevertheless, the professional stance against prenatal testing for *BRCA1/2* contrasts sharply with the nondirective ethos of genetic counseling that dictates that counselees' values and interests should determine both whether testing is undertaken and any decisions based on test results. Moreover, it seems somewhat incongruous to imply that although women have the legal right, within specified term limits, to terminate their pregnancies for no reason at all, they should not have the right to terminate a pregnancy for what is arguably a good reason—a fetus carrying a *BRCA1/2* mutation—and therefore, information about the presence or absence of those mutations should not be made available to them. This seems to conflict with the constitutionally protected right to reproductive choice.

Finally, the failure to offer genetic testing, with appropriate counseling, could give rise to liability for wrongful birth if information about the fetus's risk of developing genetic disease would have been material to a woman's reproductive decision (16). The parents of a child born with a *BRCA1/2* mutation would need to establish that a physician or genetic counselor had not told them about *BRCA1/2* testing and that if they had been informed of the genetic test for increased risk of breast and ovarian cancers, they would have had the fetus tested and would have terminated the pregnancy after learning of the presence of the mutation. Even if all of this could be established, in some states, liability would still not be imposed because the presence of the mutation merely increases the risk of cancer but does not ensure that it will occur.

A final ethical consideration that argues against prenatal testing for *BRCA1/2* pertains to the possibility of identifying these mutations in a fetus and a mother's deciding to carry the pregnancy to term anyway. Such testing would effectively result in the testing of a minor for the risk of an adult-onset condition. Genetic counselors argue that minors should not be tested for such mutations because the disease does not manifest until later in life but could immediately result in stigmatization, discrimination, changed family dynamics, survivor's guilt, and so-called vulnerable child syndrome (16). In addition to these considerations, testing of minors robs them of the opportunity to decide for themselves whether they would prefer to exercise their right not to know about their genetic makeup. Waiting until the age of majority to allow young women to decide whether to seek *BRCA1/2* testing still affords them time to engage in increased surveillance or prophylactic treatment before the onset of either breast or ovarian cancer associated with *BRCA1/2* mutations (17). In rare cases, exceptions may be justified if a minor herself desired testing. However, most minors will not be in a position to weigh the risks and potential benefits of testing in order to give informed consent. Testing of minors in an attempt to relieve parental anxiety or to inform parental decision making violates minors' potential for eventual self-determination and affords them no health-related benefit.

The Process of Informed Consent

Arising as medical paternalism gave way to increased concern for patient autonomy, the doctrine of informed consent is a cornerstone of contemporary bioethics and health law. With the dual goals of protecting patient welfare and promoting patient self-determination, the informed consent process combines concern for both the consequences and the source of patient decision making (18). To give informed consent (or refusal), a competent patient must be provided with information about the risks and potential benefits of the proposed intervention, and understand and weigh it in light of her (or his) own values. A decision that meets these criteria is an autonomous authorization of the health care professional to act on the patient's behalf (19).

What Is the Intervention?

Unlike classic informed consent contexts in which, for example, the surgeon obtains authorization to remove a patient's injured spleen, in the case of genetic testing, it may be unclear initially precisely what the patient authorizes. The drawing of blood, with its attendant risk of bruising, is not the whole of the intervention for which the patient's authorization is sought. With genetic testing, the intervention lies in creating potentially meaningful information that may have a variety of medical, psychological, social, and economic implications for the person to whom it pertains, as well as implications for those to whom the person is either genetically or emotionally related.

Disclosure of Risks and Benefits

The process of informed consent requires that the clinician disclose and explain the risks and potential benefits of the proposed intervention. Although some issues must be explained again after actual test results are obtained (if the woman decides to get tested), it is appropriate to err on the side of repetition in order to obtain as fully informed consent as possible before testing. Because risks and potential benefits vary in their probability and magnitude, because supplying too much information sometimes can inhibit rather than promote decision making, and because different people desire different amounts of information, ethics and law generally have settled on a "reasonable person standard" for determining which risks and potential benefits must form the core of such disclosure. This standard requires disclosure of those risks and potential benefits that a similarly situated reasonable person would consider material to her or his decision making (20,21). [Another standard for disclosure is the "professional standard," which requires that the clinician disclose the information that a reasonable practitioner would disclose in a similar situation (20–22). For a variety of reasons, this standard is deemed less ethically defensible than a reasonable person standard. Nonetheless, it is the legally accepted standard in about half the states.] Beyond the core disclosure, clinicians incur an ethical and legal obligation to disclose information that individual patients request or that they have reason to believe a particular patient would want.

ASCO recommends that for *BRCA1/2* testing the core disclosure should include the following elements:

1. Information about the purpose of the test, that is, to determine whether a mutation can be detected in a specific cancer-susceptibility gene
2. What can be learned from both a positive and negative test, including the most recent information on the type and magnitude of health risks associated with a positive test, as well as the risks that may remain even after a negative test
3. The possibility that no additional information will be obtained at the completion of the test
4. The options for approximation of risk without genetic testing, for example, using empirical risk tables for breast cancer given differing family histories
5. The risk of passing a mutation on to children
6. The technical accuracy of the test
7. The fees involved in both the laboratory test and the associated consultation by the health professional providing pretest education, results disclosure, and follow-up
8. The risks of psychological distress and family disruption, whether a mutation is found or not found
9. The risk of employment and/or insurance discrimination following disclosure of genetic test results
10. The level of confidentiality of results compared with other medical tests and procedures
11. The medical options and limited proof of efficacy for surveillance and cancer prevention for individuals with a positive test, as well as the accepted recommendations for cancer screening even if the genetic testing is negative (10, p. 1732)

Because of the magnitude of this information, ASCO recommends that general practitioners should consult with colleagues who have more expertise in cancer genetic testing (10) or refer patients to a cancer risk counseling (CRC) program that may be offered in conjunction with an oncology practice (12,23).

What Constitutes Risk?

Informed consent is complicated in the genetic testing context because many of the risks are not medical risks but social and psychological ones (24). "High-risk women must deal with two distinct but related problem areas: their objective physical risk and the feelings it engenders. More precisely, one must cope simultaneously on two different levels, the medical and the emotional" (6, p. 16). One important social risk is discrimination. It is difficult to forecast the likelihood of discrimination based on genetic findings because this risk depends on factors such as future employment and shifts in the economy, public policy, and social attitudes. Data on psychological sequelae of genetic testing for cancer risk are being amassed, but it is difficult to help individual patients predict which sequelae are likely outcomes for them. Finally, the risk analysis based on genetic testing yields only an epidemiologically based risk figure, the relevance of which even well-educated patients have difficulty appreciating.

The Meaning of Risk in the Context of Genetic Testing

For the patient even to understand genetic testing, the clinician should begin with educating the patient about the relationship between baseline risk and the individual risk assessment informed by genetic testing, the limitations of the meaning of test results, and the possibility of false-positive or false-negative results. The meaning of possible test results is intimately connected with the risks and possible benefits of genetic testing. Patients must understand, for example, that a negative test for *BRCA1/2* does not mean that they have no risk for breast or ovarian cancer, or even that they have no genetically related risk. Other mutations, for which no test is currently available, may increase their risk over the baseline level. Nor is a positive test result diagnostic of cancer. The possible benefits of testing, therefore, are limited by the meaning of the tests and patients' own circumstances. A positive test result can encourage patients to increase surveillance or undergo prophylactic treatment, which in turn

may decrease the risk of cancer-related morbidity and mortality. For those who discover that they do not carry a mutation, it may reduce their anxiety and possibly prevent unnecessary prophylactic interventions (6,24). One patient whose family participated in an early research project to discover breast cancer-related mutations, for example, had scheduled a prophylactic bilateral mastectomy because of her overwhelming family history of early-onset breast and ovarian cancer. One week before her scheduled surgery, she learned that she did not carry the genetic mutation and canceled the surgery (17). Women may use test results to help guide their decisions to enroll in chemoprevention studies or to seek chemoprevention as it becomes clinically available. The possible benefit of surveillance, prevention, and early treatment for any individual is constrained by her economic and emotional resources, which for some patients may limit their access to these interventions.

Some of the risks of genetic testing are also related to the limitations of the results' meaningfulness. A misunderstood negative test result could give women a false sense of security, whereas a misunderstood positive result could create great anxiety and even lead some women to cease surveillance and prevention efforts because of an unwarranted sense that they are fated to develop cancer (25). In addition to these psychological risks, patients must understand potential risks to their insurability, as discussed later. In addition to potential insurance discrimination, employers also may discriminate, whether or not legally permitted to do so under the laws discussed later in this chapter. Finally, testing may affect family dynamics, for example, if some members feel alienated from others who do not share the same level of risk or if, as discussed later in this chapter, questions of confidentiality arise.

These psychological, social, and economic risks must be explained to patients prior to testing as part of the process of informed consent. The possible benefits of testing also must be explored thoroughly to be certain that patients have realistic expectations. In particular, the possibility and limitations of benefit from a positive test result must be reviewed. These include discussion of the medical interventions available to those found to be at increased cancer risk. These interventions are reviewed later in this chapter.

Communicating the Test Results

The health care professional who will communicate genetic test results to the individual tested incurs a number of ethical and legal responsibilities. He or she must sensitively convey the results and accurately interpret them for the individual patient and must address the patient's questions, provide emotional support, and make provision for future follow-up consultation.

Communicating the Test Results

Not only must clinicians provide patients with the raw test results, they also must explain the significance of these results to the patient. This usually means going over much of the same information that was provided to the patient in order to obtain informed consent prior to testing. Although the risk of false-positive and false-negative test results must be disclosed prior to testing, when communicating the test results, this risk again must be stressed. Although there are no reliable data concerning the rates of false-positive and false-negative results, clinicians need to be familiar with the reasons for these misleading results. Testing for genetic mutations involves identification of the variation of interest against a backdrop of normal variation. Tests must be sufficiently sensitive to detect variation and sufficiently specific to identify the variation of interest. Overly sensitive tests yield false-positive results, whereas overly specific tests yield false-negative results. Both are attended by increased morbidity: False-positive results lead to unnecessary anxiety and, possibly, invasive interventions, whereas false-negative results prompt false security and may contribute to a failure to detect and treat disease.

Understanding the Test Results

In order to provide patients with accurate information, the clinician must understand the test results and their significance. Unfortunately, this is not always the case. For instance, approximately one-third of physicians who referred patients for genetic tests for a form of colon cancer incorrectly interpreted the test results (26).

Communicating Sensitively

Clinicians must be sensitive to the emotional responses of their patients and the social and familial context in which the test results will be experienced. Common emotional responses to learning of an increased risk for breast or ovarian cancer include "anger, fear of developing cancer, fear of disfigurement and dying, grief, guilt, lack of control, negative body image, altered sexual functioning and sense of isolation" (6, p. 16). These responses are often affected by "biological proximity and emotional ties to affected relatives, history of childhood abuse, major life transitions, outcomes of cancer diagnoses, and family communication styles" (12, p. 206).

Failure to recognize extreme emotional distress, including depression or a suicidal response, may provide the basis for legal liability. In addition to the potential for incurring malpractice liability for inaccurately interpreting test results, clinicians face potential liability for a patient's mental anguish if they communicate the genetic information in a negligent manner or a manner that intentionally or negligently inflicts emotional distress by engaging in extreme or outrageous conduct (27–29). While such extreme reactions to the communication of test results are rare, the possibility of their occurring must not be neglected (30,31). Some authors argue that genetic testing for familial Alzheimer disease and Huntington disease should be accompanied by extensive counseling to mitigate the risk of such negative sequelae (6,32). Such protocols also are subject to criticism for being overly paternalistic.

Finally, clinicians also must be sensitive to myriad responses that follow negative test results, including guilt about having been spared, a false sense of security, changed self-concept, or altered familial and social relationships. At the very least, clinicians should refer for psychological counseling patients who seem seriously or unusually distressed or depressed by their test results (6).

Posttest Interventions

During the process of obtaining informed consent to genetic testing and then more thoroughly after communicating test results, clinicians must disclose the risks and potential benefits of early detection and prophylactic interventions for breast and ovarian cancer. These include aggressive screening, a method of early detection, and prophylactic surgery and chemoprevention, which both seek to reduce the risk of developing disease. In light of the morbidity that attends each of these options, even patients carrying *BRCA1/2* mutations may reasonably choose simply to resume the regular course of their lives, including age-appropriate mammography screening. (Because those with negative test results still have a baseline risk of developing cancer, the importance of such screening must be stressed.) As Francis Collins admits, while "it is possible that cancer should be treated differently in women with germ-line *BRCA1* mutations, ... at present there are insufficient data to guide the surgeon or oncologist" (4, p. 187). What is clear is that "every woman at inherited risk should be provided with a thorough discussion of the most current level of information and adequate counseling regarding her particular situation before she chooses to act" (33, p. 1975). Thus the information to be disclosed must keep pace with scientific advances, and it is the clinician's responsibility to keep abreast of these developments. In this section we discuss, generically, the kinds of posttest interventions that clinicians should call to the attention of counselees or patients.

Medical Interventions for Increased Risk of Breast Cancer

Patients have several options to address an increased risk for breast cancer: They can engage in more aggressive screening, have a prophylactic mastectomy, or enroll in a chemoprevention trial.

Aggressive Screening

The least invasive option is to engage in aggressive screening to identify the onset of breast cancer in its earliest stages. This may involve the patient's starting self-examinations and mammography at an earlier age and increasing the frequency of such tests (7), and the mammography may be qualitatively different from that performed for the general population (12). Some researchers recommend that carriers of the mutation begin breast self-examinations by the ages of 18 to 21 (34). A National Institutes of Health Task Force recommended that women with *BRCA1/2* mutations begin mammography between the ages of 25 and 35 (35), although the breast tissue of women in their twenties and thirties may not be easily screened (33). Clinicians must help women to understand that none of these methods is guaranteed to detect all breast tumors in early stages and that considerable anxiety may attend such constant surveillance. Moreover, surveillance does not seek to reduce the risk of developing cancer but only the risk of serious morbidity or mortality by facilitating early treatment, which itself may not make a difference in outcome.

Prophylactic Mastectomy

Because prophylactic mastectomy involves removal of healthy breast tissue before any signs or symptoms of illness arise and entails serious morbidity, it raises a variety of concerns as a preventive intervention. Moreover, the effectiveness of this procedure in reducing the risk of cancer must still be assessed, because case studies have reported breast cancer development despite the procedure (36,37). However, one study reports a 90% decreased risk after a prophylactic mastectomy (38). The physical and potential psychological trauma of mastectomy should not be minimized, and the possibility of negative psychological sequelae of mastectomy being balanced by feelings of empowerment must be considered. Nevertheless, clinicians must stress the persistent risk (of a largely unknown magnitude) of developing breast cancer.

Chemoprevention Trials

Chemopreventive agents offer another option to reduce the risk of breast cancer (39). Nevertheless, chemoprevention cannot guarantee that cancer will not develop, nor can it be determined that a person who remains cancer-free can attribute her disease avoidance to the chemical agents used to reverse, suppress, or prevent carcinogenic progression to invasive cancer. Because of the morbidity associated with these agents, the offer of chemoprevention raises myriad ethical concerns (40). Moreover, all the ethical concerns that attend recruitment and enrollment in placebo-controlled clinical research attend chemoprevention, which is still in its research stage. Finally, because one chemopreventive agent, tamoxifen, has been shown to increase the risk of endometrial cancer, cause bone marrow suppression, promote thrombotic events, and cause other side effects in some women (41), the option of chemoprevention is fraught with both uncertainties and difficult tradeoffs.

Medical Interventions for Increased Risk of Ovarian Cancer

In addition to counseling patients about their posttest options regarding breast cancer, clinicians must disclose the risks and potential benefits of options addressing ovarian cancer risk, including general risk-reduction factors, early-detection programs, and prophylactic bilateral oophorectomy (25).

Protective Actions
Researchers note that several factors—"all of which reduce incessant ovulation"—decrease the average risk for ovarian cancer; these include having more than one full-term pregnancy, using oral contraception, and breast-feeding (35, p. 4). No studies have yet addressed the effect of these factors on patients with *BRCA1/2* mutations, but some women may give additional weight to oral contraception and breast-feeding as desirable options because of their possible effect on reducing the risk of ovarian cancer.

Early Detection Programs
Compared with breast cancer, early-stage ovarian cancer is more difficult to detect (33), and screening procedures are more invasive. Bimanual rectovaginal pelvic examination, serum tumor marker testing (CA-125), and transvaginal ultrasonography are the screening techniques in current use, with annual or semiannual screening beginning at age 25 to 35 years for women at increased risk (34,35).

Prophylactic Bilateral Oophorectomy
Because of the difficulty of early ovarian cancer detection, the National Institutes of Health (NIH) recommends prophylactic oophorectomy for those with *BRCA1* or *BRCA2* mutations after childbearing or age 35 (35). This option, however, is fraught with a difficult tradeoff, because estrogen-replacement therapy is then recommended to address the increased risk of cardiovascular disease and osteoporosis associated with prophylactic oophorectomy (35). If a patient does not have access to or cannot adhere to an estrogen-replacement program, this should be a serious consideration in her decision about whether to undergo a prophylactic oophorectomy. Moreover, the hormone-replacement therapy carries with it a concomitant increase in the risk for breast cancer (34). Finally, although an oophorectomy virtually eliminates the risk of ovarian cancer (33), there remains a minimal risk of peritoneal carcinomatosis.

Negative Test Results

Posttest counseling for those with a negative *BRCA1/2* test result must stress that only 5% to 10% of breast cancer is familial, and therefore, patients may still develop breast or ovarian cancer. That is, they still share the general population's level of risk. In addition, because of the risk of errors in testing, clinicians should encourage patients with a negative test to have another confirmatory test. Accurate interpretation of negative results is as important as for positive findings. Tests differ significantly in what they can detect. "Tests for specific mutations leave undetected any other mutations."

Informing Family Members

If patients learn that they carry a *BRCA1/2* mutation, some may convey this information to other family members not only to seek emotional support for themselves but also so that those relatives may be motivated to seek counseling and possible genetic testing. Clinicians are obligated to inform their patients of the relevance that genetic information may have for patients' relatives. However, for various reasons, some patients may not wish to convey genetic information about themselves to their family members. Ethical and legal questions then arise for their clinicians: Is it permissible to breach the confidence of these patients to inform their relatives, or is there even a duty to do so?

Ethical Considerations

Some commentators suggest that the real "patient" in the context of genetics is the family and not a specific individual (42–44). However, there is a long tradition of privacy and individuality in medicine, a tradition the gives rise to a reasonable expectation of confidence-keeping on the part of patients who seek genetic testing. A clinician's ethical obligation to the patient rarely permits breach of that confidentiality. In fact, some states have adopted genetic confidentiality laws that allow a patient to sue a physician for revealing genetic information (45–47). These statutes do not make allowances for clinicians wishing to reveal genetic information to relatives who also may carry the mutation.

Guidelines governing genetic research also suggest that patient confidentiality in genetic testing almost always should override family members' interests in knowing a patient's genetic information. Guidelines from the Office of Protection from Research Risks (which, technically, apply only in the research setting) state that each person within a family is an individual and deserves to have information about him or her kept confidential (48). Under this standard, a clinician would only reveal a patient's genetic information to that individual's family members in rare circumstances. Likewise, the President's Commission for the Study of Ethical Problems in Medicine and Biomedical and Behavioral Research established stringent conditions that must be met before a patient's confidentiality may be overridden:

> ... first, reasonable efforts to elicit a voluntary consent have failed; second, there is a high probability both that harm will occur if the information is withheld and that the disclosed information will actually be used to avert harm; third, the harm that identified individuals would suffer is serious; and finally, if third parties are warned, appropriate precautions are taken to ensure that only the genetic information needed for diagnosis and treatment of the disease in question is disclosed [49, p. 44].

These guidelines do not impose a duty to breach confidentiality but merely set out strict criteria under which it may be permissible to do so. Furthermore, the second and third criteria are exceedingly difficult to meet. Disclosure in breach of confidentiality is not permissible for diseases that are neither treatable nor preventable (50). In this case, it is difficult to assess the magnitude of possible harm for relatives (i.e., the actual risk of cancer). In addition, it is difficult to predict that the relatives will avail themselves of the opportunity for genetic counseling and testing, that they actually would use the results of testing to attempt to avert harm (i.e., engage in surveillance and preventive interventions), and that their attempts would be successful. Moreover, members of families with a history of breast or ovarian cancer, as well as members of ethnic groups in which *BRCA1/2* mutations occur with increased prevalence, may seek to be tested on the basis of this information alone. Their relative who carries a *BRCA1/2* mutation is generally not the sole source of motivation for them to seek counseling and testing. In effect, they are on the same general notice to seek testing as is the tested relative.

Although clinicians may justifiably encourage their patients to inform their relatives and should explain the potential benefit to family members of knowing this genetic information, their patients are under no obligation to disclose the information. In addition, informing family members entails imposing on them some of the risks attendant on counseling and testing. Among these are anxiety, as well as the possibility of discrimination in insurance and employment. Given current actuarial treatment of family history data, the risk of being denied insurance (or charged higher premiums) because one knows of a relative with a *BRCA1/2* mutation is probably not greater than the risk of incurring the same consequences simply because of a family history of disease. As discussed later in this chapter, however, insurance industry practices evolve to keep pace with scientific developments. Therefore, caution is advisable in imposing potentially unwanted information on individuals who have not sought it. This caution and a professional duty to "safeguard patient confidences within the constraints of the law" (51, p. xxii) combine to support the clinician's respecting the confidentiality of genetic findings.

Legal Considerations

Courts have shown substantial ambivalence about permitting breaches of confidentiality for the benefit of third parties. The strongest precedent for such breaches is the 1973 California case of *Tarasoff* v. *Regents of University of California*, which has been followed in several dozen other states. *Tarasoff* did not deal with disclosure of genetic information but rather arose in the psychotherapy context. The California Supreme Court held that when the patient of a psychotherapist makes a credible threat of harm to an identifiable victim, the therapist has a legal duty to take reasonable measures to protect that person, which may include providing a warning (52).

In contrast to the context of *BRCA1/2* testing, however, the situation in *Tarasoff* was immediately life-threatening. Nevertheless, the rationale of *Tarasoff* has been applied recently to the context of genetic information in *Safer* v. *Pack* (53). In *Safer*, a woman sued the estate of her father's physician 26 years after her father's death, alleging that the physician breached a duty to inform her of her father's hereditary colon cancer and multiple polyposis. She alleged that she was thereby prevented from availing herself of surveillance and early treatment interventions. The court held that a physician has a duty to warn individuals "known to be at risk of avoidable harm from a genetically transmissible condition" and concluded that genetic predispositions are not unlike communicable diseases because the "individual or group at risk is easily identified, and substantial future harm may be averted or minimized by a timely and effective warning" (53, p. 1192).

The ruling in the *Safer* case is far from definitive. On relatively similar facts, the only other case, *Pate* v. *Threkel*, held that the physician's duty was discharged by informing the patient of the familial implications of her hereditary condition (53a). It found no duty to seek out and warn members of the patient's family. The court noted, however, that the trial court would have to reconsider the balance of harms that may have resulted from a failure to inform the patient's

relative (daughter) against the harms that may have resulted from such disclosure.

Thus some commentators believe a trend is evolving toward expanding the clinician's duty to inform beyond the patient to the patient's relatives (50). Others urge caution in finding such a duty and emphasize the possible harms that may result from such disclosures, the limited benefits of testing that currently may be foreseen, the reasonable limits of professional responsibility to identify and contact potentially interested third parties, and finally, the shared responsibility of those who would benefit from testing and surveillance to seek such interventions on the basis of knowledge of family history of disease, as well as general knowledge about the availability of testing (21,54,55). If disclosure to relatives becomes the professional or legal norm, or if a clinician anticipates breaching confidentiality for whatever reason, that clinician should disclose the possibility of this breach during the informed consent process.

Insurance Coverage and Insurance Discrimination

A genetically related increased risk for breast and ovarian cancer may affect the terms of coverage or even eligibility for life, disability, and health insurance. In addition, patients who have such an increased risk may be concerned about whether particular surveillance techniques or preventive interventions will be covered under their health insurance policies and whether, based on such genetic information, insurers may lawfully increase their premiums or cancel their coverage. Although clinicians do not need to convey detailed information about insurance coverage and discrimination to patients as a part of informed consent, they should inform patients in general terms that having genetic testing for cancer, especially if it yields positive results, may make obtaining life, disability, and health insurance more difficult or more costly in the future.

Insurance Coverage

The terms of coverage under various insurance policies depend, in part, on the definition and interpretation of such terms as *disease, genetic predisposition, medical necessity,* and *preexisting condition.* Many insurance policies only cover the treatment of disease; therefore, one must determine whether genetically related risk for breast and ovarian cancer would fall within policies' definitions of disease. If genetic risk for cancer is defined as a disease, then even prophylactic surgery may be covered under such policies (56,57). However, insurance companies may seek to deny coverage for posttesting prophylactic surgeries, surveillance screenings, or treatment by considering the genetic mutation to be a preexisting condition (58,59). Even in those group contracts where a preexisting condition exclusion holds only for a limited time, insurers may still attempt to deny coverage based on the argument that the deleterious gene is not a disease and thus the contemplated interventions are not "medically necessary." Policies may still cover annual mammography but not more aggressive surveillance, even though it would seem to be in the best interest of companies for patients to discover cancer in its earliest stage to avoid more expensive, protracted treatment. If increasing numbers of patients undertake expensive surveillance and prevention regimens, however, the financial implications for insurers are unclear.

Insurance Discrimination

Of potentially greater concern than companies' failure to reimburse for surveillance and preventive interventions is the risk that insurers will deny all coverage or charge exceedingly high premiums for life, disability, or health insurance to those who are at a genetically related increased risk for breast or ovarian cancer (60). Clinicians should be aware of these concerns because patients may ask them not to record information about referral for genetic testing and test results in their medical record; some patients may even wish to use pseudonyms to obtain the tests.

Nevertheless, when applying for insurance, patients must respond truthfully to insurers' questions about personal and family medical histories; failure to do so may result in a later forfeiture of coverage. Some patients may decline genetic testing for fear of becoming ineligible

for life, disability, or health insurance coverage. Because future insurability, or insurability at standard rates, may be jeopardized by having undergone genetic testing, especially if the result is positive, clinicians should disclose these possibilities to patients as part of the initial informed consent process.

Federal Law

The Health Insurance Portability and Accountability Act (HIPAA) provides some protection against health insurance discrimination based on genetic information for individuals in group medical plans (61). This law imposes narrow restrictions on the conditions under which a group health insurance plan may exclude a person from coverage or charge a higher premium based on a preexisting condition. For present purposes, more important is the fact that the law does not consider "genetic information" to be a preexisting condition (61). In other words, sponsors of group insurance plans such as employers, unions, and insurers are prohibited by HIPAA from establishing eligibility criteria based on genetic information. They cannot consider a genetic predisposition, whether based on the results of genetic testing or on other information, as a preexisting condition, and thus individuals cannot be denied participation in group health plans because they are *BRCA1/2* carriers. A preexisting condition of cancer, for which insurance discrimination can occur legitimately, exists only when a clinician can reasonably diagnose the particular cancer.

State Law

All states have long-standing laws that prevent unfair discrimination by life and health insurers. They typically define unfair discrimination as discrimination not justified by actual risk. Because an increased risk does exist for those with *BRCA1/2* mutations, it is uncertain whether these general laws provide any protection. Newer state laws, however, may cover this gap in legal protection. The majority of states recently have passed laws preventing health maintenance organizations and health insurance companies from charging higher premiums for individuals who have a genetic mutation (62). Most of these state initiatives focus on health insurance, although some apply to life and disability insurance (63,64). The laws vary in their provisions and their susceptibility to unforeseen exceptions. Moreover, while these state laws generally seek to provide comprehensive protection from insurance discrimination based on genetic information, one broad exception may exist. Employers whose plans are self-insured may be largely exempt from these state laws under the federal ERISA statute and judicial decisions interpreting it (65).

Employment Discrimination

Employers, like insurance companies, may have an interest in knowing information about an employee's health status, including whether an employee has sought testing for genetic disease and the results of those tests. Thus patients also may be justifiably concerned about whether an employer may use genetic information about them to refuse to hire, to fire, or to discriminate against them in compensation, promotion, job assignments, and other terms and conditions of employment. Clinicians who refer for or perform genetic testing therefore have a responsibility, as a part of the pretesting informed consent process, to provide patients with the general information that having genetic testing, especially if it yields positive results, may affect their employability or employment status.

Federal Law

The Federal Rehabilitation Act (FRA) (66) and the Americans with Disabilities Act (ADA) (67) probably prohibit employers from discriminating against people who have disease-related genetic mutations (68). The congressional debates surrounding the enactment of the ADA cited genetic discrimination as one of the purposes for its enactment (69). However, the regulations promulgated to interpret the ADA explicitly provide that a "characteristic predisposition to illness or disease" is not a disability under the ADA (70). In addition, the FRA prohibits discrimination (by all entities receiving federal funds) against someone who may not currently have an impairment but who is "regarded as having" a disability (71). This has been interpreted

to include those regarded as being handicapped by purely latent conditions, such as having an asymptomatic congenital back anomaly that an employer believes to pose a heightened risk of injury or having asymptomatic HIV infection. The Equal Employment Opportunity Commission (EEOC) — the federal agency that enforces the ADA, which applies to all employers with 15 or more employees — employs a similar interpretation of the ADA. Both the FRA and the ADA allow preemployment medical examinations, but they prohibit an employer from using the results to refuse employment unless the exclusion is shown to be job-related, consistent with business necessity, and not amenable to reasonable accommodation (70,72,73). Simply having a genetically related increased risk for disease would not currently limit an employee's ability to perform and thus would not be a basis for refusing employment under these two laws.

State Law

All states have laws that prohibit employment discrimination on the basis of handicap, and some of these laws may be sufficiently broad to prohibit discrimination on the basis of genetic risk for breast and ovarian cancer. Some states use the FRA as a model for their laws and thus would prohibit discrimination on the basis of a perceived, as well as an actual, disability (74–95). Several states also have directly prohibited employers, along with insurance companies, from requiring genetic testing as a condition of employment and from discriminating based on genetic information (96–101).

Conclusion

Clinicians may be faced with one or all of the foregoing issues in the genetic testing context. With case and statutory law just beginning to emerge in these areas, it is necessary to extrapolate from similar contexts to predict the boundaries of clinicians' legal liability. Similarly, by examining analogous contexts, for example, of informed consent and of confidence-keeping, clinicians can glean ethical guidance in this unfamiliar territory of genetic testing. To this general legal and ethical guidance must be added the proviso that clinicians' duties evolve in response to changes in science and in social context. As new surveillance and prevention interventions are developed, for example, or as new data about genetic testing emerge, clinicians must alter the core disclosure of the informed consent process to reflect these developments. Because the risks and potential benefits of genetic testing are affected not only by scientific advance but also by policy development, new regulations, and changing social climates, these changes in social context also influence the content of clinicians' disclosures and discussions with patients. Consultation with specialist colleagues and referral of patients for professional genetic counseling, as well as for psychological counseling and support, will remain sound legal and ethical options for clinicians seeking to act responsibly in the face of rather daunting complexities.

Acknowledgments We thank Ellen Conser for her assistance in preparing the references.

References

1. Lerman C, Daly M, Masny A, Balshem A. Attitudes about genetic testing for breast-ovarian cancer susceptibility. J Clin Oncol 1994;12:843–850.
2. Easton DF, Bishop DT, Ford D, Crockford GP, and The Breast Cancer Linkage Consortium. Genetic linkage analysis in familial breast and ovarian cancer: results from 214 families. Am J Hum Genet 1993;52:678–701.
3. Easton DF, Ford D, Bishop DT. Breast and ovarian cancer incidence in *BRCA1* mutation carriers. Am J Hum Genet 1995;56:265–271.
4. Collins FS. *BRCA1*: lots of mutations, lots of dilemmas. New Engl J Med 1996;334:186–188. Editorial, comment.
5. American Cancer Society. Cancer Facts and Figures. New York: American Cancer Society, 1995.
6. Peters JA. Familial cancer risk: II. Breast cancer risk counseling and genetic susceptibility testing. J Oncol Manage 1994;Nov–Dec:14–22.
7. Genetic testing for susceptibility to breast cancer. In: Hayes' Directory of New Medical Technologies Status, sec. 103.03; available in WESTLAW, Hayes-Med database.
8. Pegalis SE, Wachsman HF. American Law of Medical Malpractice. 2d ed., sec. 3:6 Deerfield, IL: Clark, Boardman, Callaghan, 1992.
9. Louisell DW, Williams H. Medical Malpractice, par. 8.05[1]. New York: Mathew Bender, 1997.
10. Statement of the American Society of Clinical Oncology (ASCO) on genetic testing for cancer susceptibility, adopted on February 20, 1996. J Clin Oncol 1996;14:1730–1740.
11. Statement of the American Society of Human Genetics (ASHG) on genetic testing for breast and ovarian cancer predisposition. Am J Hum Genet 1994;55:i–iv.
12. Peters J. Breast cancer genetics: relevance to oncology genetics. Cancer Control 1995;May–June:195–208.
13. Elias S, Annas GJ. Generic consent for genetic screening. New Engl J Med 1994;330:1611–1613.
14. Parker LS. Ethical concerns in the research and treatment of complex disease. Trends Genet 1995;11:520–523.
15. Bloch M, Hayden MR. Opinion: predictive testing for Huntington's disease in childhood—challenges and implications. Am J Hum Genet 1990;46:1–4.
16. Wertz DC, Fanos JH. Genetic testing for children and adolescents: who decides? JAMA 1994;272:875–881.
17. Breo DL. Altered fates: counseling families with inherited breast cancer. JAMA 1993;269:2017–2022.
18. Appelbaum PS, Lidz CW, Meisel A. Informed Consent: Legal Theory and Clinical Practice. New York: Oxford University Press, 1987.
19. Faden R, Beauchamp TL. A History and Theory of Informed Consent. New York: Oxford University Press, 1986.
20. Frantz LB. Annotation: Modern status of views as to general measure of physician's duty to inform patient of risks of proposed treatment, 88 A.L.R. 3d 1008-44, secs. 4–5 (1978 & Suppl. 1995).
21. Pelias MZ. Duty to disclose in medical genetics: a legal perspective. Am J Med Genet 1991;39:347–354.
22. *Green* v. *Hussey*, 262 N.E.2d 156, 161 (Ill. App. Ct. 1970).
23. Peters JA. Familial cancer risk: I. Impact on today's oncology practice. J Oncol Manage 1994;Sept–Oct:18–30.
24. Schaler RR, Benderly BL. Challenging the Breast Cancer Legacy: A Program of Emotional Support and Medical Care for Women at Risk. New York: Harper Collins, 1992.
25. Bombard AT, Fields AL, Aufox S, Ben-Yishay M. The genetics of ovarian cancer: an assessment of current screening protocols and

recommendations for counseling families at risk. Clin Obstet Gynecol 1996;39:860–872.

26. Giardiallo FM, Brensinger JD, Petersen GM, et al. The use and interpretation of commercial *APC* gene testing for familial adenomatous polyposis. New Engl J Med 1997;336:823–827.

27. Restatement (Second) of Torts, sec. 46 St. Paul: American Law Institute, 1965.

28. Luepke EL. Note: HIV misdiagnosis: negligent infliction of emotional distress and the false positive. Iowa Law Review 1996;81:1229–1248.

29. Allen DM. Annotation: Recovery for emotional distress resulting from statement of medical practitioner or official, allegedly constituting outrageous conduct, 34 A.L.R. 4th 688–691 (1984 & Suppl. 1995).

30. Kolata G. Tests to assess risks for cancer raising questions. New York Times, March 27, 1995, p. A(1).

31. Becker CL. Note: Legal implications of the G-8 Huntington's disease genetic marker, 39 Case W. Res. L. Rev. 273–305, 282.

32. Post SG. Genetics, ethics, and Alzheimer disease. J Am Geriatr Soc 1994;42:782–786.

33. King MC, Rowell S, Love SM. Inherited breast and ovarian cancer: what are the risks? What are the choices? JAMA 1993;269:1975–1980.

34. Burke W, Daly M, Garber J, et al. Recommendations for follow-up care of individuals with an inherited predisposition to cancer: II. *BRCA1* and *BRCA2* — Cancer Genetics Studies Consortium. JAMA 1997;277:997–1003.

35. National Institutes of Health (NIH). Ovarian cancer: screening, treatment, and followup. NIH Consensus Statement Online 1994;April 5–7:1–30.

36. Goodnight JE, Quagliana JM, Morton DL. Failure of subcutaneous mastectomy to prevent the development of breast cancer. J Surg Oncol 1984;26:198–201.

37. Mies C. Recurrent secretory carcinoma in residual mammary tissue after mastectomy. Am J Surg Pathol 1993;17:715–721.

38. Stephenson J. Study shows mastectomy prevents breast cancer in high-risk women. JAMA 1997;277:1421–1422. News.

39. Henderson M. Current approaches to breast cancer prevention. Science 1993;259:630–631.

40. Vogel VG, Parker LS. Ethical issues in chemoprevention clinical trials. Cancer Control 1997; 4:142–149.

41. O'Shaughnessy JA. Chemoprevention of breast cancer. JAMA 1996;275:1349–1353.

42. Pelias MZ, Blanton SH. Genetic testing in children and adolescents: parental authority, the

rights of children, and duties of geneticists. University of Chicago Law School Roundtable 1996;3:525–543.

43. Wertz DC, Fletcher JC. Ethics and genetics: an international survey. Hastings Center Report 1989;July–Aug(suppl):20–24.

44. American Society of Human Genetics (ASHG) Ad Hoc Committee on Genetic Counseling. Genetic counseling. Am J Hum Genet 1975;27: 240–242.

45. N.Y Civ. Rights Law, sec. 79-1 (McKinney Suppl. 1997).

46. Or. Rev. Stat. Secs. 659.700 to .720 (Suppl. 1997).

47. Tex. Lab. Code Ann., sec. 21.403 (West Suppl. 1997).

48. U.S. National Institutes of Health, Office for Protection from Research Risks. Protecting Human Research Subjects: Institutional Review Board Guidebook. Washington: U.S. Government Printing Office, 1993.

49. President's Commission for the Study of Ethical Problems in Medicine and Biomedical and Behavioral Research. Screening and Counseling for Genetic Conditions: A Report on the Ethical, Social, and Legal Implications of Genetic Screening, Counseling, and Education Programs. Washington: The Commission, 1983.

50. American Society of Human Genetics (ASHG), Social Issues Subcommittee on Familial Disclosure. ASHG statement: professional disclosure of familial genetic information. Am J Hum Genet 1998;62:474–483.

51. American Medical Association (AMA) Council on Judicial Affairs. Code of Medical Ethics: Current Opinions with Annotations, 1996–1997 ed. Chicago: AMA, 1996.

52. *Tarasoff* v. *Regents of Univ. of Cal.*, 551 P.2d 334 (1976).

53. *Safer* v. *Pack*, 677 A.2d 1188 (N.J. Super. Ct. App. Div. 1996).

53a. *Pate* v. *Threkel*, 661 so. 2d 278 (Fla. 1995).

54. Hecht F. Duty to disclose to family member in medical genetics. Am J Med Genet 1992;42:758. Letter.

55. Pelias MZ. The duty to disclose to family members in medical genetics: response to Dr. Hecht. Am J Med Genet 1992;42:759–760. Letter.

56. *Katskee* v. *Blue Cross Blue Shield*, 515 N.W. 2d 645, 647–648 (Neb. 1994).

57. Glazier AK. Genetic predispositions, prophylactic treatments and private health insurance: nothing is better than a good pair of genes. Am J Law Med 1997;23:65–68.

58. Ad Hoc Committee on Genetic Testing/ Insurance Issues. Background statement: genetic testing and insurance. Am J Hum Genet 1995;56:327–331.

59. Kolata G. Advent of testing for breast cancer genes leads to fears of disclosure and discrimination. New York Times, February 4, 1997, p. 4.

60. Billings PR, Kohn MA, de Cuevas M, et al. Discrimination as a consequence of genetic testing. Am J Hum Genet 1992;50:476–482.

61. Health Insurance Portability and Accountability Act, Pub. L. No. 104-191 (1996) [codified as amended at 42 U.S.C., secs. 300gg to 300gg-92 (1997)]; cf. 42 U.S.C., sec. 12201(c) (1997).

62. Rothenberg, KH. Genetic information and health insurance: state legislative approaches. J Law Med Ethics 1995;23:312–319.

63. Mont. Code Ann., sec. 33-18-206 (Suppl. 1997).

64. Wyo. Stat., sec. 26-19-306 (Suppl. 1997).

65. 29 U.S.C., sec. 1144 (1997).

66. 29 U.S.C., sec. 701 et seq. (1997).

67. 42 U.S.C., sec. 12101 et seq. (1997).

68. Alper JS. Does the ADA provide protection against discrimination on the basis of genotype? J Law Med Ethics 1995;23:167–172.

69. 136 Cong. Rec. H 4623, H 4624-25, H 4637 (July 12, 1990).

70. 29 C.F.R., pt. 1630 app., sec. 1630.2(h) (1997).

71. 29 U.S.C., sec. 706(8)(B)(iii).

72. Council on Ethical and Judicial Affairs of the American Medical Association (AMA). Use of genetic testing by employers. JAMA 1991;266:1827–1830.

73. Orentlicher D. Genetic screening by employers. JAMA 1990;263:1005–1008.

74. Cal. Ins. Code, secs. 10123.3, 10140, 10147, 11512.95, 10123.31, 10123.35, 10140.1, 10140.5, 11512.96, 11512.965.

75. Cal. Health & Saf. Code, secs. 1374.7, 1374.9, 1357.52.

76. Colo. Rev. Stat. Ann., sec. 10-3-1104.7 (West Suppl. 1997).

77. Haw. Rev. Stat., sec. 431:10A-118 (Suppl. 1997).

78. Iowa Code Ann., sec. 513B.9A (West Suppl. 1997).

79. La. Rev. Stat. Ann., secs. 22:213.6, 22:213.7, 22:1214, 22:2002, 40:2207.

80. La. Rev. Stat. Ann., sec. 22:250.1(5)(p) (West Suppl. 1997).

81. S.B. 2018, 181st Leg., Reg. Sess. (Mass. 1997).

82. Minn. Stat. Ann., sec. 72A.139 (West Suppl. 1997) (1995 Minn. Laws 251).

83. H.B. 748, 89th Leg., 1st Reg. Sess. (Mo. 1997).

84. N.M. Stat. Ann., secs. 59A-23C-7.1, 59A-23E-2, 59A-23E-11, 59A-56-14 (Michie Suppl. 1997).

85. N.C. Gen. Stat., sec. 58-3-215 (Suppl. 1997).

86. N.C. Gen. Stat., sec. 58-68-30(b)(1)(b) (Suppl. 1997).

87. H.B. 2478, 45th Leg., 2d Reg. Sess. (Okla. 1996).

88. Or. Rev. Stat., sec. 746.135 (Suppl. 1997).

89. S.B. 1207, 181st Leg., Reg. Sess. (Pa. 1997).

90. H.B. 6349, S.B. 152, 1997-98 Leg., Reg. Sess. (R.I. 1997).

91. H.B. 5157, S.B. 986, 1997-98 Leg., Reg. Sess. (R.I. 1997).

92. S.B. 78, H.B. 191, 64th Leg., Reg. Sess. (Vt. 1997).

93. Va. Code Ann., sec. 38.2-508.4 (Michie Suppl. 1997).

94. Va. Code Ann., sec. 38.2-3432.1 (Michie Suppl. 1997).

95. W. Va. Code, secs. 33-15-2b, 33-16-3k (Suppl. 1997).

96. N.J. Stat. Ann., sec. 10-5-12 (West Suppl. 1997).

97. N.C. Gen. Stat. Ann., sec. 95-28.1A (Suppl. 1997).

98. N.Y. Exec. Law, sec. 296 (McKinney Suppl. 1997).

99. Or. Rev. Stat., secs. 659.036, 659.227 (Suppl. 1997).

100. R.I. Gen. Laws, secs. 28-6.7-1 to -4 (Suppl. 1997).

101. Tex. Lab. Code Ann., secs. 21.401 to .405 (West Suppl. 1997).

15

Cost-Effectiveness of the Identification of Women at High Risk for the Development of Breast and Ovarian Cancer

April Levine and Kevin S. Hughes

Recent discoveries in molecular genetics have improved our ability to identify patients who are at risk for hereditary cancer and to predict clinical outcomes for these patients. The current challenge is to design management strategies for the high-risk individual that will either prevent disease or detect it at an earlier, more treatable stage. It is incumbent on health care systems to develop a means of integrating these management strategies into the continuum of patient care.

Health care networks need to address the issues surrounding hereditary cancer for several reasons. First, the well-being of patients, both clinical and emotional, can be improved. Second, media attention to this area has greatly increased awareness of cancer genetics, and patients expect their health care system to provide these services. Third, the issue of liability has been raised regarding the absence of identification, notification, and management of familial risk. And finally, as we will try to accentuate in this chapter, addressing these issues is simply one more exemplification of the concept that providing the highest-quality medical care is the most cost-effective approach to treatment.

As this issue moves to the forefront, it will bring with it opportunities for improved medical care that eventually will save both lives and health care dollars, but the interventions required to bring this to fruition also will generate additional short-term costs. On average, however, we believe that the long-term benefits and savings will offset these additional short-term costs. What are the aspects that eventually will save lives and money, and what are the aspects that will add to cost?

Opportunities for improved medical care that eventually will save lives and health care dollars include early detection of disease by intensive surveillance and prevention of disease by chemoprevention or prophylactic surgery (1,2). Intensive screening should allow detection of disease at an earlier stage, when the disease is more likely to be curable and the treatment is less expensive (3). Taplin and colleagues (4) showed that the total costs of initial breast cancer care, as well as continuing costs, increase with stage. For example, ductal carcinoma in situ identified by intensive screening can be treated by lumpectomy and radiation therapy at a cost of approximately $10,000 (at the Lahey Clinic in 1997) and is associated with a life expectancy approaching normal (5). Conversely, invasive breast cancer with node involvement requires lumpectomy, axillary dissection, radiation, and chemotherapy at a cost of approximately $20,000 (at the Lahey Clinic in 1997) and is associated with a 5-year survival closer to 60% and the risk of requiring intensive chemotherapy and bone marrow transplantation at the time of recurrence (estimated cost, at least $28,600) (6). Prophylactic surgery or chemoprevention may decrease the incidence of cancer and therefore prevent these costs altogether. In addition, prophylactic surgery will abrogate the need for intensive surveillance. It has been estimated that the incremental cost per life-year saved for prophylactic oophorectomy, mastectomy, or combined oophorectomy plus mastectomy for women who carry a mutation in the *BRCA1* or *BRCA2* gene is between $336 and $1271 (6).

Thus the costs associated with not identifying high-risk patients may be avoided (cancers undiagnosed until higher stage, which leads to higher treatment costs, higher recurrence rates, and missed opportunities for cancer prevention), the costs associated with intensive screening of patients not at high risk may be avoided (including the cost of screening tests and the costs of false-positive results, additional tests, additional provider visits, and of additional workup and biopsies generated by false-positive test results), the cost of malpractice liability may be avoided, and the cost of poor public relations may be avoided.

To accrue these benefits, the costs of prophylactic surgery, chemoprevention, intensive screening, and genetic testing must be absorbed by the health care system. While we believe that these interventions will be medically effective and cost-effective, it is not something that can easily be proved at our current level of sophistication. While a health care system may wish to avoid these costs by ignoring the topic or attempt to hide behind the defense of unproved efficacy, this is no longer a viable option. Intensive surveillance of the high-risk individual has been accepted as the standard of care (1), and prophylactic surgery, genetic testing, and chemoprevention cannot be denied arbitrarily (7). Therefore, the opportunity for cost savings resides in our ability to limit these interventions to the highest-risk individuals by appropriate risk identification, not in refusing coverage or failing to identify high-risk individuals.

In the high-risk individual, these expensive and invasive interventions will most likely decrease the mortality of the disease and decrease the extent of treatment needed if disease develops (6). However, for the woman at average risk, these interventions are expensive, morbid, and excessive. The efficacy of screening in decreasing cancer deaths increases with increasing probability of developing breast cancer as well as increasing probability of dying from breast cancer (8). Since risk increases with genetic susceptibility, screening should be proportionately more effective in this group. Conversely, women who are at lower risk would derive little net benefit (6).

As an example, intensive surveillance of all women with a family history of breast cancer, no matter how minimal, will add tremendously to health care costs. Surveillance only of women deemed to be at high risk will add only marginally to costs while achieving the same goal of early detection, less aggressive treatment, and saved lives. Appropriate selection of women for intensive screening will limit the cost while maintaining the benefit and the cost saving.

We submit that the most cost-effective way to incorporate identification of the high-risk individual into a system and therefore reap the benefits of improved patient care is to begin with the development of a comprehensive approach to the hereditary breast/ovarian cancer syndrome. The choice of breast and ovarian cancer susceptibility as the initial model is justified by the facts that breast cancer is an extremely common cancer (the most common in women and the third most common overall), that research in this area has produced a high level of understanding, that genetic testing is available and provides useful information, and that the level of popular interest is extremely high. The high profile of this hereditary syndrome and the level of knowledge and expertise that surround it make this a natural area in which to begin. Extension of this model to other hereditary cancer syndromes as they reach maturity will be relatively simple and inexpensive, further justifying the initial investment, and eventually will provide a health care system with a comprehensive approach to cancer genetics.

We believe that a comprehensive approach to hereditary breast/ovarian cancer syndrome can best be accomplished through the development of a risk assessment clinic. A risk assessment clinic provides consultation regarding difficult or high-risk patients. However, of equal importance, it serves as the repository and resource of hereditary cancer information, as the developer of guidelines for identification and treatment of patients at high risk for hereditary cancer, and as the responsible agent for educating primary care providers in dealing with patients who have a family history of cancer. This chapter explains why this approach may be the most effective and the most cost-effective method of providing quality care.

We will limit the scope of this chapter primarily to hereditary breast/ovarian cancer syndrome. Other risk factors for breast cancer will be addressed briefly at the end of this chapter.

We will begin by looking at both the costs and the differential costs of the various approaches.

Screening Recommendations for Average and High-Risk Individuals

For the general population, current American Cancer Society recommendations (Table 15-1) for breast cancer screening include yearly mammography after age 40 (9). The American Cancer Society recommendations for ovarian cancer screening are a yearly pelvic examination as part of cervical cancer screening (9). Women at high risk for the development of breast and ovarian

cancer require more intensive screening to detect cancer at an early stage. A workshop (1) convened by the National Cancer Institute has made recommendations for intensive screening for this group. The report specifically states that any women whose family history suggests that she may harbor a mutation in *BRCA1* or *BRCA2* should undergo this intensive screening program unless definitive genetic testing proves she is not a carrier.

Patients who are at the highest risk for the development of breast cancer should have a breast examination every 6 months beginning between the ages of 25 and 35 (at Lahey Clinic, we begin at age 25) and an annual mammogram beginning between the ages of 25 and 35 (we begin at age 25). (Women who are pregnant or attempting to become pregnant should not have the mammogram.) Patients who are at the highest risk for ovarian cancer should have a pelvic examination every 6 months beginning between the ages of 25 and 35 (we begin at age 30), a transvaginal sonogram every 6 months beginning between the ages of 25 and 35 (we begin at age 30), and serum CA-125 level determinations every 6 months beginning at age 25 to 35. The high false-positive rate of CA-125 in premenopausal patients most likely abrogates any benefit in this population; therefore, many centers do not begin until age 50 or after menopause (Michael Muto, Brigham and Women's Hospital, Boston, personal communication, 1997). (At Lahey, we begin at menopause.)

Table 15-1. Screening recommendations and cost

Screening (Age)	Average Risk (Number of Exams)	High Risk (Number of Exams)	Number of Additional Studies Over Routine Screening	Cost per Unit	Lifetime Additional Cost for Intensive Screening
Physical exam (25–70)	Yearly (45)	Every 6 months (90)	45	$98	$4,410
Mammography (25–39)	0	Yearly (15)	15	$108	$1,612
Mammography (40–70)	Yearly (30)	Yearly (30)	0	$108	0
TVS (30–70)	0	Every 6 months (80)	80	$103	$8,240
CA-125 (25–49)	0	0	0	0	0
CA-125 (50–70)	0	Every 6 months (40)	40	$15	$600

Additional Costs of Intensive Screening

What are the additional costs generated for a patient who undergoes intensive screening compared with routine screening (Table 15-2)? In terms of breast screening, since yearly examinations during routine visits are the norm, the recommendation for examination every 6 months will add one additional examination per year between the ages of 25 and 70, or an additional 45 examinations. At a cost of $98 per visit (at the Lahey Clinic in 1997), the cost of 45 examinations will add up to approximately $4410. For mammography, since the norm is yearly mammograms beginning at age 40, yearly mammograms beginning at age 25 will add 15 additional mammograms between the ages of 25 and 40. At a cost of $108 each (at the Lahey Clinic in 1997), the cost of 15 mammograms will add up to $1612. The total screening cost thus would be $6022 per patient.

These costs are not limited to the testing itself, but also to the workup of false-positive results. Elmore and colleagues (10) have shown eloquently that false-positive results of mammography and clinical breast examination will add about 33% to the cost over 10 years of routine screening. In their study, 2400 women aged 40 to 69 underwent a median of four mammograms and five clinical breast examinations within a 10-year period. Of the women screened, 23.8% had at least one false-positive mammogram, 13.4% had at least one false-positive clinical examination, and 31.7% had at least one false-positive result for either test. A *false-positive result* was defined as a test in a woman who does not have cancer that generated an additional clinical visit, an additional mammogram, a breast ultrasound study, or a breast biopsy. These authors extrapolated that after 10 mammograms, the cumulative

risk of a false-positive result would be 49.1% (with a biopsy rate of 18.6%) and that after 10 clinical breast examinations, the cumulative risk of a false-positive result would be 22.3% (with a biopsy rate of 6.2%). The false-positive studies were estimated to add an additional 33% to the cost of screening.

With this in mind, the additional 15 mammograms generated by intensive screening in the 25- to 40-year-old age group and the 45 additional breast examinations will add at least 33% to the cost of screening. Since the cost of the intensive screening adds $6030 per patient, the additional cost of false-positive studies would be $1989.90. This brings the lifetime additional cost of intensive surveillance relative to the breast to $8019.90.

These are very conservative cost estimates considering the fact that the threshold for breast biopsy may be lower for this group than for women in the general population. In addition, the false-positive rate may be higher in women under 40 years of age, since the per-test rate of false-positive results was age-dependent. Women aged 40 to 49 years had a false-positive mammography rate of 7.8% and a false-positive clinical examination rate of 6%, whereas women aged 70 to 79 years had a false-positive mammography rate of 4.4% and a false-positive clinical examination rate of 2.2%.

In terms of ovarian cancer screening, as the American Cancer Society guidelines (9) call only for yearly pelvic examination as part of cervical screening; all costs for transvaginal sonography (TVS) and serum CA-125 determinations are additional costs. Using the intensive surveillance suggested (1), 80 TVSs will be performed between the ages of 30 and 70, and 40 CA-125 level determinations will be performed between the ages of 50 and 70. At a cost of $103 per TVS and $15 per CA-125 determination (at the Lahey Clinic in 1997), intensive surveillance will add $8840 per patient.

Costs also include the workup of all false-positive tests. Here we need to extrapolate because data are scarce. A CA-125 level of greater than 35 units has been identified in about 1.6% of women 50 years of age or older (11) who underwent screening. One could estimate that over a 20-year period of CA-125 determination

Table 15-2. Additional lifetime costs for patients of intensive screening

	Breast	Ovary
Cost of intensive screening	$6,022.00	$8,840.00
Cost of false positive	1,989.90	1,036.35
Total	$8,011.90	$9,876.35

every 6 months (40 tests), 1.6% of 40, or 0.64 tests per patient will be abnormal (64% of patients will have an abnormal test at some time). To be conservative, let us assume that the rate is only half that number and that only 32% will have an elevated CA-125 level at least one time. All women with an elevated CA-125 level (32%) will come to a repeat test, and perhaps one-third (10% of all patients) will go on to oophorectomy.

If 100 women undergo CA-125 testing every 6 months for 20 years (40 × 100 × $15 = $60,000), 32% have a repeat test done (32 × $15 = $480), and 10% have an oophorectomy (10 × $4811 = $48,110) (6), the total cost will be $108,590 for 100 patients, or $1,085.90 per patient (including the cost of false-positive studies of $485.90 per patient).

Van Nagell and colleagues (12) found that 9.2% of premenopausal women had an abnormality detected on TVS, and all had a repeat study. More than one-third of these women had a persistent abnormality (3.8% of premenopausal patients screened), and surgery was recommended. Thirteen of 16 women agreed to surgery, and all the women were found to have normal ovaries or benign disease. This finding was from a single screen, and it would be reasonable to assume over 20 years (between the ages of 30 and 50) of TVS every 6 months, twice as many women in total (18.4%) would have an abnormal TVS at some point and would undergo CA-125 determination and repeat TVS, and perhaps one-third of them (6%) would go on to oophorectomy.

In postmenopausal women, 11 patients (2.4%) went to surgery because of an abnormal TVS. Ten patients had benign disease, and one patient had metastatic colon cancer. This finding also was from a single screen, and it would be reasonable to assume over the 20 years (between the ages of 50 and 70) of TVS every 6 months, twice as many women in total (4.8%) would progress to oophorectomy.

If 100 premenopausal women undergo TVS testing every 6 months for 20 years (40 × 100 × $103 = $412,000), 18 have a repeat TVS (18 × 103 = $1854) and a CA-125 determination (18 × 15 = $270), and 6% have an oophorectomy (6 × $4811 = $28,866), the total cost is $442,990 for 100 patients, or $4429.90 per patient.

Table 15-3. Cost per patient by syndrome

Syndrome	Cost of Intensive Screening
Hereditary breast cancer	$8,019.90
Hereditary breast/ovarian cancer	$17,896.25

If 100 postmenopausal women undergo TVS testing every 6 months for 20 years (40 × 100 × $103 = $412,000) and 4.8% have an oophorectomy (5 × $4811 = $24,055), the total cost is $436,055 for 100 patients, or $4360.55 per patient. This brings the total cost of ovarian screening by TVS to $8790.45 (which includes the cost of false-positive results of $550.45 per patient).

Putting these data together, the additional cost of intensive screening with CA-125 plus TVS will be about $9876.35 ($1085.90 + $8790.45) per patient screened. Total cost will be slightly less because women who experience ovarian cancer, women who have prophylactic oophorectomy, and women who have an oophorectomy generated by a false-positive test will stop being screened.

Owing to the high probability of a *BRCA1* or *BRCA2* mutation in women with familial ovarian cancer, every patient undergoing intensive ovarian cancer screening will most likely also undergo intensive breast cancer screening at a lifetime cost of about $8019.90 (Table 15-3). The total cost of breast cancer screening plus ovarian cancer screening for these patients will be about $17,896.25.

Chemoprevention

Approaches to the prevention of breast and ovarian cancer take on added significance as we refine our ability to identify the highest-risk patients. For ovarian cancer, chemoprevention by the use of oral contraceptives (OCs) has been shown to be effective in the general population (13,14) and may be effective in patients at hereditary risk. Because of the low morbidity associated with OCs, every woman believed to be at increased risk should begin to take OCs as early as possible, even in the absence of documentation of risk. OCs should be continued for at least 10 years or through menopause (excluding pregnancy time) or until definitive information is available regarding duration of use.

Tamoxifen has been shown to be effective in decreasing the incidence of estrogen receptor (ER)–positive breast cancer in a high-risk population (15). However, since hereditary breast cancers caused by *BRCA1* mutations tend to be ER-negative, the efficacy of tamoxifen in hereditary cancer families requires confirmation. If proven efficacious, we may ask patients at risk for the development of hereditary cancer to begin this drug while still premenopausal. Since the side effects of tamoxifen are significant, it may be prudent to document actual risk by genetic testing before starting this medication.

Costs of Breast Chemoprevention

The Breast Cancer Prevention Trial (15) has found that tamoxifen will decrease the rate of breast cancer by about half in a high-risk population. While it is not yet clear that tamoxifen will be effective in patients at risk for hereditary breast cancer, the data should be available in the near future. If it is determined that tamoxifen is effective, then women who are at high risk of experiencing hereditary breast cancer probably should receive this drug. How long tamoxifen should be taken or at what age it should be started is unknown.

The cost of tamoxifen itself for 5 years is about $3500. Health care provider visits to monitor the drug can be absorbed into the ongoing 6-month visits in this population and do not add additional cost. The rate of life-threatening side effects in the premenopausal population is small, and costs therefore will be limited. Side effects that are unpleasant but not life-threatening, such as hot flashes or vaginal dryness, may generate a small number of additional visits or phone calls and may generate prescriptions for nonhormonal therapies, but in general, the costs for these will be minimal. Smith and Hilner (15a) indicate that the cost of tamoxifen is $8479 per additional year of life, and the lifetime cost-effectiveness is approximately $50,000 per year of life saved, a common benchmark.

Whereas it is not unreasonable to begin OCs in any woman with even a vague suspicion of increased risk of ovarian cancer, this approach is not appropriate with regard to tamoxifen. Because this is an expensive drug with significant side effects, and because tamoxifen has no beneficial effects in the premenopausal patient at average risk, use of this drug should be selective. Therefore, it may be reasonable to encourage a premenopausal woman at high risk of hereditary breast cancer to undergo genetic testing if tamoxifen is being considered. This would mean that 1) patients who carry a mutation would have tamoxifen prescribed, 2) patients who do not carry a mutation would not receive the drug (and intensive screening would be stopped), and 3) patients who have an equivocal test would have recommendations made on the basis of analysis of family history. This complex undertaking would be handled most appropriately within the context of a risk-assessment clinic. The cost savings relative to decreased screening and avoidance of tamoxifen should more than offset the cost of genetic testing, but more important, avoiding this medication in women at average risk is good medical care.

Ovarian Chemoprevention

Essentially every premenopausal patient identified as potentially at risk for hereditary ovarian cancer should be encouraged to take OCs. While it is not documented that this medication is effective in preventing hereditary ovarian cancer, a strong suggestion exists that this is the case. At what age this therapy should be started is unknown, but it appears that the earlier it is started, the better. How long it should be continued is also not known. While there may be a theoretical concern regarding an increased risk of breast cancer caused by OCs in this population, no data support this. Owing to the virtual absence of significant side effects, it is not unreasonable to recommend beginning OCs in the teens and continuing them until age 50 or until additional information regarding the most effective duration becomes available. The cost of each 10 years of OCs would be approximately $3000, including the medication. The cost of physician visits is not an additional cost, since these women are already being seen every 6 months. The differential cost would be related to the number of women in this age group who normally would be taking

OCs versus having all women at risk take OCs. The differential savings would be related to the number of ovarian cancers prevented.

Genetic Testing

Tests for *BRCA1* and *BRCA2* genes have now been developed for commercial use and are being offered to women with a strong family history of breast cancer or ovarian cancer or both. Options that are available for women who test positive for *BRCA1* or *BRCA2* mutations include prophylactic mastectomy, intensive surveillance (6), or chemoprevention (2). Prophylactic mastectomy is thought to reduce the risk of breast cancer by 90% (16), and prophylactic oophorectomy reduces the risk of ovarian cancer by at least 50% (17). Prophylactic surgery should increase survival as well as prevent cancer (6). Prophylactic oophorectomy and prophylactic mastectomy most likely will be effective in preventing cancer and saving lives in high-risk individuals but should not be used without documentation of risk status by genetic testing.

Costs of Genetic Testing

The costs of genetic testing include the costs of pretest counseling, posttest counseling, contacting relatives who also may require testing, and retrieving documentation of medical care and pathology reports from relatives and the cost of the test itself. Pre- and posttest counseling have been discussed elsewhere in this book (see Chap. 6). For patients who are found to be inappropriate candidates for testing, or for those who do not want testing, the total time spent could be about 1 hour. Patients who undergo testing will require pre- and posttest counseling, normally requiring a total of about 3 hours. The cost for a risk-assessment clinic to do this will vary with the personnel involved. At our risk-assessment clinic, the nurse practitioner and social worker see and evaluate the patient, with a total cost for counseling of about $200. Obtaining documentation of medical conditions of relatives can take an average of 1/2 hour of administrative time per patient. We would suggest that the expertise residing in a risk-assessment clinic will make it more cost-effective to handle this situation than

to have each primary care provider develop his or her own system for this undertaking.

It is more complicated to estimate the cost of the actual blood test. For the non-Jewish woman, the current practice is to test a living affected relative first to identify the family-specific mutation. The cost for this testing will vary by laboratory, but, as an example, full gene sequencing costs about $2400 (Myriad Genetics, Salt Lake City, Utah). When the family-specific mutation is known, the cost of testing additional family members will be around $300 each (Myriad Genetics). Assuming that both the unaffected patient and her affected relative are covered under the same health plan, the cost will be $2700. But how will costs be assigned if your unaffected patient wants to be tested and her affected sister is covered under a different health plan? Additionally, in our mobile society, it is not unusual for the affected relative to live in another state. For her to be tested will require that she receive counseling and testing in her local area and that the results be communicated to you. Part of the function of a risk-assessment clinic is to develop a network of contacts with other risk-assessment clinics throughout the country to facilitate this process. In the absence of a risk-assessment clinic, will each of your providers need to develop their own network of contacts?

Therefore, the total cost of testing the affected family member plus testing the unaffected member will be about $3100 ($2700 for the two blood tests and $400 for the two counseling sessions).

For the Jewish patient, it is not unreasonable to test the patient for the three common mutations without testing an affected relative (counseling $200 and blood test $450; Myriad Genetics). If no mutation is found, testing an affected family member for the three common mutations is a reasonable option (counseling $200 and blood test $450). If the affected relative carries a mutation, the chance of the patient having a mutation drops dramatically. If the relative tests negative, either full gene sequencing can be done ($2400, with an expected low yield), or the patient can be counseled based on the family history. Therefore, testing of an Ashkenazi woman can be estimated to cost around $650, with the testing of a few patients costing $1300 or more if a relative is pursued after a negative test.

Cost savings of a risk-assessment clinic reside in the expertise that moves this time-consuming problem out of the primary care practice (leaving time for other patient care issues) and in the avoidance of inappropriate testing. Most women who believe that they are at high risk actually are not and often can be dissuaded from intensive screening or genetic testing. No useful estimates are currently available, but it is reasonable to assume that most women who come to a risk assessment clinic seeking genetic testing can be reassured, avoiding the cost of the test and also avoiding the cost of intensive screening.

Costs of Prophylactic Surgery

A certain number of women at risk of hereditary breast or ovarian cancer will opt for prophylactic surgery, as discussed elsewhere in this book (see Chapters 6 and 11). The choices of procedures follow: For ovarian cancer, three types of prophylactic surgery are possible: bilateral salpingo-oophorectomy by laparoscopy, bilateral salpingo-oophorectomy by laparotomy, and hysterectomy plus bilateral salpingo-oophorectomy by laparotomy (laparoscopic-assisted hysterectomy is a less common option). The cost for these types of surgery averages $4811 to $6200 (6). For purposes of this discussion, we will use $5000. For breast cancer, four current prophylactic procedures are common: bilateral mastectomy with free transverse rectus abdominis musculocutaneous (TRAM) flap reconstruction, bilateral mastectomy with rotation TRAM flap reconstruction, bilateral mastectomy with implant reconstruction, and bilateral mastectomy without reconstruction. The average cost for procedures with TRAM flap reconstruction is about $9000 per surgery, and the average cost for mastectomy without reconstruction is about $5200. For purposes of this discussion, we will use $7000 per surgery.

Prophylactic surgery is an aggressive approach to prevention of breast and ovarian cancer, and therefore, we would recommend that any patient considering prophylactic surgery undergo genetic testing first. One-third to one-half of these patients will test negative for a mutation in *BRCA1* or *BRCA2* and can be spared this procedure.

Patients may choose oophorectomy, mastectomy, or both. Six patients choosing oophorectomy would cost $30,000, six choosing mastectomy would cost $42,000, and six choosing both mastectomy and oophorectomy would cost $72,000. If six non-Ashkenazi women present for prophylactic surgery and undergo genetic testing, the cost of six tests would be $18,600 (6 × $3100). It is reasonable to assume that one-third will have a mutation, one-third will not have a mutation, and one-third will have an equivocal test. We will make the assumption subsequently that the one-third with a mutation have surgery, that the one-third without a mutation do not have surgery, and that 50% of the one-third with an equivocal test have surgery and 50% do not. Therefore, if six patients considering oophorectomy underwent genetic testing (6 × 3100 = $18,600), and then only three women had the procedure ($15,000), the cost would be approximately $30,600 compared with $30,000 if all six patients had oophorectomy. Although representing no real difference in cost, this approach spares three patients a procedure that is not indicated.

If six patients considering prophylactic mastectomy underwent genetic testing ($18,600) and then only three had the procedure ($21,000), the cost would be $39,600 compared with $42,000 if all had mastectomy. If six patients considering both prophylactic mastectomy and prophylactic oophorectomy underwent genetic testing ($18,600), and then only three patients had the procedure, the cost would be about $54,600 compared with $72,000 if all six patients had the procedure.

The Risk Assessment Clinic as an Approach to High-Risk Identification

We would submit that the development of an approach to the identification of women at high risk for the development of hereditary breast and ovarian cancer is cost-effective in itself. It becomes most cost-effective when considered in the context of developing a model that can be extended to other hereditary cancers as other cancer genes are identified and clinical relevance is found.

Laissez-Faire Approach

A health plan may take the laissez-faire approach and hope that health care providers accrue enough information about hereditary cancer to make an appropriate determination regarding which patients are at risk. While this is the approach used by most health plans today, we believe that the field of cancer genetics is developing too rapidly and that there are too many issues and too many practitioners to make this a practical approach. This approach most likely will lead to average-risk women being intensively screened, high-risk women not being intensively screened, genetic testing being done for inappropriate patients, inappropriate counseling being offered to women seeking genetic testing, genetic tests being misinterpreted, and the use of prophylactic surgery for the wrong patients.

In addition, expecting the primary care provider to provide complete risk assessment and counseling for all members of his or her panel is unreasonable. A thorough risk assessment of a single patient can take more than an hour. Assessment and counseling for genetic testing for a single patient often can take 2 to 3 hours. It is highly unlikely that a busy primary care provider will have time within his or her schedule to provide this time-intensive service.

Risk Assessment Clinic Approach

The approach that we would recommend is the development of a risk assessment clinic, as defined elsewhere in this book (see Chapter 10). The purpose of this clinic would be to see high-risk patients for the purpose of better defining their risk, to serve as a central repository of information regarding hereditary cancer, to develop guidelines for testing and management, and to educate patients and primary care providers. This strategy will help to minimize the number of patients who undergo intensive screening, prophylactic surgery, or chemoprevention and therefore minimize costs.

The clinic would see all women requesting genetic testing and undertake the extensive

counseling process necessary. This will help to limit testing to only the highest-risk woman, in whom the test may provide clinically relevant information. This will greatly decrease the number of women undergoing testing and therefore decrease cost. Taking on the responsibility of providing the intensive counseling necessary prior to and following genetic testing removes this time-consuming task from the primary care provider's office, again saving money.

The use of OCs as a chemopreventive agent is safe and can be left to the primary care provider (when informed appropriately). However, the clinic would see all women requesting chemoprevention of breast cancer and would undertake the extensive counseling process necessary. This would help to limit the number of women taking controversial chemopreventive agents to only those at highest risk, in whom they may provide some clinical utility. In addition, it would be incumbent on the risk assessment clinic to be involved in clinical trials that aim to define the activity of new agents. Patients who participate in these trials are often provided free or discounted medications. For example, the second National Surgical Adjuvant Breast Project (NSABP) prevention trial (15) will randomize patients to receive either raloxifene or tamoxifen. The cost of 1 year of tamoxifen is $700, and the cost of 1 year of raloxifene is about $720. On the trial, these medications will be provided free of charge.

For patients who would consider tamoxifen outside the study, appropriate counseling within the context of the risk assessment clinic will limit its use to the highest-risk woman. Under the influence of intensive media barrage, many women feel that tamoxifen or raloxifene is the answer to preventing breast cancer. It would take an extremely well-informed primary care provider with an inordinate amount of time to dissuade a woman from this notion. The result could be many women receiving prescriptions for the sake of expediency. Conversely, the risk-assessment clinic is designed to have the expertise and time needed to educate the patient and most often can prevent the average-risk woman from unnecessarily taking one of these drugs. In terms of dollars, dissuading an average-risk woman from taking tamoxifen will save $700 per year, or about $3500 over 5 years.

The risk assessment clinic also serves as the responsible agent for educating primary care providers in dealing with patients who have a positive family history. Communication back to the referring provider after each consultation will serve as an educational process that increases the ability of the provider to differentiate high- from average-risk patients. The educated primary care provider will then be better able to identify the highest-risk patients for referral to the risk-assessment clinic and to reassure average-risk patients. By improving the ability of the primary care provider to identify high-risk patients, more high-risk women will be identified, and fewer average-risk women will be referred to the risk assessment clinic for intensive evaluation or screening, eventually decreasing costs. The clinic also would serve as a repository and resource of hereditary cancer information for the primary care provider and would develop guidelines for the identification and treatment of patients at high risk for hereditary cancer.

Savings Generated by the Risk Assessment Clinic Approach

In calculating the costs of developing this approach to the identification of women at high risk for breast and ovarian cancer, the alternative must be considered. In this case, the alternative would be the cost of not developing a risk assessment clinic and not providing an intensive educational effort. Costs will be multiplied for every patient in whom risk is not properly assigned. Patients at risk who do not receive intensive screening likely will experience more advanced cancer before it is detected, which will be more expensive to treat and less curable. Patients who are not at risk and are misclassified as at high risk will receive expensive intensive screening to no purpose. In addition, they will decrease the overall relative risk of the screened population and therefore increase the absolute number of false-positive results, again increasing costs. Assuming that providers are currently identifying high-risk women based on the current level of understanding, it is likely that some

low-risk women are receiving intensive screening that they do not need and that some high-risk women are not being adequately screened.

General Estimates

Having developed general estimates for the cost of intensive surveillance, chemoprevention, prophylactic surgery, and genetic testing, the next step is to place this in the context of a clinical practice. This requires an estimation of the number of women with a family history of breast or ovarian cancer or both, the significance of that history, and the ease of categorization of that history (how obvious it is that the family history of that patient is or is not significant).

To this end, we have examined information gathered from various sources in our practice, and we have tried to synthesize a cohesive picture.

A group of 129 nurses at Lahey Clinic under the age of 40 years were queried regarding their family history as part of a study of breast cancer risk (18). Family history of breast cancer was reported in 31% of these women. This information was combined with a larger series looking at all history. In a separate series of 477 women undergoing mammography at Lahey Clinic who had a family history of breast or ovarian cancer, 86% had a family history of breast cancer only, 5% had a family history of breast cancer and ovarian cancer, and 9% had a family history of ovarian cancer alone. When the family histories of these patients were reviewed by experts (Constance Roche, M.S.N., R.N., C.S., Lahey Clinic, Peabody, Massachusetts; and Marie Wood, M.D., UVM, Burlington, Vermont), 62 of the 412 patients (15%) with a breast-cancer-only family history were believed to require further evaluation for hereditary syndrome, 9 of the 44 patients (20%) with an ovarian-cancer only family history were believed to require further evaluation for hereditary syndrome, and 10 of the 21 patients (48%) with an ovarian-cancer-only family history were felt to require further evaluation for hereditary syndrome. If we consider ovarian cancer alone or in combination with breast cancer to represent the breast/ovarian cancer syndrome, then 19 of 65 women (29%) would require further evaluation for a hereditary breast/ovarian cancer syndrome.

By combining this information, we can extrapolate that of all women under 40 years of age, 34% would have a family history of breast cancer, ovarian cancer, or both, with 29% of all women having a family history of breast cancer only, 2% of all women having a family history of breast and ovarian cancer, and 3% of all women having a family history of ovarian cancer alone (5% having a family history of ovarian cancer with or without breast cancer).

Extrapolating the expert categorization, 4% (0.15 × 29%) of all women would require further evaluation for a hereditary breast cancer syndrome, and 1.5% (0.29 × 5%) of all women would require further evaluation for a hereditary breast/ovarian cancer syndrome (Fig. 15-1). Since this was determined by expert review of family history, it is reasonable to assume that primary care providers may overestimate who is at risk. For our purposes, let us place this estimate at 50%. If so, we would expect that primary care providers would feel that 4% × 1.5, or 6%, of all women would be considered part of hereditary

breast cancer syndrome, and 1.5% × 1.5, or 2.25%, of all women would be considered part of hereditary breast/ovarian cancer syndromes (Fig. 15-2).

What would be the screening cost per 100 women under these two scenarios? In an integrated network with a risk assessment clinic, 4 of 100 women would undergo intensive breast screening at a cost of $8019.90 per patient (total = $32,079.60), and 1.5 women per 100 would undergo intensive breast and ovarian cancer screening at a cost of $16,810.35 per patient (total = $25,215.52). The total cost of intensive screening per 100 women would be $57,295.12.

Using the laissez-faire approach, 6 of 100 women would undergo intensive breast screening (cost = $48,119.40), and 2.25 would undergo intensive breast and ovarian screening (cost = $37,823.29). The total cost of intensive screening per 100 women would be $85,942.69.

Having a risk assessment clinic potentially would save $28,647.57 per 100 women. If your health plan has 200,000 covered lives and half

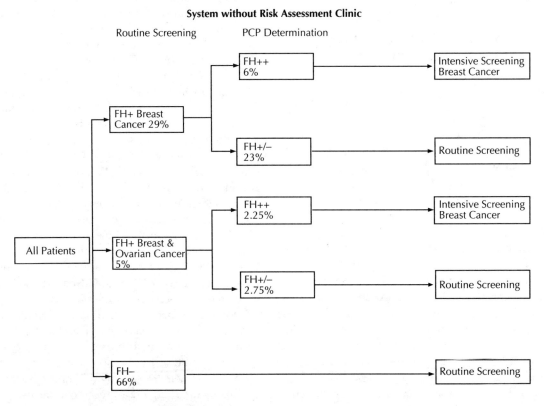

System without Risk Assessment Clinic

Routine Screening   PCP Determination

Figure 15-1. System without risk assessment clinic.

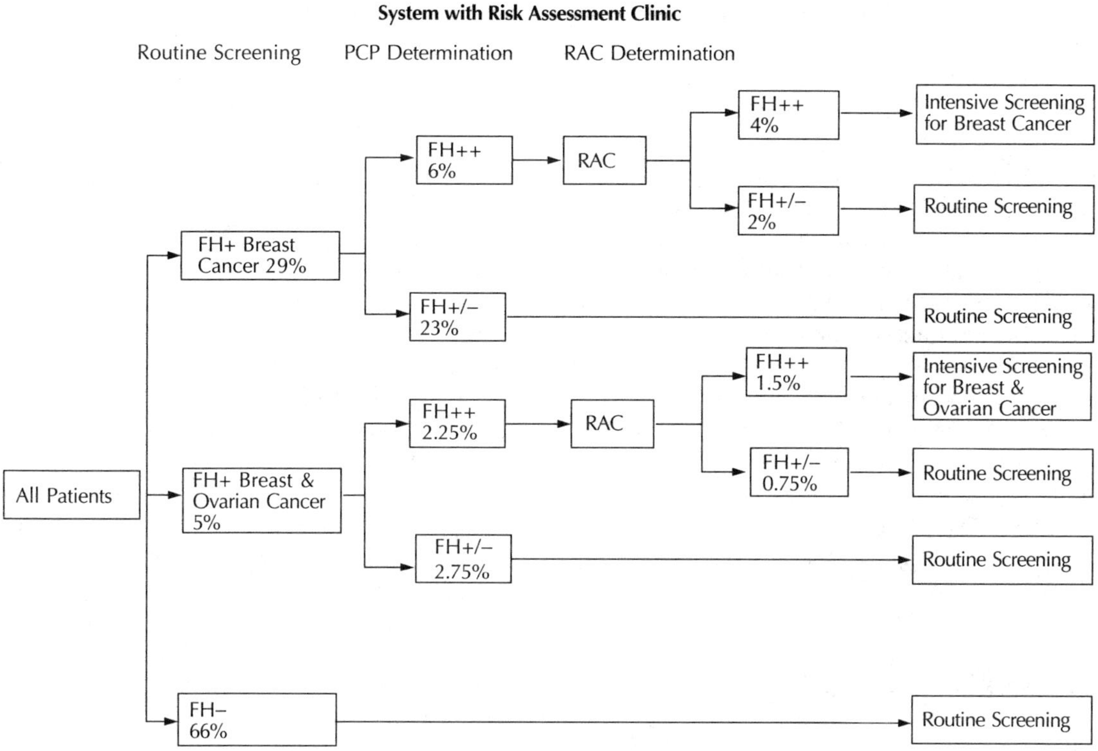

System with Risk Assessment Clinic

Figure 15-2. System with risk assessment clinic.

are women, the cost savings could be up to $28,647,570 (100,000 × $28,647.57/100).

A Suggested System-Wide Approach

A potential system-wide approach to the management of hereditary breast or breast/ovarian syndrome could be as follows:

1. Undertake an intensive educational effort of all primary care providers and patients regarding this area, and seek to identify all high-risk women.
2. Average-risk women can be reassured by their primary care providers, and truly high-risk women will be sent to the risk assessment clinic.
3. At the risk assessment clinic, an intensive risk assessment will weed out more average-risk women who will be advised to resume standard screening.

Moderate Risk

Women at moderate risk of hereditary breast cancer syndrome will undergo intensive breast screening and be considered for future chemoprevention trials. Women at moderate risk of breast/ovarian syndrome will be encouraged to use OCs while premenopausal and to undergo intensive breast/ovarian screening.

High Risk

Women believed to be at very high risk of hereditary breast cancer syndrome will undergo intensive screening and be considered for chemoprevention trials. Genetic testing would be strongly considered, and the patient who tests positive for a mutation would be informed of the option of prophylactic mastectomy and also would most likely move into the high-risk breast/ovarian syndrome category (assuming all *BRCA1* and *BRCA2* mutations increase the risk of ovarian cancer). Women who definitely test negative can resume average-risk screening, whereas women who have equivocal tests should continue intensive screening.

Women believed to be at high risk for breast/ovarian cancer syndrome will undergo intensive screening and be encouraged to use OCs. If over age 40, we would encourage this group to undergo incidental oophorectomy if any other abdominal procedure is planned. We would encourage genetic testing because such testing will affect management. If the patient carries a mutation, she should be informed of the pros and cons of prophylactic mastectomy and also should be encouraged to have prophylactic oophorectomy after childbearing is complete.

We submit that this template for a system-wide approach may be useful in answering the question: "Yes, but will it affect patient management?" The answer should be a resounding, "Yes."

Other Risk Factors

There is a distinct role for a risk assessment clinic for the identification and management of women with at high risk of being part of hereditary breast/ovarian cancer families. In the Risk Assessment Clinic at Lahey Clinic (see Chap. 10), 80% of the patients we see fall into this group.

Why is the risk assessment clinic approach ideal for this population? Consider that risk factors can be categorized based on three characteristics: 1) proportion of the population that carries the factor, 2) degree of effect of that factor, and 3) ease with which women with that factor can be identified. Also consider that the role of the risk assessment clinic is to 1) identify the woman at high risk and reassure the woman at average risk, 2) counsel the woman regarding her risk, and 3) develop a management strategy. Lets look at three examples:

1. Early menarche as defined by Gail (19) affects a tremendous portion of the population [74% of the population in one study (20)] but carries with it a minuscule effect on risk [relative risk 1.099–1.207 (1)]. Identification of women with this factor is relatively easy, and therefore, you do not need a risk assessment clinic to identify

these patients. Counseling at a risk assessment clinic for this factor makes little sense, and the effect on the population is so small that one would not change management strategy based on this factor. It is unlikely the risk assessment clinic will be cost-effective in this instance.

2. Atypical hyperplasia or lobular carcinoma in situ are factors that affect a very small population (about 1% of breast biopsies show this change), but the risk these factors carry is very large (see Chapter 12). In general, patients with these factors are easy to identify if the pathologist is well trained (the pathology report either shows one of these diagnoses or not). One would recommend a different management strategy for this population with more intensive breast screening. A risk assessment clinic is not needed to identify the woman at high risk (easily discerned from the pathology report) but may be useful in developing an individualized management strategy (all require a similar method of intensive screening, and the use of tamoxifen as a chemopreventive agent must be addressed). The risk assessment clinic also helps in educating and counseling these patients regarding risk. In this situation, the risk assessment clinic could be considered cost-effective if it moves the education and counseling process out of the primary care provider's office and it addresses the issue of chemoprevention.

3. Many women have a family history of breast cancer, but very few women actually carry a mutation in one of the susceptibility genes. The effect of family history on risk is small to nonexistent unless a woman carries a mutation in one of the breast cancer–susceptibility genes. Identification of a woman with a family history of breast cancer is relatively simple, but as described in this chapter, discerning who is at risk of carrying a susceptibility gene is not trivial. Management strategies are diverse and individualized, ranging from normal screening, to intensive breast screening with or without ovarian screening, to prophylactic surgery. As such, the value and cost-effectiveness of a risk assessment clinic are easier to establish. Evaluating the woman with a family history and determining if she is at average risk or high risk for breast cancer or at high risk for breast and ovarian cancer can be a major undertaking. Understanding the subtleties and nuances comes with a large volume that individual primary care providers seldom see. Counseling of the patients at high risk and reassurance of those at average risk are time-consuming and require a thorough knowledge of genetics, screening, cancer care and diagnosis, and psychological techniques. The development of a management strategy is extremely individualized.

A risk assessment clinic is cost-effective in dealing with hereditary cancer issues, probably is cost-effective in dealing with individuals with atypical hyperplasia or lobular carcinoma in situ, and adds only marginal value regarding lesser risk factors except as a source of information to primary care providers, who should deal with the majority of these patients.

Summary

The age of hereditary cancer is upon us, and health plans must prepare. We submit that the development of a risk assessment clinic as an entity in itself and as the responsible agent for instituting a comprehensive, system-wide approach will decrease costs by preventing cancer (i.e., appropriate use of chemoprevention and prophylactic surgery), by decreasing the stage of cancer detected (i.e., appropriate use of intensive screening), and by decreasing the inappropriate use of expensive interventions in average-risk women (i.e., preventing chemoprevention, intensive screening, prophylactic surgery, and genetic testing in women at average risk).

The alternative of ignoring the situation and hoping that primary care providers can figure it out for themselves is an expensive alternative.

References

1. Burke W, Daly M, Garber J, et al. Recommendations for follow-up care of individuals with an inherited predisposition to cancer: II. *BRCA1* and *BRCA2*. Cancer Genetics Study Consortium. JAMA 1997;277(12):997–1003.
2. Hughes KS, Papa MZ, Whitney T, McLellan R. Prophylactic mastectomy and inherited cancer predisposition. Cancer 1999;86:1682–1696.
3. Brown ML, Fintor L. Cost-effectiveness of breast cancer screening: preliminary results of a systematic review of the literature. Breast Cancer Res Treat 1993;25:113–118.
4. Taplin SH, Barlow W, Urban N, et al. Stage, age, comorbidity, and direct costs of colon, prostate, and breast cancer care. J Natl Cancer Inst 1995;87(6):417–426.
5. Hughes KS, Lee AK, Rolfs A. Controversies in the treatment of ductal carcinoma in situ. Surg Clin North Am 1996;76(2):243–265.
6. Grann VR, Panageas KS, Whang W, et al. Decision analysis of prophylactic mastectomy and oophorectomy in *BRCA1*-positive or *BRCA2*-positive patients. J Clin Oncol 1998;16(3):979–985.
7. *Katskee v. Blue Cross/Blue Shield of Nebraska*, Nebraska Supreme Court No. S-92-1022 (1994).
8. Eddy DM, Hasselblad V, McGivney W, Hendee W. The value of mammography screening in women under age 50. JAMA 1988;259(10):1512–1519.
9. Based on scientific research and expert opinion, the ACS has established recommendations to detect cancer early in asymptomatic people (without symptoms of cancer). American Cancer Society Web Site: http://www2.cancer.org/prevention/more_detection.cfm
10. Elmore JG, Barton MB, Moceri VM, et al. Ten-year risk of false positive screening mammograms and clinical breast examinations. New Engl J Med 1998;338(16):1089–1096.
11. Einhorn N, Sjovall K, Knapp RC, et al. Prospective evaluation of serum CA-125 levels for early detection of ovarian cancer. Obstet Gynecol 1992;80(1):14–18.
12. van Nagell JR Jr, Higgins RV, Donaldson ES, et al. Transvaginal sonography as a screening method for ovarian cancer: a report of the first 1,000 cases screened. Cancer 1990;65(3):573–577.
13. Hankinson SE, Colditz GA, Hunter DJ, et al. A quantitative assessment of oral contraceptive use and risk of ovarian cancer. Obstet Gynecol 1992;80(4):708–714.
14. Gross TP, Schlesselman JJ. The estimated effect of oral contraceptive use on the cumulative risk of epithelial ovarian cancer. Obstet Gynecol 1994;83(3):419–424.
15. Fisher B, Costantino JP, Wickerham DL, et al. Tamoxifen for prevention of breast cancer: report of the National Surgical Adjuvant Breast and Bowel Project P-1 study. J Natl Cancer Inst 1998;90(18):1371–1388.
15a. Smith TJ, Hilner BE. Tamoxifen should be cost-effective in reducing breast cancer risk in high-risk women. J Clin Oncol 2000;18:284.

16. Hartman L, Jenkins R, Schaid D, et al. Prophylactic mastectomy (PM): preliminary retrospective cohort analysis. Proc Am Assoc Cancer Res 1997;38:1123. Abstract.

17. Streuwing JP, Watson P, Easton DF, et al. Prophylactic oophorectomy in inherited breast/ovarian cancer families. Nat Cancer Inst Monogr 1995;17:1529–1533.

18. Gil F. Hereditary breast cancer risk: factors associated with the decision to undergo *BRCA1* testing. Eur J Cancer Prev 1996;5(6):488–490.

19. Gail MH, Brinton LA, Byar DP, et al. Projecting individualized probabilities of developing breast cancer for white females who are being examined annually. J Natl Cancer Inst 1989;81:1879–1886.

20. Mackarem G, Roche CA, Hughes KS: The effectiveness of the Gail model in estimating risk for development of breast cancer in women under 40 years of age. Breast J 2000 (in press).

16

Population-Based Prevention Strategies

Amy Trentham-Dietz, Richard R. Love, and Polly A. Newcomb

Unlike some chronic diseases, such as lung cancer or AIDS, breast cancer does not appear to have a single cause or exposure that leads to its development. The complex and incompletely understood biology of breast cancer makes potential prevention approaches difficult. When well-studied preventive interventions are efficacious, their successful application to the general population will depend on the degree to which they are acceptable, easily reproducible, limited in their adverse side effects, and inexpensive. Interventions with these characteristics have been difficult to define. Here we summarize possible strategies and their feasibility to prevent breast cancer.

Theoretical Feasibility of Breast Cancer Prevention

The differences in incidence rates among and within populations, and on migration of populations, provide compelling evidence that breast cancer should be preventable. Substantial variations in breast cancer rates are seen in different countries (1); in the United States and Canada, the incidence rates of breast cancer are over four times greater than those in Africa, China, or Japan (2,3). In general, however, differences in incidence rates among countries are becoming smaller (4). Incidence of breast cancer more than doubled in Japan during the period 1970–1985 (4). In the United States, incidence rates increased remarkably around 1974 and again in the 1980s, primarily due to a rapid increase in the numbers of mammographic screening–detected cancers (5,6). Independent

of these surges in rates, long-term breast cancer incidence has been slowly increasing in the United States at about 0.5% to 1.0% per year since the 1930s (4). These changes in incidence rates within populations, prior to screening, suggest that environmental/lifestyle factors are important in this disease (4,7). Similarly, decreases in breast cancer mortality rates in younger women during the 1970s and early 1980s preceded widespread use of effective screening and adjuvant therapies and so must also be consequent to other factors important in disease development and biology (5,8).

Studies of migrant populations demonstrate how breast cancer incidence rates change along with changes in environmental factors. Migrants from countries with lower incidence rates of breast cancer to countries with higher incidence rates tend to assume the cancer risk of their new homes within two or three generations (7,9) (Fig. 16-1). The speed at which incidence rates change varies among ethnic groups and may depend on the pace of acculturation (4). For example, Japanese born in the United States have breast cancer rates similar to their Caucasian counterparts, whereas Japanese born in Japan and migrating later experience a small increase in breast cancer incidence rates (10). This and other migrant studies show that factors in early life (3,10) and in adulthood (11) can have an impact on breast cancer risk. In summary, different incidence rates among populations and the specific lifestyle and environmental factors responsible for these differences suggest that prevention of breast cancer is possible.

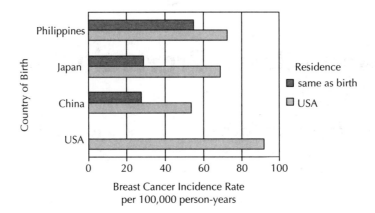

Figure 16-1. Breast cancer incidence rates according to migration pattern. Age-standardized breast cancer incidence rates for women aged 20 to 54 years according to country of residence and birth, 1983–1987. [Data from Ziegler et al. (9).]

Components of a Comprehensive Model of Breast Cancer Development and Prevention

Prevention of breast cancer clearly should be based on an understanding of etiology. A comprehensive model of breast cancer development and prevention should address three related and overlapping components (Fig. 16-2). These components depend on a framework of three landmark hormonal events: menarche, pregnancy, and menopause. The first model component stresses the structures of the breast.

Undifferentiated breast structures are the origin of most ductal breast cancers (12). Increases in hormone levels and the rate of cell division during pregnancy appear to coincide with differentiation of most breast lobular cells, so lobular maturation and differentiation of breast terminal end buds appear to be critical events in susceptibility to breast malignancy in both animals and humans (12,13). In particular, terminal differentiation protects against the formation of precancerous lesions as a result of DNA damage or the lack of DNA repair mechanisms (14). After a transiently increased risk after first pregnancy (15), the differentiation

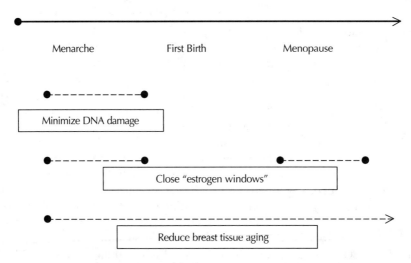

Figure 16-2. Strategies for breast cancer prevention according to relevant time periods across the female lifespan.

of end buds ultimately leads to a lifelong reduction of breast cancer risk (12,16). Based on these data, prevention strategies should minimize exposures causing DNA damage during the early but critical time in a young woman's life between the ages at menarche and the first full-term pregnancy and make the duration of this time as short as practical (17).

A second model component was first described by Korenman as the "estrogen window hypothesis" (18,19). Korenman argued that exposure to unopposed estrogen, such as periods of low progesterone, increases the susceptibility of breast tissue to tumor induction by environmental carcinogens. He stressed the importance of the duration of the time window rather than the level of unopposed estrogen in the body. Therefore, measures to prevent breast cancer following this component focus on reducing the length of time when estrogen is present without progesterone, that is, shortening the perimenarcheal and perimenopausal times when menstrual cycles are unpredictable and avoiding potentially harmful exposures during this time.

A third aspect of a comprehensive model acknowledges that breast tissue age is not simply calendar age — that exposure to estrogen and progesterone accelerates the pace of aging (20). Breast tissue ages most rapidly during exposure to ovulatory menstrual cycles and, in particular, to the luteal phase of the cycle, during which cell proliferation is increased in response to the presence of both estrogen and progesterone (21). Increased luteal phase cell proliferation occurs along with a greater chance of replication of DNA mutations that lead to breast cancer (22). Strategies that address this third element focus on reducing the number of ovulatory menstrual cycles over the course of a woman's lifetime by delaying menarche, moving forward the onset of menopause, or suppressing ovulation. Other strategies, such as avoiding alcohol, weight gain, and possibly physical inactivity, aim to reduce hormone levels even after menopause or block hormonal effects at the cellular level (as with antiestrogen therapy).

A broad model of breast cancer prevention incorporates strategies from all three components: minimize DNA damage while breast tissue is especially vulnerable to cancer initiation,

shorten the time frame when the breast is particularly susceptible to damage, and lower the levels of hormones that occur in the presence of tumor initiation and promotion. While strategies to address these are definable, their feasibility, effectiveness, toxicity, and acceptability to large populations of women make some worth pursuing and others impractical.

Potential Interventions

A number of modest risk factors for breast cancer, including parity and age at menarche and first birth, have been described for decades and contribute substantially to the model of breast cancer development and prevention discussed earlier.

Reproductive Risk Factors

Two reproductive factors are consistently associated with increased risk of breast cancer: later age at first full-term pregnancy and lower (or null) parity. Earlier age at first birth should reduce the length of time that the breast tissue is vulnerable to malignant initiation due to environmental exposures (23). While an early pregnancy (or pseudopregnancy) appears to be a desirable event from the standpoint of breast cancer risk, no easy way to simulate the effects of pregnancy on the breast in humans has been defined, and the long-term risks associated with such possible interventions are unknown.

Colditz and Frazier (17) have proposed a "social strategy" that promotes early and closely spaced childbearing for breast cancer control in the United States. It is not clear that such a social agenda would lead to improved overall health and well-being for women. Secular changes, such as expanding employment and educational opportunities, and the availability of effective contraceptives have led to dramatic changes in childbearing practices. While about 15% of women born in the late 1930s were nulliparous or had their first child after age 29, this percentage nearly doubled for women born in the early 1950s (24). Increases in the availability of convenient and affordable day care may occur, along with more flexible work schedules and the acceptance of prolonged lactation, all of which

Table 16-1. Breast cancer prevention strategies for healthy women

Factor	Strategy	Feasibility
Definitely effective		
Antiestrogen therapy	Reduce effect of estrogen on the breast	Uncertain for healthy women
Radiation	Avoidance	High
Probably effective		
Fruit and vegetable intake	Increase consumption	High
Obesity	Weight loss, avoid weight gain	High
Physical activity	Regular vigorous exercise	High
Lactation	Early, exclusive and long-term breast-feeding	High
Alcohol	Avoidance/moderation	High
Age at first birth	Early childbearing	Low
Age at menarche	Delay	Low
Age at menopause	Early surgical or chemotherapy-induced menopause	Low
Possibly effective		
Oral contraceptives	Avoidance	High
Hormone replacement therapy	Avoidance	High
Chemoprevention	Suppression of ovulation	Low
Uncertain effectiveness		
Tobacco	Avoidance/cessation	High
Gene therapy	Limit genetic susceptibility	Uncertain
Fat intake	Reduce consumption	Uncertain

may help to increase the numbers of women able to choose to have children at younger ages. Such societal support, however, cannot influence the emotional readiness of individual women to bear children. In sum, while studies of these two reproductive factors — parity and age at first birth — have helped to elucidate the biology of breast cancer, modification of behavior related to these factors appears likely to be unacceptable to many women and is therefore unlikely to have a substantial effect on breast cancer incidence in the United States (25,26) (Table 16-1).

Age at Menarche

Numerous studies have confirmed that early age at menarche increases the risk of breast cancer (16). Each 1-year delay in the age at menarche is associated with a 5% decreased risk of breast cancer (16). Exposure to carcinogens during the critical but vulnerable time between menarche and the age at first birth may be especially relevant (17,23).

Several studies have examined determinants of menarche to achieve a better understanding of how this event may be delayed through intervention. One such determinant is early-life body weight. At a given age, higher-weight girls are more likely to have an earlier age at menarche than girls who weigh less (27–32). Higher body fat and greater height have also been shown to predict earlier menarche (29,30,33). Limited data have suggested that increased participation in sports activities is associated with delayed menarche, whereas increased time being physically inactive, such as while watching television, is associated with accelerated menarche (29,30). Additionally, international variations in diet may partially account for differences in average ages at menarche and, in turn, different rates of breast cancer. In particular, Chinese girls tend to experience first menses at an average of 17 years, African-American girls at 12.2 years, and white American girls at 12.8 years (26,34). Lifestyle factors such as body weight, physical activity, and diet most likely have contributed to a decline in the age of menarche in the United States from 17 years two centuries ago to a current average of 12.8 years (35), and in turn, this may be contributing to the gradual increase in breast cancer incidence over the last several decades.

While, from the perspective of breast cancer prevention, an intervention to delay menarche seems worth investigating, insufficient data exist on the feasibility of modifying the timing of menarche. Further, interventions to delay menarche may be accompanied by adverse effects on bone mineral density and other measures of health. Efforts for children, both girls and boys, to eat a well-balanced diet and to lead an active lifestyle are certainly warranted for good health in general.

Stature

Diet affects not only the timing of menarche and maintenance of menses but also height attainment, so adult height reflects to some extent childhood and adolescent nutrition (35,36). Height, and the nutritional level height represents, may affect breast cancer risk through acceleration of growth hormone release and increased insulin-like growth factor levels (37) or increased follicular phase plasma estradiol peaks (38). However, genetic factors are more likely than nutritional factors to influence variability in height for most white women in the United States (36). As reviewed by Hunter and Willett (39), many studies have described null associations between height and breast cancer risk. Since that review, other studies have reported significant increases, of 40% to 100%, in risk (40,41). Absent or more modest increases in risk are perhaps due to limited variation in height among study participants. Avoidance of childhood obesity is obviously desirable to reduce the risk of heart disease and diabetes. But again, dietary restriction as a means to reduce height attainment in children is also obviously not an acceptable, or even feasible, method to prevent breast cancer, and it is not otherwise at all evident how to use this association to intervene in disease frequency.

Age at Menopause

Later age at menopause increases the risk of breast cancer (16). Each 5-year delay in the age

at menopause increases the risk of breast cancer by about 17% (42), whereas bilateral oophorectomy prior to age 40 years reduces the risk by as much as 45% (43). The cumulative number of menstrual cycles and the associated higher estrogen levels may be important determinants of breast cancer risk. While surgical castration for healthy women at average risk of breast cancer is not a medically or socially acceptable intervention, oophorectomy (along with pharmacologic treatment of the adverse effects of early menopause) in women at increased risk of breast cancer is probably an effective intervention in women undergoing major gynecologic surgery for other indications.

Modifiable Lifestyle Interventions

Several changes in lifestyle factors have been consistently associated with decreased risk of breast cancer. While broad changes are certainly possible, long-term behavior modification is very difficult for people to achieve. As the battles against tobacco-associated disease have taught us, major permanent behavior changes are tremendously challenging even though they lead to large benefits in terms of averting or delaying disease development.

Diet

Ecologic and laboratory studies demonstrate an association of fat intake with increased risk of breast cancer (23,39,44,45), and several biologic mechanisms are suggested to explain a promoting role of fat in breast cancer (46). However, individual-level data from cohort studies do not consistently support this relation (47,48) (Fig. 16-3). Case-control studies more frequently provide results supporting the association. One summary analysis suggests a 46% increase in the risk of breast cancer among women with the highest intake of saturated fat (49), while another summary of 25 case-control studies found a 28% increase in risk for the highest category of total fat consumption (50). Null associations in epidemiologic studies are attributed to the difficulty associated with assessing diet and measuring fat intake, and the homogeneity of study participants' diets (46). Support for a fat/breast cancer

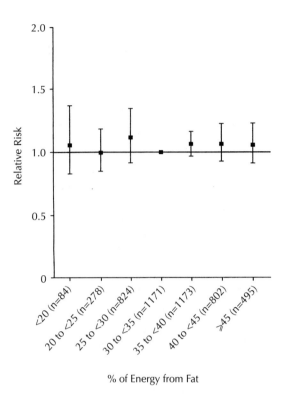

% of Energy from Fat

Figure 16-3. Pooled relative risks and 95% confidence intervals of breast cancer for various levels of energy from fat. Estimates from seven cohort studies with a level of 30% to less than 35% of total energy from fat designated as the reference category. N denotes the number of breast cancer cases in each category. [Reprinted by permission of the publisher from Hunter et al. (48). Copyright © 1996, Massachusetts Medical Society. All rights reserved.]

hypothesis was sufficient to include a low-fat dietary intervention in the Women's Health Initiative, a nationwide randomized controlled trial in 48,000 women (45). Some investigators doubt that this trial will elucidate the role of fat intake in breast cancer development (7,39).

Increasing intake of some specific dietary components may reduce the risk of breast cancer. Evidence is suggestive that carotenoids protect against breast cancer (39). Beta-carotene intake has been associated with significant 45% to 55% reductions in risk in case-control studies (51,52). Other beneficial dietary factors include potentially phytoestrogens, fiber, vitamin C, vitamin E, and selenium (39,50). In epidemiologic studies, it is often difficult to separate the effects of specific

dietary components, whole fruits and vegetables, and reduced total caloric intake through lower consumption of fat. In a summary of the evidence, an international panel of experts concluded that increased intake of fruits and vegetables probably decreases the risk of breast cancer, finding no convincing evidence to link any dietary constituent, food, or nonalcoholic drink with risk (53). Regardless of the strength of associations between dietary factors and breast cancer risk, following recommendations to increase fruit and vegetable consumption is beneficial for overall health, not just for breast cancer risk reduction.

Obesity

The association of weight with breast cancer risk is not always consistently described in studies, yet emerging data suggest that individual weight gain patterns may be most strongly associated with risk. Generally, most case-control studies of the relationship between body weight and risk of postmenopausal breast cancer report elevated estimates (39). However, cohort studies tend to show attenuated or no increased risk (40,54). The explanation for this inconsistency is not clear (39). The findings of our large population-based case-control studies (41,55), as well as those of other case-control studies, suggest that recent weight gain may be an important determinant of risk. Women in the highest category of weight (or body mass index) appear to have a 30% to 75% increased risk of postmenopausal breast cancer as compared with women in the lowest weight category (39,41,55). Since cohort studies often evaluate body size far in advance of diagnosis, they may find an attenuated association. A positive association, however, was not found in the Nurses' Health Study, where weight was updated every 2 years during 8 years of follow-up (54,56). Conversely, in the Iowa Women's Health Study — a cohort of older women with relatively short follow-up (6 years) — weight was positively associated with breast cancer risk (57). The relation of study design (case-control versus cohort) to the association found with breast cancer risk appears not to be a simple function of how long before diagnosis the weight data apply.

Most studies to date (54,56–62) — but not all (40,63) — have observed an increased risk of breast cancer in postmenopausal women who gained weight since young adulthood. This association may be attenuated in women who use hormone-replacement therapy (54) (Fig. 16-4). The apparent reduction in risk after weight loss supports the role of weight as a tumor promoter (64), as does the consistent finding that obesity (or weight) is associated with poor prognosis (65–69).

Estrogens derived from androgenic steroids in adipose tissue (70) may account for the increased risk of breast cancer in postmenopausal obese women (23). Obese postmenopausal women have higher serum levels of estrone and estradiol than women of normal weight (64,71–73). The lower levels of sex hormone–binding globulin in heavier women also may increase cancer risk by raising the serum free estradiol level (74–77).

Women do not generally believe that obesity is a potential cause of breast cancer (78). Yet, as indicated by population attributable risk estimates, at least 10% to 16% of postmenopausal breast cancer cases may be accounted for by obesity and weight gain (54,79). Optimal weight maintenance or weight loss may provide for all women an opportunity for breast cancer control.

Physical Activity

While an association between high levels of strenuous physical activity and a 12% to 60% reduced risk of breast cancer is observed quite consistently, there is a limited understanding of many aspects of this association (80,81) (Fig. 16-5). Recreational exercise (82,83) and, to a lesser extent, occupational physical activity (84,85) have received much study. Activities of daily living, such as those experienced by homemakers, are difficult to quantify and have received very little evaluation in relation to breast cancer risk. Other undefined parameters, including the types of activities, intensity levels, frequencies and durations of activity, and time periods (e.g., early life, recent, or both), are relevant to risk, as is the issue of whether protection is conferred on all women or certain subgroups according to menopausal status or some other exposure. It is not clear whether a

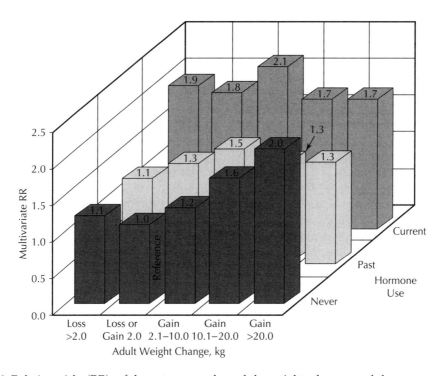

Figure 16-4. Relative risk (RR) of breast cancer by adult weight change and hormone use among postmenopausal women. [Used with permission from Huang et al. (54). Copyright © 1997, American Medical Association.]

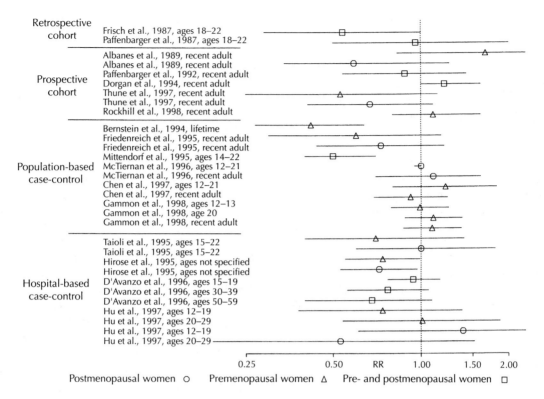

Figure 16-5. Relative risks and 95% confidence intervals of breast cancer from studies included in a comprehensive review of the literature on physical activity. [Used with permission from Rockhill and Colditz (80). Copyright © 1998, Oxford University Press.]

dose-response relationship or a threshold effect exists between physical activity and risk. In addition, the contributing effects of nutrition and body size may be important but have not yet been defined.

A biologic mechanism explaining why increased levels of physical activity influence breast cancer risk is unclear. Physical exertion may affect breast tissue exposure to estrogen by decreasing serum hormone levels (81) and/or by reducing the total number of lifetime ovulations (86). Early-life physical activity can delay menarche, which also may lead to lifetime reduced exposure to ovarian hormones (29,87,88), whereas physical activity later in life may moderate weight gain and decrease fat stores (89). Moderate exercise may promote optimal immune function (81). Much remains to be understood, and guidelines regarding specific activity interventions are yet to be defined, but the underlying message — that physical activity may decrease the risk of breast cancer — is

widely supported by women and health care providers.

Lactation

Evidence that lactation, like other reproductive experiences, is associated with a modest reduction in breast cancer risk is of great interest. Overall, the reduction in risk appears to be about 20% for those who have ever breast-fed and is even greater for women with histories of prolonged lactation or who initiate breast-feeding at young ages (90,91) (Fig. 16-6). Although not consistently demonstrated, the risk reduction may be limited to premenopausal women (90,92,93). It appears unlikely that this inverse association is attributable to a biased proportion of breast cancer patients who used lactation suppressants or who had difficulty either starting or continuing breast-feeding (90,94). Breast-feeding may reduce risk through direct physical effects on the breast, such as the complete differentiation of the

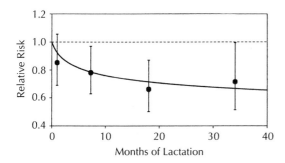

Figure 16-6. Relative risks and 95% confidence intervals of breast cancer among premenopausal women according to the cumulative duration of lactation. Both log-transformed and categorical variables were used in analyzing the data; the curve shows the results of the logarithmic model, and the solid symbols those of the categorical model. [Reprinted by permission of the publisher from Newcomb et al. (90). Copyright © 1994, Massachusetts Medical Society. All rights reserved.]

lobules, as well as through beneficial hormonal changes (12).

While a strong or consistent protective effect of lactation on breast cancer risk has not been observed in some large and well-conducted studies (95,96), this likely reflects the limited breast-feeding practices among modern women. If early, exclusive, and extended breast-feeding is necessary to achieve a breast cancer risk reduction, future studies among U.S. women may be unable to clarify this association. Lactation as a possible means of reducing the risk of breast cancer is one of many reasons for women to follow the American Academy of Pediatrics' recommendation to nurse their infants during the first year (97).

Chemoprevention

Since chemoprevention is addressed in depth in Chapter 12, strategies to prevent breast cancer using pharmaceuticals in the general population are discussed only briefly here. A pharmacologically based approach to breast cancer control faces many challenges, independent of questions of efficacy. The effects on multiple organ systems—both adverse (e.g., endometrial cancer)

and beneficial (e.g., bone preservation)—argue for careful risk consideration on an individual basis. The benefits of a chemopreventive agent depend on each woman's true and perceived risks. Indeed, this approach is likely only appropriate in high-risk individuals.

Luteinizing hormone–releasing hormone agonists (LHRHAs) inhibit ovulation and eliminate ovarian estrogen and progesterone production, essentially producing chemical castration (98). A preliminary study of a regimen including LHRHAs, low-dose estrogen, progesterone, and testosterone in a sample of high-risk women found favorable mammographic density changes (99). This complex therapy attempts to remove the negative effects of estrogen and progesterone on the breast while preserving the positive effects of estrogen on other tissues in the body, including the ovary, endometrium, bone, and heart. Such a delicate physiologic balancing act is complex and challenges the efforts of investigators to develop a drug that prevents breast cancer. Even people taking aspirin, a relatively safe and inexpensive drug, for the prevention of heart attack are advised to decrease blood pressure, avoid stress, and lose extra weight. Thus, while drug trials are producing promising results, drug therapy alone without lifestyle change most likely will not prevent breast cancer for the majority of women in the near future.

Prevention by Proscription
Exogenous Hormones

Since exposure to endogenous estrogens increases breast cancer risk, exogenous estrogens also have received much investigation in relation to risk. To address these very common and important potential sources of increased breast cancer risk, the Collaborative Group on Hormonal Factors in Breast Cancer (100,101) gathered data from over 50 studies in 20 countries concerning oral contraceptives and postmenopausal hormone-replacement therapy. Combined, these studies included over 50,000 breast cancer patients and 100,000 control individuals without breast cancer. The Collaborative Group (100) found that current users of oral contraceptives experienced a small increase in the risk of breast cancer [relative risk (RR) 1.24, 95% confidence interval (CI) 1.15–1.33]. The excess risk disappeared within 10 years of cessation of use. Breast cancer diagnosed in oral contraceptive users tended to be less advanced clinically than cancer diagnosed in those who had never used oral contraceptives.

Use of postmenopausal hormone replacement therapy (HRT) appears to increase the risk of breast cancer by about 2% for each year of use (RR 1.023, 95% CI 1.011–1.036) (101). The effect of HRT is attenuated with increasing body weight and diminishes greatly within 5 years of cessation of use. While the Collaborative Group did not report elevated risks according to subgroups of women, such as consumers of alcohol or users of estrogen-progesterone combination therapy instead of estrogen alone, isolated studies have suggested increased risks for these users (74,102,103). As with oral contraceptives, stage of disease in cancer patients who reported use of HRT was less advanced as compared with stage of disease in never users. Women may choose to avoid oral contraceptives and HRT in order to avert a potential increase in their risk of breast cancer, yet the benefits and convenience of these medications are responsible for their widespread use by women.

Alcohol

Pooled analyses of both case-control (39,104) and cohort (105) studies have found consistent increases in the risk of breast cancer with alcohol consumption. Women who consume at least two drinks per day experience a 20% to 70% increase in risk (39,104,105) (Fig. 16-7). Certain subgroups may experience a higher risk, such as women who use postmenopausal HRT or women with smaller body mass (106). It is not clear whether consumption early in life (e.g., teens and twenties) or in later decades is more strongly related to risk (39,107).

The biologic mechanism linking alcohol with breast cancer is not clear. Alcohol may increase endogenous estrogen levels in both premenopausal and postmenopausal women (108–110). However, not all studies have observed this association (72,111,112). Alcohol also may increase the risk of breast cancer through

increased cell proliferation in the breast or indirect effects of ethanol on cells outside the breast (104).

The public is not well informed about the role of alcohol in breast cancer etiology. One interview study of women with and without breast cancer queried women on what they considered to be potential causes of breast cancer (113); only 3.4% of patients and 2.9% of controls listed alcohol. Although a public health message that clearly balances the beneficial and detrimental effects of alcohol on breast cancer and competing health risks would be difficult to structure, researchers have an obligation to allow women to make informed decisions regarding their health (107). A population-wide reduction in alcohol intake probably would reduce breast cancer incidence (53), but the feasibility of this reduction depends on the ability of women to act on their understanding of the risks and benefits of consuming alcohol.

Tobacco

In general, the association between cigarette smoking and the risk of breast cancer has been weak. Initially, MacMahon and colleagues (114) hypothesized that cigarette smoking may reduce the risk of premenopausal breast cancer by lowering estrogen levels in the luteal cycle. A review of the published studies on this topic did not support this theory (115). Continuing study has revealed divergent results. Brunet and colleagues (116) reported a 54% reduction in risk among women with *BRCA1* or *BRCA2* mutations who smoked at least 4 pack-years. Conversely, two case-control studies conducted in the United States and Canada found that smoking during adolescence increased breast cancer risk by 70% to 80% (117); the authors suggested that the developing breast is particularly vulnerable to cancer initiation by cigarette smoke. Furthermore, the relation between risk of breast cancer and smoking may be modified jointly by menopausal status and N-acetyltransferase-2 genotype (118–120). Thus tobacco does not influence the risk of breast cancer in the general population, but isolated studies have reported increased (and decreased) risks for smokers in certain subgroups.

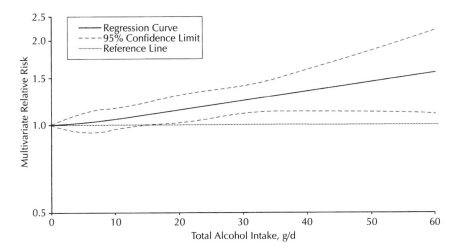

Figure 16-7. Nonparametric regression curve for the relationship between total alcohol intake and breast cancer. Model derived using the combined data from six prospective studies, with cubic polynomials fit between four prespecified knot positions at 1.5, 5.0, 15.0, and 30.0 g/d of alcohol. [Used with permission from Smith-Warner et al. (105). Copyright © 1998, American Medical Association.]

Radiation

Irradiation is clearly an initiating factor in breast cancer, especially for women exposed in the first four decades of life (121,122) (Fig. 16-8). The practical conclusion is that breast irradiation should be avoided, particularly in young women and children. In the past, chest radiation was given as treatment for thymus enlargement, acne, and asthma. While radiotherapy is no longer prescribed in these situations, the extent to which radiation from low-dose diagnostic exposures is associated with breast cancer risk is not known. Extrapolating data from epidemiologic studies of high-dose exposures suggests that yearly mammograms during the ages 40

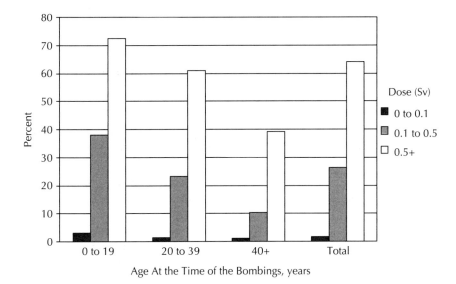

Figure 16-8. Estimated percentage of breast cancer cases related to radiation among atomic bomb survivors according to age at the time of the bombings and radiation dose, 1950–1985. [Data from Land (121).]

to 49 will result in one extra breast cancer case per 10,000 women (123). Women heterozygous for the ataxia telangiectasia gene, or possibly other major susceptibility genes, may have an increased risk of breast cancer, an elevated sensitivity to ionizing radiation, and an even greater risk for breast cancer when exposed to diagnostic or therapeutic radiation to the chest (124,125). Screening mammography reduces the risk of death from breast cancer for women over 50 years of age, but younger women and women with inherited or acquired defects in DNA repair mechanisms should avoid radiation except when the risk of death (e.g., from malignancy) definitely outweighs the risk of breast cancer.

Targeted Interventions

Since a substantial portion of women who develop breast cancer do not have an identifiable risk factor, all women must be considered at risk (126,127). Some estimates suggest that modifiable lifestyle factors could be responsible for a substantial portion of cases (1,79,126). The feasibility and probable effectiveness of behavior changes for breast cancer prevention vary (see Table 16-1). If 30% of cases were prevented, as many as 54,000 fewer women would suffer from breast cancer each year in the United States.

Education

Girls, their parents, and young women may be especially important targets for breast cancer prevention efforts for two main reasons. First, the time before age at first birth may have a large impact on lifetime breast cancer risk in terms of age at menarche and exposure of breast tissue to hormones and cancer initiators (12,17,23,98,128). Second, healthy habits fostered in primary and secondary school aged children may be sustained throughout the lifetime. Mezzetti and colleagues (79) estimate that 33% of all breast cancer cases can be attributed to low intake of beta-carotene, high alcohol consumption, and physical inactivity. We need to resist efforts to reduce education budgets by eliminating health, food science, and physical fitness programs in schools.

Screening

Secondary prevention by mammography for women 50 years of age and over reduces the risk of breast cancer mortality by 25% to 30% (129,130). Age is the strongest predictor of breast cancer risk, so as women age, routine breast cancer screening increases in importance. The age-adjusted incidence rate of female breast cancer for women under age 65 is 74 per 100,000, whereas the rate for women aged 65 and over is 443 per 100,000 (131). Although the efficacy of mammography for women in their forties is controversial, guidelines support mammography for women in this age group (123,132). (See Chap. 7 for a more lengthy discussion of screening for younger women.) Data from clinical trials are not available to support mammographic screening for women over 74 years of age, yet mammography is probably warranted for women without substantial competing comorbidities and for whom treatment for breast cancer would be done if cancer were discovered. Of particular concern is the detection of breast carcinoma in situ — lesions with uncertain malignant potential — especially in this age group. Older women are less likely than younger women to obtain regular screening tests, even though their risk of disease is much greater (133). Effective programs to promote mammographic screening for women in their sixties, and most likely their seventies, would prevent a substantial portion of breast cancer mortality.

Implementation

The adoption of any one of these potential prevention strategies on an individual or population level depends on many factors. In general, individuals will make decisions about reproduction, diet, and other lifestyle factors based on the societal and medical support available to them. Physicians will play a key role in these decisions not only by dispensing preventive drugs but also by assisting women in understanding their risk status and providing counseling about change, such as weight loss, and screening. On a population level, a promising general social strategy for breast cancer prevention would include (134): 1) mandated physical and health education in all school grades, 2) competition against unhealthy food advertising, 3) assistance for people to close the gap between knowledge and behavior (e.g., alcohol risk), and 4) training for physicians to communicate healthy diet and exercise messages and secondary prevention recommendations to their patients. These strategies would need to be tailored to their target groups, since the social context of the intended audience is a key consideration, especially when people have limited access to sites where they can exercise or obtain affordable, high-quality food from supermarkets (135).

Summary

Breast cancer rates have increased because of lifestyle changes. Most of this increase is attributable to reproductive and nutritional changes that have improved the overall quality of life for women, and society should be unwilling (and indeed unable) to modify these behaviors. However, there are potentially important and acceptable interventions available today for breast cancer prevention. These include eating well, losing or maintaining body weight, and being physically active and are all components of a healthy lifestyle in general. These are also the most difficult changes to make and require substantial social and medical support. Chemoprevention as a strategy for high-risk women is an emerging reality, whereas secondary prevention through routine screening is appropriate for women of all risk profiles. Breast cancer prevention may necessitate no less than a change in social norms. These strategies to change social norms would lead to a reduced incidence not only of breast cancer but probably of other cancers, cardiovascular disease, and diabetes as well.

Acknowledgments The assistance of Felicia Roberts and Patrick Remington is gratefully acknowledged.

References

1. Doll R, Peto R. The causes of cancer: quantitative estimates of avoidable risks of cancer in the United States today. J Natl Cancer Inst 1981;66:1191–1308.

2. Muir CS, Nectoux J. International patterns of cancer. In: Schottenfeld D, Fraumeni JF, eds. Cancer Epidemiology and Prevention. 2nd ed. New York: Oxford University Press, 1996:141–167.

3. Henderson BE, Pike MC, Bernstein L, Ross RK. Breast cancer. In: Schottenfeld D, Fraumeni JF, eds. Cancer Epidemiology and Prevention. 2nd ed. New York: Oxford University Press, 1996:1022–1039.

4. Kelsey JL, Horn-Ross P. Breast cancer: magnitude of the problem and descriptive epidemiology. Epidemiol Rev 1993;15:7–16.

5. Chu KC, Tarone RE, Kessler LG, et al. Recent trends in U.S. breast cancer incidence, survival and mortality rates. J Natl Cancer Inst 1996;88:1571–1579.

6. Lantz PM, Remington PL, Newcomb PA. Mammography screening and increased incidence of breast cancer in Wisconsin. J Natl Cancer Inst 1991;83:1540–1546.

7. Kelsey JL, Bernstein L. Epidemiology and prevention of breast cancer. Annu Rev Public Health 1996;17:47–67.

8. Bailar JC, Gornick HL. Cancer undefeated. New Engl J Med 1997;336:1569–1574.

9. Ziegler RG, Hoover RN, Pike MC, et al. Migration patterns and breast cancer risk in Asian-American women. J Natl Cancer Inst 1993;85:1819–1827.

10. Shimizu H, Ross RK, Bernstein L, et al. Cancers of the prostate and breast among Japanese and white immigrants in Los Angeles County. Br J Cancer 1991;63:963–966.

11. Thomas DB, Karagas MR. Migrant studies. In: Schottenfeld D, Fraumeni JF, eds. Cancer Epidemiology and Prevention. 2nd ed. New York: Oxford University Press, 1996:236–254.

12. Russo J, Russo IH. Toward a physiological approach to breast cancer prevention. Cancer Epidemiol Biomark Prev 1994;3:353–364.

13. Love RR, Vogel VG. Breast cancer prevention strategies. Oncology 1997;11:161–168.

14. Russo J, Russo IH. Influence of differentiation and cell kinetics on the susceptibility of the rat mammary gland to carcinogenesis. Cancer Res 1980;40:2677–2687.

15. Lambe M, Hsieh C, Trichopolous D, et al. Transient increase in the risk of breast cancer after giving birth. New Engl J Med 1994;331:5–9.

16. Kelsey JL, Gammon MD, John EM. Reproductive factors and breast cancer. Epidemiol Rev 1993;15:36–47.

17. Colditz GA, Frazier AL. Models of breast cancer show that risk is set by events of early

life: prevention efforts must shift focus. Cancer Epidemiol Biomark Prev 1995;4:567–671.

18. Korenman SG. Oestrogen window hypothesis of the aetiology of breast cancer. Lancet 1980;1:700–701.

19. Korenman SG. The endocrinology of breast cancer. Cancer 1980;46:874–878.

20. Pike MC, Krailo MD, Henderson BE, et al. "Hormonal" risk factors, "breast tissue age" and the age-incidence of breast cancer. Nature 1983;303:767–770.

21. Henderson BE, Ross RK, Judd HL, et al. Do regular ovulatory cycles increase breast cancer risk? Cancer 1985;56:1206–1208.

22. Pike MC, Spicer DV, Dahmoush L, Press MF. Estrogens, progestogens, normal breast cell proliferation, and breast cancer risk. Epidemiol Rev 1993;15:17–35.

23. Kuller LH. The etiology of breast cancer — from epidemiology to prevention. Public Health Rev 1995;23:157–213.

24. White E. Projected changes in breast cancer incidence due to the trend toward delayed childbearing. Am J Public Health 1987;77: 494–497.

25. Stoll BA. Asking the right questions. In: Stoll BA, ed. Reducing Breast Cancer Risk in Women. Boston: Kluwer Academic Publishers, 1995:237–242.

26. Harris JR, Lippman ME, Veronesi U, Willett WC. Breast cancer (first of three parts). New Engl J Med 1992;327:319–328.

27. Cooper C, Kuh D, Egger P, et al. Childhood growth and age at menarche. Br J Obstet Gynecol 1996;103:814–817.

28. Soriguer FJ, Gonzalez-Romero S, Esteva I, et al. Does the intake of nuts and seeds alter the appearance of menarche? Acta Obstet Gynaecol Scand 1995;74:455–461.

29. Merzenich H, Boeing H, Wahrendorf J. Dietary fat and sports activity as determinants for age at menarche. Am J Epidemiol 1993;138: 217–224.

30. Petridou E, Syrigou E, Toupadaki N, et al. Determinants of age at menarche as early life predictors of breast cancer risk. Int J Cancer 1996;68:193–198.

31. Meyer F, Moisan J, Marcoux D, Bouchard C. Dietary and physical determinants of menarche. Epidemiology 1990;1:377–381.

32. Maclure M, Travis LB, Willett W, MacMahon B. A prospective cohort study of nutrient intake and age at menarche. Am J Clin Nutr 1991;54:649–656.

33. Graber JA, Brooks-Gunn J, Warren MP. The antecedents of menarcheal age: heredity, family environment, and stressful life events. Child Dev 1995;66:346–359.

34. Herman-Giddens ME, Slora EJ, Wasserman RC, et al. Secondary sexual characteristics and menses in young girls seen in office practice: a study from the Pediatric Research in Office Settings network. Pediatrics 1997;99:505–512.

35. Wyshak G, Frisch RE. Evidence for a secular trend in age of menarche. New Engl J Med 1982;306:1033–1035.

36. Willett WC. Nutritional Epidemiology. New York: Oxford University Press, 1990:311–340.

37. Stoll BA. Does extra height justify a higher risk of breast cancer? Ann Oncol 1992;3:29–30.

38. Dorgan JF, Reichman ME, Judd JT, et al. The relation of body size to plasma of estrogens and androgens in premenopausal women (Maryland, United States). Cancer Causes Control 1995;6:3–8.

39. Hunter DJ, Willett WC. Diet, body size, and breast cancer. Epidemiol Rev 1993;15:110–132.

40. van den Brandt PA, Dirx MJM, Ronckers CM, et al. Height, weight, weight change, and postmenopausal breast cancer risk: the Netherlands Cohort Study. Cancer Causes Control 1997;8:39–47.

41. Trentham-Dietz A, Newcomb PA, Storer BE, et al. Body size and risk of breast cancer. Am J Epidemiol 1997;145:1011–1019.

42. Hsieh CC, Trichopoulos D, Katsouyanni K, Yuasa S. Age at menarche, age at menopause, height and obesity as risk factors for breast cancer: associations and interactions in an international case-control study. Int J Cancer 1990;46:796–800.

43. Brinton LA, Schairer C, Hoover RN, Fraumeni JF. Menstrual factors and risk of breast cancer. Cancer Invest 1988;6:245–254.

44. Freedman LS, Clifford C, Messina M. Analysis of dietary fat, calories, body weight, and the development of mammary tumors in rats and mice: a review. Cancer Res 1990;50:5710–5719.

45. Prentice RL, Kakar F, Hursting S, et al. Aspects of the rationale for the Women's Health Trial. J Natl Cancer Inst 1988;80:802–814.

46. Wynder EL, Cohen LA, Muscat JE, et al. Breast cancer: weighing the evidence for a promoting role of dietary fat. J Natl Cancer Inst 1997;89:766–775.

47. Willett WC, Hunter DJ, Stampfer MJ, et al. Dietary fat and fiber in relation to risk of breast cancer. JAMA 1992;268:2037–2044.

48. Hunter DJ, Spiegelman D, Adami H-O, et al. Cohort studies of fat intake and the risk of breast cancer—a pooled analysis. New Engl J Med 1996;334:356–361.
49. Howe GR, Hirohata T, Hislop TG, et al. Dietary factors and risk of breast cancer: combined analysis of 12 case-control studies. J Natl Cancer Inst 1990;82:561–569.
50. Clavel-Chapelon F, Niravong M, Joseph RR. Diet and breast cancer: review of the epidemiologic literature. Cancer Detect Prev 1997;21:426–440.
51. Freudenheim JL, Marshall JR, Vena JE, et al. Premenopausal breast cancer risk and intake of vegetables, fruits, and related nutrients. J Natl Cancer Inst 1996;88:340–348.
52. Longnecker MP, Newcomb PA, Mittendorf R, et al. Intake of carrots, spinach, and supplements containing vitamin A in relation to risk of breast cancer. Cancer Epidemiol Biomark Prev 1997;6:887–892.
53. World Cancer Research Fund, American Institute for Cancer Research. Breast. In: Food, Nutrition and the Prevention of Cancer: A Global Perspective. Menasha, WI: World Cancer Research Fund/American Institute for Cancer Research, 1997:252–287.
54. Huang Z, Hankinson SE, Colditz GA, et al. Dual effects of weight and weight gain on breast cancer risk. JAMA 1997;278:1407–1411.
55. Trentham-Dietz A, Newcomb PA, Egan KM, et al. Weight change and risk of postmenopausal breast cancer (United States). Cancer Causes Control 2000;11:(in press).
56. London SJ, Colditz GA, Stampfer MJ, et al. Prospective study of relative weight, height and risk of breast cancer. JAMA 1989;262: 2853–2858.
57. Barnes-Josiah D, Potter JD, Sellers TA, et al. Early body size and subsequent weight gain as predictors of breast cancer incidence (Iowa, United States). Cancer Causes Control 1995;6:112–118.
58. Paffenbarger RS, Kampert JB, Chang H. Characteristics that predict risk of breast cancer before and after the menopause. Am J Epidemiol 1980;112:258–268.
59. Le Marchand L, Kolonel LN, Earle ME, Mi M-P. Body size at different periods of life and breast cancer risk. Am J Epidemiol 1988;128:137–152.
60. Folsom AR, Kaye SA, Prineas RJ, et al. Increased incidence of carcinoma of the breast associated with abdominal adiposity in postmenopausal women. Am J Epidemiol 1990;131:794–803.

61. Chu SY, Lee NC, Wingo PA, et al. The relationship between body mass and breast cancer among women enrolled in the Cancer and Steroid Hormone Study. J Clin Epidemiol 1991;44:1197–1206.
62. Brinton LA, Swanson CA. Height and weight at various ages and risk of breast cancer. Ann Epidemiol 1992;2:597–609.
63. Kyogoku S, Hirohata T, Takeshita S, et al. Anthropometric indicators of breast cancer risk in Japanese women in Fukuoka. Jpn J Cancer Res 1990;81:731–737.
64. Enriori CL, Reforzo-Membrives J. Peripheral aromitization as a risk factor for breast and endometrial cancer in postmenopausal women: a review. Gynecol Oncol 1984;17:1–21.
65. Tretli S. Height and weight in relation to breast cancer morbidity and mortality: a prospective study of 570,000 women in Norway. Int J Cancer 1989;44:23–30.
66. Ewartz M. Survival of breast cancer patients in relation to factors which affect the risk of developing breast cancer. Int J Cancer 1991;49:526–530.
67. Mohle-Boetani JC, Grosser S, Whittemore AS, et al. Body size, reproductive factors, and breast cancer survival. Prev Med 1988;17:634–642.
68. Goodwin PJ, Boyd NF. Body size and breast cancer prognosis: a critical review of the evidence. Breast Cancer Res Treat 1990;16:205–214.
69. Seine RT, Tosen PP, Rhodes P, et al. Obesity at diagnosis of breast carcinoma influences duration of disease free survival. Ann Intern Med 1992;116:26–32.
70. Siiteri PK. Adipose tissue as a source of hormones. Am J Clin Nutr 1987;45:277–282.
71. Ota DM, Jones LA, Jackson GL, et al. Obesity, non-protein-bound estradiol levels, and distribution of estradiol in the sera of breast cancer patients. Cancer 1986;57:558–562.
72. Cauley JA, Gutai FP, Kuller LH, et al. The epidemiology of serum sex hormones in postmenopausal women. Am J Epidemiol 1989;129:1120–1131.
73. Hankinson SE, Willett WC, Manson JE, et al. Alcohol, height, and adiposity in relation to estrogen and prolactin levels in postmenopausal women. J Natl Cancer Inst 1995;87: 1297–1302.
74. Ewertz M. Influence of non-contraceptive exogenous and endogenous sex hormones on breast cancer risk in Denmark. Int J Cancer 1988;42:832–838.

75. Judd HL, Shamonki IM, Frumar AM, LaGasse LD. Origin of serum estradiol in postmenopausal women. Obstet Gynecol 1982;59:680–686.

76. Moore JW, Key TJ, Bulbrook RD, et al. Sex hormone binding globulin and risk factors for breast cancer in a population of normal women who had never used exogenous sex hormones. Br J Cancer 1987;56:661–666.

77. Enriori CL, Orsini W, del Carmen Cremona M, et al. Decrease of circulating level of SHBG in postmenopausal obese women as a risk factor in breast cancer: reversible effect of weight loss. Gynecol Oncol 1986;23:77–86.

78. Brinton LA, Malone KE, Stanford JL, et al. Re: Should we consider a subject's knowledge of the etiologic hypothesis in the analysis of case-control studies? Am J Epidemiol 1994;140:1054–1055.

79. Mezzeti M, La Vecchia C, Decarli A, et al. Population attributable risk for breast cancer: diet, nutrition, and physical exercise. J Natl Cancer Inst 1998;90:389–394.

80. Rockhill B, Colditz GA. Re: Physical activity and breast cancer risk in a cohort of young women. J Natl Cancer Inst 1998;90:1909.

81. Gammon MD, John EM, Britton JA. Recreational and occupational physical activities and risk of breast cancer. J Natl Cancer Inst 1998;90:100–117.

82. Mittendorf R, Longnecker MP, Newcomb PA, et al. Strenuous physical activity in young adulthood and risk of breast cancer (United States). Cancer Causes Control 1995;6:347–353.

83. Bernstein L, Henderson BE, Hanisch R, et al. Physical exercise and reduced risk of breast cancer in young women. J Natl Cancer Inst 1994;86:1403–1408.

84. Thune I, Brenn T, Lund E, Gaard M. Physical activity and the risk of breast cancer. New Engl J Med 1997;336:1269–1275.

85. Coogan PF, Newcomb PA, Clapp RW, et al. Physical activity in usual occupation and risk of breast cancer. Cancer Causes Control 1997;8:626–631.

86. Friedenreich CM, Rohan TE. A review of physical activity and breast cancer. Epidemiology 1995;6:311–317.

87. MacMahon B, Trichopoulos D, Brown J, et al. Age at menarche, urine estrogens and breast cancer risk. Int J Cancer 1982;30:427–431.

88. Apter D, Reinila M, Vihko R. Some endocrine characteristics of early menarche, a risk factor for breast cancer, are preserved into adulthood. Int J Cancer 1989;44:783–787.

89. McTiernan A. Exercise and breast cancer—time to get moving? New Engl J Med 1997;336:1311–1312.

90. Newcomb PA, Storer BE, Longnecker MP, et al. Lactation and a reduced risk of premenopausal breast cancer. New Engl J Med 1994;330:81–87.

91. Newcomb PA. Lactation and breast cancer risk. J Mam Gland Biol Neoplasia 1997;2:311–318.

92. Byers T, Graham S, Rzepka T, Marshall J. Lactation and breast cancer: evidence for a negative association in premenopausal women. Am J Epidemiol 1985;121:664–674.

93. Yang CP, Weiss NS, Band PR, et al. History of lactation and breast cancer risk. Am J Epidemiol 1993;138:1050–1056.

94. Brinton LA, Potischman NA, Swanson CA, et al. Breastfeeding and breast cancer risk. Cancer Causes Control 1995;6:199–208.

95. Kvale G, Heuch I. Lactation and cancer risk: is there a relation specific to breast cancer? J Epidemiol Commun Health 1988;42:30–37.

96. Michels KB, Willett WC, Rosner BA, et al. Prospective assessment of breastfeeding and breast cancer incidence among 89,887 women. Lancet 1996;347:431–436.

97. American Academy of Pediatrics Work Group on Breastfeeding. Breastfeeding and the use of human milk. Pediatrics 1997;100:1035–1039.

98. Pike MC, Ross RK, Lobo RA, et al. LHRH agonists and the prevention of breast and ovarian cancer. Br J Cancer 1989;60:142–148.

99. Spicer DV, Ursin G, Parisky YR, et al. Changes in mammographic densities induced by a hormonal contraceptive designed to reduce breast cancer risk. J Natl Cancer Inst 1994;86:431–436.

100. Collaborative Group on Hormonal Factors in Breast Cancer. Breast cancer and hormonal contraceptives: collaborative reanalysis of individual data on 53,297 women with breast cancer and 100,239 women without breast cancer from 54 epidemiologic studies. Lancet 1996;347:1713–1727.

101. Collaborative Group on Hormonal Factors in Breast Cancer. Breast cancer and hormone replacement therapy: collaborative reanalysis of data from 51 epidemiologic studies of 52,705 women with breast cancer and 108,411 women without breast cancer. Lancet 1997;350:1047–1059.

102. Colditz GA, Stampfer MJ, Willett WC, et al. Prospective study of estrogen replacement therapy and risk of breast cancer in postmenopausal women. JAMA 1990;264:2648–2653.

103. Bergkvist L, Adami HO, Persson L, et al. The risk of breast cancer after estrogen and

estrogen-progestin replacement. New Engl J Med 1989;321:293–297.

104. Longnecker MP. Alcoholic beverage consumption in relation to risk of breast cancer: meta-analysis and review. Cancer Causes Control 1994;5:73–82.

105. Smith-Warner SA, Spiegelman D, Yaun S-S, et al. Alcohol and breast cancer in women: a pooled analysis of cohort studies. JAMA 1998;279:535–540.

106. Schatzkin A, Longnecker MP. Alcohol and breast cancer: where are we now and where do we go from here? Cancer 1994;74:1101–1110.

107. Willett WC, Stampfer MJ. Sobering data on alcohol and breast cancer. Epidemiology 1997; 8:225–227.

108. Gavaler JS, Love K, Van Thiel D, et al. An international study of the relationship between alcohol consumption and postmenopausal estradiol levels. Alcohol Alcoholism Suppl 1991;1:327–330.

109. Gavaler JS, Deal SR, Van Thiel DH, et al. Alcohol and estrogen levels in postmenopausal women: the spectrum of effect. Alcohol Clin Exp Res 1993;17:786–790.

110. Reichman ME, Judd JT, Longcope C, et al. Effects of alcohol consumption on plasma and urinary hormone concentrations in premenopausal women. J Natl Cancer Inst 1993; 85:722–727.

111. London S, Willett W, Longcope C, McKinlay S. Alcohol and other dietary factors in relation to serum hormone concentrations in women at climacteric. Am J Clin Nutr 1991;53:166–171.

112. Newcomb PA, Klein R, Klein BEK, et al. Association of dietary and life-style factors with sex hormones in postmenopausal women. Epidemiology 1995;6:318–321.

113. Swanson CA, Coates RJ, Malone KE, et al. Alcohol consumption and breast cancer risk among women under age 45 years. Epidemiology 1997;231–237.

114. MacMahon B, Trichopoulos D, Cole P, Brown J. Cigarette smoking and urine estrogens. New Engl J Med 1982;307:1062–1065.

115. MacMahon B. Cigarette smoking and cancer of the breast. In: Wald N, Baron J, eds. Smoking and Hormone-Related Disorders. New York: Oxford University Press, 1990:154–166.

116. Brunet JS, Ghadirian P, Rebbeck TR, et al. Effect of smoking on breast cancer in carriers of mutant *BRCA1* or *BRCA2* genes. J Natl Cancer Inst 1998;90:761–766.

117. Palmer JR, Rosenberg L, Clarke EA, et al. Breast cancer and cigarette smoking: a hypothesis. Am J Epidemiol 1991;134:1–13.

118. Ambrosone CB, Freudenheim JL, Graham S, et al. Cigarette smoking, *N*-acetyltransferase-2 genetic polymorphisms, and breast cancer risk. JAMA 1996;276:1494–1501.

119. Millikan RC, Pittman GS, Newman B, et al. Cigarette smoking, *N*-acetyltransferases 1 and 2, and breast cancer risk. Cancer Epidemiol Biomark Prev 1998;7:371–378.

120. Hunter DJ, Hankinson SE, Hough H, et al. A prospective study of NAT2 acetylation genotype, cigarette smoking, and risk of breast cancer. Carcinogenesis 1997;18:2127–2132.

121. Land CE. Studies of cancer and radiation dose among atomic bomb survivors. JAMA 1995;274:402–407.

122. Tokunaga M, Land CE, Yamamoto T, et al. Incidence of female breast cancer among atomic bomb survivors, Hiroshima and Nagasaki, 1950–1980. Radiat Res 1987;112:243–272.

123. Gordis L, Berry DA, Chu SY, et al. National Institutes of Health Consensus Development Conference Statement: Breast cancer screening for women ages 40–49, January 21–23, 1997. J Natl Cancer Inst 1997;89:1015–1026.

124. Swift M, Morrell D, Massey RB, Chase CL. Incidence of cancer in 161 families affected by ataxia-telangiectasia. New Engl J Med 1991;325:1831–1836.

125. Swift M, Reitnauer PJ, Morrell D, Chase CL. Breast and other cancers in families with ataxia-telangiectasia. New Engl J Med 1987; 316:1289–1294.

126. Seidman H, Stellman SD, Mushinski MH. A different perspective on breast cancer risk factors: some implications of the nonattributable risk. CA 1982;32:301–313.

127. Madigan MP, Ziegler RG, Benichou J, et al. Proportion of breast cancer cases in the United States explained by well-established risk factors. J Natl Cancer Inst 1987;87:1681–1685.

128. DeWaard F, Trichopoulos D. A unifying concept of the aetiology of breast cancer. Int J Cancer 1988;41:666–669.

129. Fletcher SW, Black W, Harris R, et al. Report of the International Workshop on Screening for Breast Cancer. J Natl Cancer Inst 1993;85:1644–1656.

130. Kerlikowske K, Grady D, Rubin SM, et al. Efficacy of screening mammography: a meta-analysis. JAMA 1995;273:149–154.

131. Ries LAG, Kosary CL, Hankey BF, et al., eds. SEER Cancer Statistics Review, 1973–1994,

National Cancer Institute. NIH Pub. No. 97-2789. Bethesda, MD, 1997:124.

132. Marwick C. Final mammography recommendation? JAMA 1997;277:1181.

133. Costanza ME. The extent of breast cancer screening in older women. Cancer 1994;74:2046–2050.

134. Vanchieri C. Lessons from the tobacco wars edify nutrition war tactics. J Natl Cancer Inst 1998;90:420–422.

135. Sorensen G. Population-level change in risk factors for cancer. Cancer Causes Control 1997;8:S43–S45.

Index

Note: Page numbers followed by f indicate figures; those followed by t indicate tables.

UCSF LIBRARY MATERIALS MUST BE RETURNED TO:

THE UCSF LIBRARY

530 Parnassus Ave.

University of California, San Francisco 94143-0840

**Borrowers are responsible for keeping track of
due dates and overdue items are subject to penalties.
Refer to the Borrower's Policy for details.**

Items may be renewed within five days <u>prior to</u> the due date

in person, by phone (415-476-2335), or online at

http://ucsfcat.ucsf.edu/patroninfo/

All items are subject to recall after 7 days.

28 DAY LOAN

28 DAY

JAN 2 - 2003

RETURNED

JAN - 2 2003

28 DAY

APR 1 4 2003

RETURNED

MAR 2 4 2003